THE HE...R

A GUIDE TO SYM...

CONDITION

RESOLUTION

| A |
| B |
| C |

7A. THE NAME
The word agreed upon to summarize the Symptom (6A), that historically was also presumed to cause it.

RUNG 7

7B. SOCIAL SUPPORT
At RUNG 7B, everyone can support you better when they know The Name (7A) that summarizes your symptoms.

6A. SYMPTOM
The expression of RUNGS 1A–5A at a level that can be perceived or measured.

RUNG 6

6B. TREATMENT
RUNG 6B Treatment is symptom-focused: surgery, drugs and some manual modalities are all designed to suppress the Symptom (6A).

5A. LOCATION
The regions of the body that manifest the stress from RUNGS 1A–4A, often below the awareness threshold.

RUNG 5

5B. THERAPY
RUNG 5B Therapy is support-focused: vitamins, supplements, herbs and some manual modalities attempt to heal the Location (5A).

4A. FUNGUS / VIRUS
Fungus: your best friend, helps you break down Bad Bacteria (2A).
Virus: your worst enemy, thrives in an environment of Metal Toxicity (3A).

RUNG 4

4B. ANTIFUNGAL / VIRAL
Anti-fungals: overlook the fact that fungi play a vital role in health.

Anti-virals: don't generally provide a long-term solution.

3A. METAL TOXICITY
Elements in their non-bioavailable form adhere to you when Bad Bacteria (2A) absorb them for cellular metabolism.

RUNG 3

3B. METAL DETOX
RUNG 3B Metal Detox can minimize the Symptom (6A) by starving Bad Bacteria (2A) of the Metals (3A) that they metabolize.

2A. BAD BACTERIA
At some stage all Bad Bacteria (2A) come from a Parasite (1A). Once excreted into your body they circulate everywhere, causing inflammation and tissue damage.

RUNG 2

2B. BAD BACTERIA
Probiotics: temporarily replace good bacteria but don't eliminate Bad Bacteria (2A) from Parasites (1A).
Antibiotics: kill off Bad Bacteria (2A) but never Parasites (1A).

1A. PARASITES
Various Parasites (1A) inhabit your body. They deplete nutrients, damage tissue and excrete Bad Bacteria (2A). Best eliminated by Frequency Therapy (1B).

RUNG 1

1B. FREQUENCY THERAPY
Eliminates all species of Parasites (1A) from all locations. Clean, quick, comprehensive and free of side effects, it is **the future of human healthcare.**

0A. THE VECTOR
All animals in nature are the primary or intermediate hosts to various species of Parasites (1A), many of which can infect humans.

RUNG 0

0B. AWARENESS
Educate yourself. Start by reading *Experiments in Muscle Testing* by Leonard Carter. Then, apply what you learn.

↖ Start Here

www.TheHealthLadder.com

EXPERIMENTS IN
MUSCLE TESTING

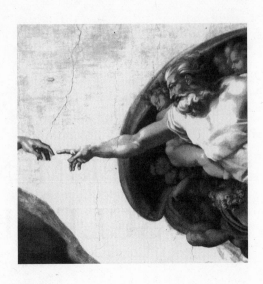

A Note on the Cover Art

Artist: Michelangelo Buonarroti (1475–1564)
Died at: 89
Artwork: *The Creation of Adam*, 1511, fresco
Current location: Sistine Chapel, Vatican City

Called Buonarroti by his patrons the Medici family, Michelangelo had already chiseled what would become two of the most famous sculptures in history, the *Pietà* and *David*, before the age of thirty.

The ceiling of the Sistine Chapel was a major commission for him, partly because he wasn't a painter. There was no guarantee that it would turn out well. Instead of a modest first try, what emerged from five years of neck-breaking labour arguably became the most famous painting in history: a marvel of light, color, subtlety and perspective that, though painted in the dark, looked like it had been touched by the hand of God.

The detail that appears on this book cover is the iconic *Creation of Adam* where the actual hand of God reaches out toward the hand of Adam—never quite touching but always there, always within reach.

In the same way, muscle testing has the capacity to connect the bodies we live in with the Truth of the Mind of the Creator.

Gloria in excelsis Deo.

THE COMPLETE MUSCLE TESTING SERIES:
BOOK 1

EXPERIMENTS IN
MUSCLE TESTING

*A Universal Guide to Health,
Wellness and Longevity*

Leonard Carter

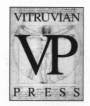

VITRUVIAN
VP
PRESS

Cover design, book design and typesetting by Vitruvian Press
All image permissions are held by the publisher
www.VitruvianPress.com
Edited by Cassandra Filice
Printed in Canada

Disclaimer: Legal and medical disclaimer is found on page 418. Your
use of this book and any information herein implies your knowledge,
understanding and acceptance of this disclaimer.

ISBN: 978-0-9868996-0-7
Title: Experiments in Muscle Testing
Subtitle: A Universal Guide to Health, Wellness and Longevity
Author: Leonard Carter
Publisher: Vitruvian Press

SECOND EDITION

with colored Health Ladder

Published July 2021

For Niki and Buddy

*without whose helping hands (and paws)
I couldn't have brought this
philosophy to the world*

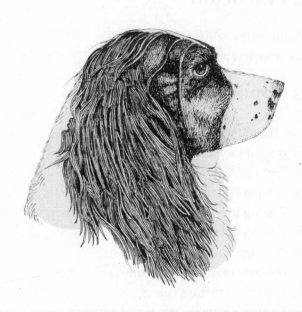

v

TABLE OF CONTENTS

ACKNOWLEDGEMENTS

I am not the creator of muscle testing. It is a continent of thought that others discovered. Nor was I among the first explorers here but rather a latecomer to this New World that lay across an ocean of knowledge, time and understanding.

Indeed, my understanding of this field has evolved considerably over the years, and I must acknowledge with gratitude the patience and open mindedness of all the people I shared my ideas with when they were in a less developed form. I hope that this book will set the record straight on many conversations that were, at the time, necessarily incomplete. I am also grateful to about 3000 people, many of whom travelled from great distances and helped me in one way or another to come to the bulk of the realizations outlined here.

I was inspired by Dr. George Goodheart, who first developed muscle testing, and by some of his students, doctors of Applied Kinesiology who defined my early understanding of the field. I am indebted to Dr. David R. Hawkins for his life's work in consciousness research. I never met him, but after 20 years of studying his works, I am still a student, sitting at his feet, marveling at every word.

I am the beneficiary and the product of the Judeo-Christian West with its roots in classical civilization and the intellectual heritage that this entails.

There are a handful of people who deserve specific mention. Jeff Presley for the Buddy sketches, Sarah Black for research assistance, Alejandra Flores for modeling, Logan Dube for project management, Claudia Tavernese for art consulting, Natassja Fong at Elle Studios, my editor Cassandra Filice at www.writetotheend.ca, and of course Buddy the springer, who helped out more than I could ever explain.

I couldn't have brought about this book at all without my wife Niki, who patiently assisted me with hundreds of thousands of muscle tests over more than a decade.

And I am grateful to you, my reader, for taking the time to learn this material and for caring about the truth. Thank you.

INTRODUCTION

Looking back on the history of humanity we can identify a series of transformative realizations:

Flint technology, the discovery and mastery of fire, that we would live longer if we cooked our meat, that metal could be melted out of rocks; of language, of story telling, of agriculture, of the city, of mathematics, music, art, philosophy and logic; that we have a soul, and the awareness that reality and time emanate from an energetic substrate that can be called the Creator, Divinity or God.

A pivotal technology was the development of writing, so that all those memories could stop being lost to the mists of time.

From there we began to stand on the shoulders of giants and discovered the principles of universal gravitation, electricity, the microscopic world, periodic chemistry, flight, radio waves, the atom, subatomic particles, relativity and the universe, stretching across vast parsecs in artistic filaments, nebulae, voids and galaxy clusters.

We living souls have danced through this history, surrounded by family, pets, friends, food and memories, with such a brief span of years to learn the most important lessons: be grateful, tell the truth, follow our path and leave the world better than we found it. After that, medical conditions manifest and we die.

In all of this time we have overlooked the technology of muscle testing. It so simple that the Neanderthals could have used it. Yet, it is complex enough to lead us to a series of realizations that are missing from the resumé of humanity: that our bodies have a bioelectric field; that parasites cause medical conditions; that electromagnetism can be used to treat them; and that we need a new mathematics, a new chemistry and a new science to work with living, dynamical systems.

An awareness of these principles can be said to usher in a stage of civilization thought of as space age medicine. The future is now and it is yours to realize.

Leonard Carter
Vancouver, 2021

Part 1: Clarification

Contents of Part 1:

Part I:

Clarification

1

Why We Need Muscle Testing

Look, but it cannot be seen—it is invisible.
Listen, but it cannot be heard—it is inaudible.
Reach out, but it cannot be touched — it is intangible.
By these three alone, it cannot be known;
By these together, it emerges as the One.

–Lao Tzu
Tao Te Ching, **1:14**

(English translation © Vitruvian Press)

A ll of humanity has in common the need to be healthy. This is perhaps the most universal basis for understanding one another. But how can we understand health when it is buried deep within the senses? The ancient healing systems are out of date with the modern world, the old masters speak in metaphors.

The above words of Lao Tzu echo across the centuries, anticipating a theme that subsequent philosophers, spiritual teachers and modern-day neuroscientists have continued to grapple with: that there is an age-old disconnect between our five senses and the ultimate reality in which we exist. From Dōgen and Huang Po to Plotinus, Meister Eckhart and Maharishi, the message is the same: that The Field of awareness is a Oneness that each of our senses perceives inadequately and that we fail to fully comprehend.

We assume that our senses provide a complete picture of reality but they do not. It is well known that we can observe less than 1 trillionth of the spectrum of light and hear less than 1 trillionth of the spectrum of sound; taste only a fraction of the molecules in any food and smell the barest minimum of odors; that we exist in an extraordinarily narrow range of pressure, temperature, gravitation and radiation. Our perception is further limited by cognitive capacity, memory, emotional interpretation, fear, personal agenda and spiritual awareness, as well as the unconscious biases of culture, age, language, profession and our perception of time.

We make major decisions based on the assumption that what we perceive with our senses is all we need to know. Then, since assumptions are things we don't know we're making, we're not even aware that this is happening and call it reality.

These assumptions are at the core of our health problems. We don't know what we don't know, and assuming that we do know it reinforces the disconnect between our senses and the reality that we need to understand. Our bodies become the metaphorical monkey in the middle and the results are sickness, pain and premature aging. More recently, we have seen this in our global response to viruses, manifested in fear, panic and the biggest lockdowns in human history. 2020 is a year few will forget.

We need a sixth, more accurate sense to understand health.

This book is not about the Ultimate Reality. It is about how we can use muscle testing as a sixth sense to enhance our existing five senses, improve our health, minimize pain and make our lives better, more productive, potentially longer and hopefully, a bit more sane.

Who Should You Follow?

Being stuck with only five senses is like being lost in the middle of a great desert. You don't know which direction to go and there are sand dunes for as far as the eye can see. Walking on your own in any direction only gets you more lost. Luckily, you're with four friends and one of them does know the way out. But which one? They're all going in a different direction. Their names are Nobody, Everybody, Anybody and Somebody. Who should you follow?

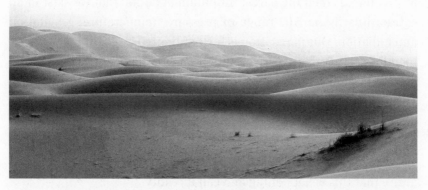

Nobody knows where he's going. In fact, Nobody knows everything, but you can't follow Nobody.

Everybody seems to know where he's going, but he has a reputation for ending up right back where he started, so you've decided not to follow Everybody this time.

Anybody might know where he's going, but Anybody can get lost, so you won't follow Anybody.

Somebody has to know where he's going, so he's your best bet. But sometimes it's hard to know who Somebody is because although he's not Everybody, he could be Anybody and he might be Nobody.

It would be best if you and Everybody followed Somebody because if Everybody followed Anybody, Everybody would get lost and Somebody would have to go after him. Then you would have Nobody to follow. And you can't follow Nobody. Do you follow this?

This play on language illustrates the problem of trying to use the conscious mind, which is fundamentally trapped by the senses and the biases of sense perception, to find a way out of the limitations that consciousness itself is defined by. This is why we instinctively look to other people for a reality check, why group opinions matter to us and why philosophers and sages have been grappling with the problem of what actually constitutes truth for thousands of years.

Truth in this case is primarily concerned with biological truth. The concept of **being lost in a desert** is an allegory for our understanding of our own health. Whether we're sick or healthy, worried about viruses or carefree, we have no idea what's really going on at a physiological level. Because our nervous systems aren't wired to communicate to our conscious minds the information we need to know to be in control of our health, we need to follow Somebody else.

In a desert world like this, the person with a compass automatically becomes the leader, they automatically become Somebody. Muscle Testing (MT) is like a compass for the five senses. MT is the sixth sense that Somebody can use to lead us out of the desert of our five senses. But even with a compass, Somebody needs to understand what direction to take. What's out there?

Where Should You Go?

There are bad things out there. Pesticides, heavy metals, parasites, pathogenic fungi, bacteria, viruses, super-bugs, industrial chemicals, paints, petroleum by-products, air pollution, water pollution, soil contamination, toxic clothing fibers, household chemical fumes, smoke, smog, carcinogens, toxic waste and radiation.

And then, there are the effects these things may have on our bodies: cancer, heart disease, liver toxicity, kidney failure, pancreatic problems, diabetes, gall bladder swelling, gall stones, thyroidism (hyper- and hypo-), splenic inflammation, adrenal disorders, bladder infections, lung conditions, stomach ulcers, irritable bowel syndrome, diarrhea, colitis, cysts, tumors, lipomas, constipation, colon polyps, food allergies, prostate inflammation, period cramps, neck pain, vision problems, hearing dysfunction, brain tumors, tooth decay, skin rashes and hair loss, not to mention sleep disorders, mood swings, irritability, addiction, depression and psychiatric conditions.

You certainly don't want to go to any of those places. Instead, the goal destination is some form of treatment.

But which treatment?

You could see a medical doctor, get an MRI, bone scan, X-ray, do blood work, urine tests, stool tests. Be referred to a cardiologist, run on a treadmill, check your cholesterol. See a urologist, a rheumatologist, an endocrinologist, get your brain chemistry checked. Look up a psychiatrist, try some antidepressants.

If none of that helps, you could go alternative: get a chiropractic adjustment, see a naturopathic doctor, try homeopathy or the kind of massages you have to learn how to pronounce first: tuina, rolphing, myofascial release. Or try the more subtle route: craniosacral therapy, osteopathy or neurolink. Take an herbal metal chelator for a while. Do a dozen diets: South Beach, Mediterranean, eat in the zone, buy organic, go paleo, raw, vegetarian or vegan. Put butter in your coffee, but only grass-fed butter. Take lots of vitamins, minerals, enzymes, probiotics, protein powders, amino acids and essential fatty acids. Drink fish oil by the tablespoon. Get acupuncture, acupressure or moxicombustion.

In case your symptoms are just stress-related, try exercise: cardio, weights, a personal trainer, aerobics or spinning. Stretch. Try different types of yoga, see which one works best for you: hatha, ashtanga or kundalini? Try essential oils and Bach flower remedies. Soak in mineral salts, sit under healing lights, use pulsed magnets, play cleansing frequencies and binaural beats.

Explore the energy end of things, look up the latest guru all your friends are seeing. Try tapping, SRT, reiki, tai chi, chi kung, yogic breathing. Maybe you just need a laughter-induced endorphin high: try going to comedy clubs for a while. Learn to live in acceptance, be in the moment, make peace with your inner child, find the power of the now. If none of that works, consult a spiritual guide, maybe it's unresolved karma from another lifetime. Get your chakras cleansed, meditate, forgive, do a past-life regression and learn to let it all go.

There is an anxiety to this searching for health that can leave one feeling frustrated, exhausted and depressed. Health problems linger that no approach seems to permanently resolve. The search goes on, it becomes a lifestyle and there are two lingering, unanswered questions: Why do we get sick? How do we get healthy?

It is a legitimate approach to take a spiritual view of all this and in his masterpiece *Letting Go* (Hawkins, 2012), Dr. David Hawkins outlines a psychological and spiritual technique (the letting go technique) that may indeed be the ultimate resolution to all spiritual challenges. However, even people who choose to pursue a spiritual path as their end goal will experience illness in their lives and the danger of equating it with spirituality lies in mistakenly assuming that illness is therefore a necessary component of spiritual growth. This can result in unnecessary suffering (e.g., mistakenly assuming you're sick because you're evolving) and even spiritual guilt, where sickness is interpreted as karmic punishment for lack of spiritual progress.

And there are many more people that don't want to follow a spiritual path, either from lack of time, aptitude or interest. At the end of the day, this group believes, health is grounded in the here and now. And why shouldn't it be?

One way or the other, if your focus is on your health then MT can help. Whether you feel like you're lost in a desert or think you know where you're going, the content that follows is designed to get you to your destination.

Chances are this isn't the first time you've heard this sort of claim, so who should you follow when Everybody makes the same claim? Who is right? Is Anybody right? So many opinions, perspectives, interpretations and agendas can lead to information overload.

Life needs to be simpler.

This book provides a simple roadmap and MT is the compass. It is designed to teach you to think for yourself. It is designed to teach you how to be the change that you want to see in the world.

Outthinking Thought

As soon as we try to think for ourselves, we encounter the problem that biologically speaking, we can't.

There are internal problems that we simply aren't wired to be able to interpret: aging, imbalances, deficiencies and dysfunctions in the organs, glands, brain, eyes and ears; the nose, throat, sinuses, teeth, bones, scalp and hair; the skin, circulatory, pulmonary and skeletal systems, and the more subtle aspects of brain chemistry like awareness, memory, mood and cognition that all register their own unique vitamin, mineral, protein and fat requirements, metal toxicities, enzyme deficiencies, circulatory capacity, inflammatory levels, parasite load, bacterial balance, and fungal and viral levels.

And then there are external problems: foods we may be reactive to, parasites and metal toxicities in food and water, toxic cosmetics, chemical preservatives, industrial chemicals, air and water pollution, chemicals in plastics, perfumes and household cleaners, electromagnetic pollution, wifi, 4G, 5G, radio waves, microwaves and artificial lighting. And viruses. It's a wonder any of us is alive.

We cannot force our thoughts about these problems when we lack the sensory organs to give us conscious access to information about them, and because we aren't directly aware that its absence is a problem, it has been traditional to ignore this sensory disconnect, write it off as insignificant or clothe it in impressive diagnostic medical jargon, summarized as thousands of diseases, disorders, conditions, syndromes, dystrophies, sclerosises, -plasias, -itises, allergies, acronyms and cancers. In the 20th century, more medical conditions were defined than in all the preceding centuries combined. In that time, there wasn't a corresponding cure discovered for a single one of them. But the symptoms are real and the fear is real.

It is the tension between these opposing perspectives, the proliferation of medical conditions and the complete absence of a single cure, that is our starting point. This is the heart of the matter.

We need a different way of thinking about this issue.

Historical Blind Spots

Our subjugation to medical conditions over the centuries (e.g., the 2400 year tradition of diagnostic medicine) has culminated in the general, largely unconscious assumption that the word agreed upon to summarize the symptom is itself the cause of the symptom. This is both a logical fallacy, since a thing cannot cause itself (e.g., diabetes cannot cause diabetes) and a major blind spot in understanding.

Acknowledging that the circular argument inherent in diagnostic medicine is a blind spot will strengthen comprehension of the solution. Seeing it contrasted with other **historical blind spots** will place it in the context of the development of scientific thought.

Examples of historical blind spots are:

1. Geocentrism (the assumption of Earth at the center of the universe)
2. Flat Earth (the fear that ships would sail off the edge of the world)
3. Static continents (the lack of awareness of deep time, continental drift)
4. Outer space made of ether (no concept of astrophysics)
5. Base elements as earth, air, fire, water (no periodic chemistry)

Each of these ideas was so unquestioningly accepted that for hundreds or sometimes thousands of years it was an assumption nobody even realized they were making. A comparison with the blind spot of diagnostic medicine will illuminate the current discussion:

6. Diagnosis (the implicit assumption that a name causes a symptom)

The symptom is real but is our thinking about it accurate? If not, how can we think differently? The human race overcame the other historical blind spots when new technologies were introduced. Can MT be a learned thinking process that sets us free from the diagnostic perspective? Or can we use MT to develop a new technology that frees us from the conceptual impasse of the problem of diagnosis?

The problem of diagnosis is that a description is not also a cure. If there is a way out of this problem, it is not to be found at the level of thinking that created the description. It is the philosophy of diagnosis that we need to outthink. What we need are some cures.

The Cure

There is no question that the world needs cures. This was painfully apparent to billions of people around the world in 2020, locked down in their homes, afraid of getting a virus that had no cure. There is no lack of love for life and in fact there is no shortage of questions about why life gets derailed by disease. The same questions keep coming up:

Why do only some people die from viruses?	see Pt3-Ch9
What causes illness?	see Pt3-Ch13
What is the auto in autoimmune?	see Pt3-Ch13
Does organic mean it's good for you?	see Pt3-Ch10
Does GMO mean it's bad for you?	see Pt3-Ch10
What causes food allergies?	see Pt3-Ch11
Why do supplements make some people feel worse?	see Pt3-Ch3
Are fish full of mercury?	see Pt3-Ch4
Is candida the problem?	see Pt3-Ch9
Is your heart healthy?	see Pt3-Ch2
What causes degeneration in the elderly?	see Pt3-Ch15
What is the secret to longevity?	see Pt3-Ch22
What can help a sick child?	see Pt3-Ch14
Is our drinking water safe?	see Pt3-Ch24
Are raw diets good for our pets?	see Pt3-Ch16
How can we identify a parasite picked up on a trip?	see Pt3-Ch21
Can a parasite cause a medical condition?	see Pt3-Ch5
Can parasites be treated with frequencies?	see Pt3-Ch6

At some point you will ask yourself all these questions and many more. These are questions that Anybody and Everybody have answers to, and Somebody must have the right answers, but there is so much disagreement as to what the answers are that it often seems like Nobody has the answers, and this gets us even more stuck.

The hope, of course, is that we can use MT to find better answers and think our way out of the desert, but this gives rise to the obvious question: why hasn't this been done already? What sorts of things could go wrong when we try to interpret a MT?

Getting Even More Lost: Hulda Clark

When trying to interpret advanced scientific information, which is what we are doing when we use MT to evaluate the body's bioelectric field, there are two main things that can go very wrong and if either of them does we will get even more lost: logic and ethics.

1. **Logic** At face value, data from MT is only factual. To interpret the data we must use logic. Basic logic is simple but the advanced logic required to draw scientifically coherent conclusions about health is not simple: it is complex, layered and nuanced. We will spend most of this book learning what the nuances are.

2. **Ethics** When interpreting MT data, it is necessary to have accountability to the truth foremost in mind and the wellbeing of the patient foremost at heart. What are the consequences to ourselves or others if we are wrong? This needs to be factored into all MT feedback.

There is a scenario where interpretation, when applied without logic or ethics, can do more harm than good. We see this clearly in the case of Hulda Clark (1928-2009), an alternative healing cult figure that was a visionary but possibly also the biggest charlatan of the 20th century.

In theory, she was correct: we can evaluate the body's bioelectric field, parasites do cause illness and frequencies can eliminate them. However, in practice, her claims were either wrong (that all parasites autopopulate inside of us; that hand-held Parasite Zappers work and that specific frequencies are needed for different parasite species, thus perpetuating the myth about Rife frequencies), absurd (that every surface in every house is covered in pigeon tapeworm eggs; that all cancer is caused by the sheep liver fluke), or grossly unethical (that if patients drank a single glass of black walnut tincture, their cancer would be cured and they should cancel their chemotherapy appointments; that she could diagnose AIDS and cure it, too, but that the patient needed to come back again and again for expensive treatments or else it would return). The final nail in the coffin of her disastrous legacy was that she published a book titled *The Cure for All Cancers* (Clark, 1993) and in the end, died of cancer (2009).

Without logic and ethics, we can become far more lost.

Experiments in Muscle Testing

When used logically and ethically, MT greatly accelerates information processing in biological and medical experimentation. While the essence of diagnosis is summarized by the process of guess, wait, and see, MT is immediate.

A diagnostic mentality that depends upon guessing, waiting, and seeing can extend experimentation over months, years and even centuries, whereas MT provides the ability to consider hundreds of variables in minutes; then hundreds more; then hundreds more. A major scientific discovery that would at one time have required a century of distinctions can take place in an afternoon. This is because the evaluation of the impact of a stimulus on the body can be determined before the fact as opposed to after the fact.

This evolution away from the need to guess, wait, and see changes how we can approach health experimentation. By acting as a sifting mechanism, MT can be used to ascertain which experiments are likely to have a positive outcome, eliminating time spent running unnecessary experiments and often bypassing prevailing misconceptions.

Applied to pharmaceutical chemistry, this could be to the development of new medicines and antibiotics what the flint stone was to the development of fire.

Applied to food allergies it allows for the recognition that numerous other identifiable causes (bacterial and parasitic) underlie them, the elimination of which may hold the promise of the elimination of the allergy itself, something that is unheard of under the current diagnostic paradigm where no cures are available.

Applied to virology, this could provide us with information that eliminates the need for quarantines, lockdowns and chaos.

Applied to medical conditions, it is the future of healthcare.

We are already experimenting. We always have been. What you will find if you learn how to perform **experiments in muscle testing** is that it will make your consideration process quicker, more accurate and more effective: there will be no guessing, less waiting, and more seeing.

Repeatability

The experiments in MT outlined in this book are structured around the essential quality of **repeatability**. You are encouraged to verify the information presented here by repeating the MT methodology outlined relative to each claim on each page. It is by learning how to confirm or contradict these claims that the reader can have a common frame of reference and not be dependent upon their own opinion.

Statements have not been made nor conclusions drawn unless there has been extensive confirmation using repeatability as a guideline and it should be understood that all conclusions are beholden to the rules of logic. This is a universe where A is A.

Where MT appears to be inconsistent with modern scientific theory is at the margins of our understanding of mathematics, electricity and the electric field the body produces, known as the bioelectric field. Modern physics is founded on the science of electrodynamics, while for the most part biology and medicine are not.

It is through the application of bioelectrodynamics to biology and medicine that MT makes its entrance to modern science. There is limited opportunity to study this subject in a formal academic setting. The content presented here can and should act as a foundation upon which to begin building a systematic understanding of this field.

Over the years of teaching the MT methodology to students, it has been instructive to observe how both the academic and non-academic, the health professional and layman process information that hasn't traditionally been a part of mainstream learning. The information in this book is presented with that in mind and is tailored for the widespread public adoption of new content.

If the text seems overly simple at times, consider that this may be necessary when addressing a large audience. If it becomes complex in places, bear in mind that sufficient specifics are needed for the field to be understood to be in accord with logical science. However, a complete grasp of these details is not always needed to apply basic MT in most of the scenarios outlined.

Simple or complex, all MT protocols must be and are repeatable.

Core Concepts

To understand the content outlined in this book, it is suggested that you become familiar with a number of **core concepts**. To facilitate recognition, each of these is bolded as it occurs throughout the text. Some are simpler than others, but each is important.

In this chapter, for example, the core concepts are:

1. **Being lost in a desert**   5. **Ethics**
2. **Historical blind spots**   6. **Experiments in muscle testing**
3. **The problem of diagnosis** 7. **Repeatability**
4. **Logic**   8. **Core concepts**

In Appendix 1 at the end of the book, all core concepts are listed in sequence by chapter for the purposes of recollection and review. This is found on page 404.

Two Ways You Can Use This book

Readers of this material tend to fall into two main categories: active users and passive users.

Active Users want to use this content to learn how to MT or to perfect their existing technique. They may want to verify the claims made throughout this book by reproducing them and once understood, may even want to try their own experiments in MT. The supporting articles, posters and MT Kits available on the www.MuscleTesting.com website are designed with this in mind.

Passive Users may not want to learn how to MT, or perhaps can't for whatever reason (no time, no testing partner, poor motor skills, etc.), but they may still recognize the validity of the approach outlined here, and may choose to rely on this information as trusted material and as an improvement over their own best guess.

Either approach will work, as well as some combination of the two.

2

What is Muscle Testing

Straight and narrow is the path...
Waste no time.

–David Hawkins
I: Reality and Subjectivity

To be able to proceed with a common frame of reference about MT, it is necessary to clarify the two areas where people tend to go astray in their MT practice. These can be summarized as definition and perspective.

Definition entails simple differentiation of what MT is versus what it is not. This is not a matter of perspective, it is objective (i.e., applicable in all cases and true in all cases).

Perspective is more intricate in that it isn't based on a simple definition. The essence of perspective is that where we stand, so to speak, determines what we see. The hope is that we can use MT to arrive at an objective understanding of health, but depending on the parameters of the MT, the information elicited may sometimes appear subjective (i.e., not applicable in all cases).

This gives rise to an obvious concern. For MT to contribute to the science of health, or even just to get us out of whatever desert of uncertainty we're in, it needs to be accurate and repeatable. If it is, we can discuss facts and from that point of certainty we can arrive at a mutually agreed upon methodology that will allow for further use, applications and the betterment of humanity. But if instead of being repeatable, it is dependent upon perspective and therefore subjective, then there is no basis for agreement and we might as well be discussing fiction.

This, then, is the concern: To what extent does the subjectivity of perspective in MT render it unrepeatable, and therefore unreliable?

To answer this question, it is necessary to outline the means by which perspective in a MT can alter perception of the data (i.e., take what should be objective information and make it subject to other variables so that the data is unusable).

However, this understanding needs to be founded on a definition of what MT is versus is not, and so will need to wait momentarily while MT is defined.

Definition

A MT is any process whereby the strength of a muscle is evaluated by applying force to it.

On the surface, this appears quite simple until we recognize that the implication of MT is that a conclusion is being drawn based on the result of the test. So perhaps it would be more accurate to define MT as the methodology of drawing conclusions from the strong or weak responses elicited from muscles when their strength is evaluated by applying force to them.

However, this definition is also incomplete since the conclusion is being drawn not about the muscular response but about some aspect of the body, and the basis for this conclusion is an evaluation of the reaction of the muscle to some stimulus. The stimulus is what is being tested and the body is what it is being tested on. The muscle is merely the thing that connects the two.

In fact, the reaction is not thought to be on the part of the muscle itself but on the part of the body that telegraphs its reaction through the muscle. The body also telegraphs its reactions through other, less perceptible means: minute changes in pupil size, capillary dilations or the so-called blush response, minor fluctuations in heart rate, and color shifts in the invisible ranges of the electromagnetic spectrum also known as the aura, but these aren't practical to test, nor as accessible as a muscle.

The muscle, then, is the simplest indicator of the body's reaction to a stimulus. This concept is from where we derive the term indicator muscle. An **indicator muscle** is used to evaluate (because it indicates) the outgoing strength signal from the body itself, which fluctuates based on various internal and external stimuli. The most accurate **definition of MT** is:

The methodology of drawing conclusions about the effect of a stimulus on the body based on the comparative strength responses of an indicator muscle.

Seen in this way, a MT presupposes four ingredients: 1) A muscle to test with 2) A body to test on 3) A stimulus to be tested and 4) A thought process. The thought process is, of course: What will be the effect of this stimulus on this body, as evaluated via this muscle?

As stated, on the surface, this seems to be an oversimplified question, but if an accurate answer can be derived by MT any stimulus at any time, the implications are profound.

The larger significance of MT, far from merely being some new diagnostic process, is that it allows for a thinking process or sixth sense to which humans haven't ever had access due to lack of sensory information. The development of this methodology, with its corresponding provision of the missing information, has resulted in the ability to draw conclusions that are radical, innovative, pioneering and unprecedented in the history of our understanding of health.

A basic understanding of what MT is paves the way for a quick overview of what MT is not.

What Muscle Testing is Not

There are a number of practices currently in use that are presumed to provide the accuracy and reliability of MT, some of which are even called MT but that either bypass the muscle, bypass the testing or bypass logic. We can label them **false types of MT**.

A quick summary of these will help the student to recognize them. Understanding why these are not MT will save time that would otherwise be wasted on inaccuracy and blind alleys.

For organizational simplicity they are presented in chart form:

False Types of Muscle Testing		
Method		**Why this isn't Muscle Testing**
1	Pendulum swinging.	A pendulum isn't a muscle so using one isn't MT. Interpreting reality through the swing of a pendulum has no basis in linear science. There is insufficient accountability for it to be accurate.
2	Swaying forward or backward while standing up (as a response to holding a product within the bioelectric field).	Balance isn't an adequate means of MT a stimulus. First, no muscle is being tested. Then, even if balance were loosely agreed to be an indicator of muscle activation, too many muscles are involved, it's too easy to compensate and therefore not accurate. Finally, equating forward movement with a positive MT response and backward movement with a negative reveals an unconscious bias about direction that has nothing to do with biomechanics.
3	Prying your fingers apart.	Lever length of the fingers is too short, thus we can compensate too much. It also entails self-testing which is much less accurate. Combine the two at your peril.
4	Making interlocking circles with your thumbs and forefingers, then trying to pull them apart.	In addition to both reasons listed in point 3 above, this method involves momentum and is therefore highly inaccurate.

5	Lifting one finger while the hand is placed palm down on a table.	Range of motion (ROM) is not an accurate MT indicator since a weak response in a MT is not expressed as a lack of ROM in the finger extensors. Also, on principle, moving our own muscles is not the same as having someone else test our muscles, therefore this is not a MT at all.
6	Swinging an arm over the head.	Not a MT for the same reasons listed in points 4 and 5 above.
7	Self-Testing, presupposing the form is correct (e.g., self-testing one's own front deltoid).	This is not accurate for 4 reasons: 1) The deltoid fascia will tend to seize up after a few self-tests. 2) We're more likely to make a mistake of interpretation since our own brain is exerting the testing pressure and the resisting pressure. 3) There is no second person to give us a reality check, which is vital with such a fine-tuned motor skill. 4) We don't have a third hand free to manipulate the things we're MT (products or organ test points). We need to constantly cross-check and second-guess our results. In a self-test this isn't happening. Ask yourself: is there a reason you don't want it to?
8	Using an electric synchrometer or some other device to evaluate galvanic skin response.	No muscle is being tested so it's not a MT. Like MT, these devices attempt to quantify fluctuations in the bioelectric field but at the time of this writing (2021), no reliable, accurate device has been invented.
9	Truth Testing.	We must differentiate scientific MT from nonlinear Truth Testing by using the term MT to describe the first and Truth Testing to describe the second.
10	Remote MT: across the room or across the world.	This is not MT it is Truth Testing. It will be addressed below and in Pt3-Ch35. Be advised never to bet your life or health on the outcome of a Truth Test and don't believe that it is scientific MT.

Ultimately, any discussion about MT is a discussion about truth. The sole motivation for an interest in MT is to find a way to discern a truth that our senses cannot. It is the case that truth is often clouded by misconception, error and falsehood. If we use a false type of MT to try to find truth it will get us even more lost.

It is necessary for the student to be able to recognize what false types of MT are and why they are false, and then refrain from basing conclusions on them. It would also clarify matters for others if these were not referred to as MT at all.

Pendulum swinging, in Method 1 above, is focused on interpreting nonlinear reality in the same way as Truth Testing is. There is an amusing portrayal of this in *Red Rackham's Treasure* in Hergé's *Tintin* series (Hergé, 1959): Professor Calculus is seen using a pendulum for divining, much to the chagrin of his companions. In our society, this is a recipe for not being taken seriously and it has nothing to do with scientific MT.

Interestingly, dowsing for water actually does work for the same reason that pendulums don't. The rapid movement of a large volume of underground water is capable of producing an electromagnetic field that is sufficiently strong to provoke movement in an antenna such as a dowsing rod held over the flow, even dozens of feet away.

In Methods 2-7 the misconceptions are biomechanical. They have to do with balance, lever length, range of motion and neurology.

Method 8 could work if there were an accurately functioning device but as of 2021 there isn't.

In Methods 9 and 10 we encounter Truth Testing, which has layers of challenges. If it were simply a matter of using linear versus nonlinear science we might be able to fine tune the process, but the energy field that the Truth Test is responding to is a function of consciousness itself, which is dependent upon whether the participant is capable of perceiving truth to begin with. This leads to the Truth Testing paradox that we will explore in more detail below.

Having defined what MT is and is not, we can now evaluate the extent to which perspective influences the outcome of the process.

Perspective

But does it all just depend on how we look at it?

Of the four ingredients of a MT (a muscle to test with, a body to test on, a stimulus to be tested and a thought process from which to draw a conclusion) the thought process is obviously where perspective presents a concern.

The parameters of the MT thought process need to be defined so that there is a common frame of reference. On the surface at least, there are three requirements: accuracy, repeatability and logic.

Accuracy is simply a matter of using correct MT form (outlined in Pt2-Ch1), along with refraining from employing the false types of MT outlined above.

Repeatability as a concept has already been covered. It requires controlling all possible variables so that only one stimulus at a time is being MT. This, combined with accurate form, will produce the same result each time and is the hallmark of science.

Logic is the watchdog that ensures we're drawing appropriate conclusions from the data. Logic may seem simple but requires maturity, intelligence and mental discipline. A certain amount of academic training in formal logic is helpful, since scientific exploration goes wrong where logic breaks down. This is where peer review or public opinion can be invaluable since logic is often understood intuitively by others and is the basis for a reality check.

Beneath the surface, however, is a final parameter in the subject of perspective, one that is perhaps the most controversial topic of 20th century physics with implications in fields as diverse as religion, spirituality, consciousness, meteorology, turbulence, health and politics. This parameter concerns energy.

An understanding of **energy** in the context of health can be hard to arrive at since it is generally described by many different words. As an idea, energy is referred to by the terms paradigm, world view, way of seeing things, thoughts having a reality, understanding of theoretical physics, appreciation of the relationship between linear and nonlinear dynamics and level of consciousness.

As a force, it is described as a charge, a field, an aura, a manifestation, a phenomenon or a radiance.

Energy is measured in many ways including teslas (T), watts (W), volts (V), amps (A), nanometers (nm), joules (J), coulombs (C), kelvins (K), Fahrenheit (°F) and Celsius (°C). But what actually is it?

The reality of energy in the human body is that each person produces an electric field called their **bioelectric field**. This field extends a few inches outside the skin and has the tendency to telegraph both external signals inward and internal signals outward in a rapid, swirling electromagnetic exchange of information. The bioelectric field is what makes it possible for us to pick up an electric shock from a carpet. Traditionally called the aura, it can be captured on camera using Kirlian photography, and while some parties may still be holding out in their denial of its existence, as will be seen in the following two chapters, they simply don't have enough of a grounding in physics, or perhaps don't have carpets at home.

The controversial aspect of the bioelectric field is not its existence but what it telegraphs. It doesn't just telegraph biological impulses, it also telegraphs thoughts. Thoughts produce a faint electromagnetic charge, measurable on the tesla scale in picoteslas (imagine trying to capture the sound of a feather dropping on a carpet), which are projected through the body's bioelectric field along with the electric charges that everything else produces (emotions, pheromones, hormone signals, organ signals, glandular signals, immune system signals, cardiac signals, etc.).

In this way, thoughts take on an infinitesimal existence in physical reality for as long as we continue to hold them in mind. You might have noticed this if you've ever been in a room with someone who was in a bad mood. They don't need to say a thing: you can feel it. Like an old film projector, the brain is able to act as a thought projecting mechanism, though this is not widely or well understood even by physicists. Where it is not adequately understood, skepticism about the temporary physical reality of thoughts will arise.

We have arrived at the crux of the controversy of MT.

The Vanishing Point

When too many leaps are required of the student (leaps they are not accustomed to making on a good day in the fields of physics, biology, physiology, electrodynamics, biomechanics, mathematics and medicine) the average mind considers, boggles, dismisses as fantastical and then shuts down in relieved satisfaction.

MT requires a bioelectric field. Everybody has one but unfortunately, and probably because it isn't visible to the human eye, we have grown up in a culture that is unaware that anybody has one. There isn't a simple place for an idea of it in the human psyche.

However, lack of awareness of the bioelectric field is not the problem. Anyone seeking confirmation of the existence of their bioelectric field can recall a time when they got a shock from a carpet.

It requires an only slightly larger leap in imagination to realize that internal signals of the body can be telegraphed through this bioelectric field. This is also not an insurmountable concept, since we are already aware of the blush response, which we can see, and there is general awareness that we cannot see most of the spectrum of radiation. We can't see X-rays, what's going on inside an MRI or an ultrasound device. These are all based on how electricity interacts with the body and none of them is controversial.

The controversy arises when thoughts are included with everything else that can be MT. This requires a tacit acknowledgement that thoughts have a temporary physical existence, and although this can be measured, there simply hasn't been an academic precedent for it to be formally acknowledged until now.

Think of the concept of **the vanishing point** in Renaissance painting. Prior to the 1500s, if a patron had wanted art in three dimensions they would commission a sculpture. Paintings were two-dimensional. When the third dimension of depth was added (most notably by Verrocchio, DaVinci, and Michelangelo), it came as a revelation. Suddenly there was a point on the canvas where objects could disappear into a distance that hadn't existed before. It was an imaginary distance, but real things on the canvas disappeared into it. Suddenly, the perspective of the viewer rendered some things more visible (i.e., objects in the foreground), others less visible (objects in the background) and some invisible (objects past the vanishing point). Suddenly perspective mattered. At the time this was revolutionary and would have been quite disconcerting to the viewer.

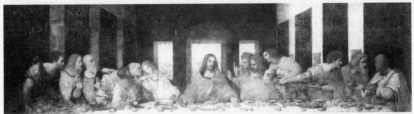

Disconcerting, perhaps, in the same way that 500 years later we denizens of the 21st century might be uneasy about acknowledging that thoughts have a physical existence that can be MT. The disquiet grows as the scientific mind leaps to the next logical step: if thoughts can be expressed in a MT, they can influence a MT. If they can influence a MT, then the results of a MT analysis are subject to perspective—they are dependent upon the thinker—and since no two people interpret experiential reality quite the same way, there arises a scenario where no two people will get the same result from a MT (i.e., lack of repeatability). If this is the case, MT cannot act as the basis for a new science due to subjectivity, which implies opinion. Opinion is the opposite of science. Science requires objectivity, or precisely the absence of opinion.

The concern is that when we introduce perspective in MT, paradoxically, logic vanishes and promptly invalidates MT itself.

Taking this dynamic to its ultimate extension brings up the dichotomy of the philosophies of **relativism versus absolutism**.

Gravity is absolute. If you step off a cliff you will fall whether it is your opinion that you will fall or not. Gravity doesn't care about your opinion, your feelings or your perspective.

Relativism implies that based on how you interpret the motion out into space, your experience of falling off a cliff can be different.

There is a notable literary example of relativism in *Tales of Power* (1974) by Carlos Castaneda, where at the end of the book his main characters jump off a high mesa, not to their deaths but into... Well, we are left to imagine. Then at the beginning of the next book in the series, *The Second Ring of Power* (1977), we find each of the characters changed, but alive and well with the implication that they survived the fall because they believed they would. This episode appears to have been designed to formally, overtly challenge the standard, absolutist interpretation of reality.

Relativism led to the concept, re-popularized in the late 20th century (it also came from the philosopher Hegel), that we can create our own reality based on our mental focus. The means by which a thought can telegraph itself out through the bioelectric field and be MT was recruited as justification or illustration of this idea. This finds its ultimate extension in the field of epigenetics, where the argument is sometimes made that mental focus can determine which genetic traits can be expressed by the human genome.

For the record, this current body of work, while not invested in "isms," is written from the perspective of absolutism: If you jump off a cliff you can create whatever reality you want on the way down, but at the bottom you're going to need to come to terms with the absolute realities of gravity, momentum and density. The relativistic proposition that we can create our own reality is a meme, a popular slogan with social and political overtones that are rooted in an anti-absolutist agenda. Rather than attempting to justify relativism by recruiting MT, proponents of that world view should acknowledge it for what it is: at the core of the clash of absolutism and relativism is the division between truth and falsehood, reality and illusion.

It is one thing to understand why the grey areas of MT are grey, it is another to feel entitled to misuse the modality of MT as a replacement for logic and accountability.

The grey areas of MT are the controversial borders where it moves from quantifying the physical to quantifying thoughts: the energy, the abstraction, the idea, the mind, the vanishing point where logic seems to vanish, the edge of reality that seems to be open to interpretation.

Thoughts Versus Truth

It necessary to make a distinction here between two types of thoughts: thoughts per se and truth specifically. In the MT world these are mistakenly considered as the same but they are in fact quite different.

Thoughts are what the mind produces during basic cognition. These can be neutral (e.g., that is a book), negative (I hate that book), or positive (I love that book), and presuppose two basic ingredients: an awareness of a thing and a reaction to it (neutral, negative or positive).

Neutral and positive thoughts generally fail to express themselves in a MT of the bioelectric field, but a negative thought both expresses itself and can be MT. This has to do with the production of stress hormones and neuropeptides that have a negative physiological effect on brain chemistry and muscle activation.

There is a precedent for this: we can measure different types of brain waves (e.g., delta, theta, alpha, beta and gamma waves) and thought patterns do show up in an EEG (electroencephalographic) reading. So why wouldn't negative thoughts express themselves in the bioelectric field? They do. Why wouldn't they be measurable? They are. **Thoughts per se** are no different for MT purposes than the blush response.

However, it is important to make the distinction that we are not measuring the truth of the thought, only its physiological effect on the nervous system in the same way that an EEG doesn't evaluate the truth of the brain waves, only their existence and functionality.

Truth entails a completely different evaluation criterion. For a thought to contain truth it must accurately correspond with absolute reality (e.g., is the book really there?).

We become aware of truth at the border between objective and subjective, linear and nonlinear, logic and intuition, matter and consciousness, science and spirituality. Since MT can be used on both sides of this boundary, it is necessary to define precisely what the boundary is.

It can be defined very simply. Everything on the canvas is objective, everything past the vanishing point is subjective. Everything up to the border is science, including MT the effect of thoughts per se, everything across the border is spirituality.

A whole system of thought has been developed around the concept of MT truth, authored by Dr. David Hawkins, the spiritual teacher and enlightened mystic who brought us the *Map of Consciousness* and his life's work in consciousness research.

In the same way that nobody speaking about drama after Shakespeare could ignore Shakespeare or of physics after Newton could ignore Newton, we can't proceed with a discussion about MT truth without orienting the conversation around Hawkins.

Hawkins: What is Truth?

The capacity for a thought to take on an existence in physical reality is already an advanced, profound concept, but the application of MT to truth brings us to the controversy. Can a MT ascertain truth?

When MT a physical stimulus, the thing being evaluated is whether the stimulus helps or hinders the body. There can be and are successive layers to this but a deliberation about good for us or bad for us is at the root of them, even when this entails thoughts per se.

When MT truth, the thing being evaluated is whether the thought is representative of absolute reality. This is a question that might seem self-evident until you consider that there is no actual way to differentiate truth from falsehood. We have ways of making a case for truth: evidence from the senses, the consensus vote, empirical experience, observation over time, logic and quantification with instruments, but these are all human constructions designed to arrive at a best guess. All knowledge is based on our best guess, even scientific knowledge. The human mind is not capable on its own of accurately differentiating truth from falsehood. That's not to suggest that there is no absolute truth—there absolutely is. But the mind can't discern it simply by thinking about it.

But what if there were a way to be certain? This is the question David Hawkins asked in the 1960s when he was first introduced to MT. It was observed early on that, astoundingly, thoughts had the capacity to express themselves in the body's bioelectric field and produce the same strong or weak MT responses that physical stimuli did. Hawkins made the conceptual leap that if thoughts per se could provoke strong or weak MT responses, truth might thus express itself as well?

The process was as simple as any other MT. A thought was held in the mind. It could have been in the mind of the tester, the person being tested or a third party and this is consistent with the principle that the thought, once produced, takes on a temporary physical existence. The questioning process in the testing was then "Is this thought true, yes or no?" The assumption was that a strong MT response corresponded with an affirmation of truth while a weak MT response indicated the absence of truth (i.e., not "yes," therefore false).

In this way the MT is thought to directly connect the tester with a field of awareness that has been called, at different times, **The Field**, the zero point field, the quantum field, the akashic field, the akashic records, the nonlinear domain, spirit, knowingness, infinity and the Mind of God.

This final intuitive leap, made possible by MT, is the formal step across the boundary of the vanishing point into **the nonlinear domain** of spirituality and consciousness research. The benefit is obvious and tantalizing: omniscience. The concern is also obvious: verifiability. In the same way that the human mind cannot know truth from falsehood to begin with, there is no way to verify that the result of the MT response about truth or falsehood is itself true or false.

There really is a response. If you try this, you may rather disconcertingly notice a strong or weak neurological response to a statement that has intrinsic truth or falsehood (e.g., in conferences, you might be invited to MT your name, then a false name). It is a much more subtle response than we might notice from a MT of an overt physical stimulus, but it is perceptible. The question here isn't whether it is noticeable, the question is whether we can trust it. Specifically, can we trust that the MT responses our bodies are exhibiting accurately correspond with truth and falsehood? That is the question.

This leads us to the **Truth Testing paradox**: Since the mind cannot discern truth from falsehood by thinking about it, and since the Truth Test is responding to the thought field that the mind creates, we cannot know that a Truth Test is correctly evaluating whether the thought field that the mind creates is true or false.

We need to be able to discern truth from falsehood to begin with, but of course once we can do that we no longer need the Truth Test. Truth Testing alone cannot be used as a brute force instrument for deriving truth. We experience truth only by experiencing it. If we can, we can, but if we can't, we can't and that's that. The capacity to experience truth is dependent upon variables other than simply wanting to be able to.

This brings us back to the matter of perspective, only this time at the deepest level. The challenge with gaining a perspective on perspective is that we have to use perspective to do it. This is **the dilemma of perspective**. It is the prison of the mind that we are already aware of, which Hawkins called the house of mirrors. Its corollary in health is trying to use the senses to understand information that the senses won't convey, which relates back to being lost in a desert of health symptoms and needing to follow Somebody out.

In the case of health, we would listen to our doctor or follow the latest health guru. In the case of consciousness, we would follow a spiritual guru, the mystic.

Throughout history, the role of the mystic has been to explore consciousness. This is done through techniques such as meditation, fasting, devotion, spiritual study, physical postures, yoga, chanting, prayer and spending time (e.g., forty days and forty nights) wandering in deserts. These traditional practices are designed to illuminate consciousness by expanding it via the process of maintaining awareness of being, but without using cognition to do so. This is the basis for the Buddhist concept of no-mind and is the opposite of philosophy, which uses only mind.

Hawkins either was a mystic to begin with or realized early on in his MT practice that the only way to transcend the dilemma of perspective, the prison of the mind, was to become a mystic. In the process of pursuing this path, he was finally successful in transcending the mind. The ultimate extent of this is a state of consciousness we know of as **Enlightenment** and Hawkins appears to have attained full Enlightenment. He describes the experience of doing so in *Letting Go* (p.190-194, 2012). The effect of this is evident in his life's work, a series of books, audiobooks, video recorded lectures and radio talks that are a testament to the power of his realization and his devotion to God. It is fascinating that we have lived in a time when a person attained this state of being. It is very rare in human history and deserves a moment's silent reflection...

Understanding Hawkins' achievement (he would have called it a realization) now puts his use of MT truth into perspective. The idea that MT can be used to solve the Truth Testing paradox is only one step removed from the vain hope that we can use perspective to solve the dilemma of perspective: we can't. The only way to transcend perspective is to transcend consciousness by attaining Enlightenment.

Outside of the attainment of Enlightenment, which solves the dilemma of perspective and mind, the concern is whether there can be a satisfactory answer to the question of verifiability when MT truth, since one can't offer as proof evidence that is itself unprovable.

Hawkins proposed a way of looking at this which is at once the simplest and most sophisticated explanation we're likely to find.

Levels of Consciousness

Understanding consciousness as Hawkins illuminates it requires a basic understanding of his *Map of Consciousness*. It is a visually simple document and any reader unfamiliar with it should look it up in Hawkins' books or on the internet when they have a moment.

A basic written outline is that consciousness can be organized into an ascending scale in a logarithmic progression from 1 to 1000 where 1 represents the lowest level of consciousness (a bacteria) and 1000 corresponds with full Enlightenment. Hawkins, using Truth Testing, assigns values on this scale, called calibrations (cal.), which are numeric representations of a **level of consciousness**.

A notable landmark on the scale is cal. 200, above which indicates honesty and below which represents the various stages of dishonesty. We all know people who feel themselves to be free from the truth so this shouldn't come as a revelation—Hawkins is simply assigning them a numeric value for ease of reference.

A major turning point is the number 500, which distinguishes the more subtle quality of perspective outlined in this chapter. At and above (cal.) 500 the nonlinear/intuitive/subjective/spiritual is a dominant orientation while at (cal.) 499 and below, the linear/logical/objective/scientific perspective is the prevailing alignment. The low 500s are the domain of the spiritual seeker, the high 500s of the saint and religious leaders like some popes and the Dalai Lama.

An additional important distinction is made at (cal.) 600, which indicates the movement out of ego and into the lower levels of Enlightenment, which continue on from 600 to 1000. This is the realm of the mystic, the sage, the prophet and the Enlightened being.

As a simple summary: cal. 1 to 199=falsehood, 200=honesty, 500=spirituality, 600=basic Enlightenment, 1000=full Enlightenment.

The impact of these tiers of consciousness on the accuracy of MT nonlinear truth (as opposed to linear thoughts) is as follows:

Hawkins makes it repeatedly clear in every book and many lectures that people who aren't at a consciousness level of 200 (people who are dishonest as a lifestyle) will not get accurate responses from Truth Testing. He even suggests that if either one of the two parties doing the Truth Test is below 200, or if the thought being tested is a non-integrous thought, the MT result won't be accurate. He goes on to quantify that a full 85% of the planet is below 200 but that the ratio is closer to 50/50 in the Judeo-Christian world. These statistics make it clear that the bulk of the world's population cannot expect to perform Truth Testing with any accuracy whatsoever.

He outlines that even above 200, from consciousness level 200-499, there will still only be partial accuracy and only at 500-599 will a more general, progressive level of accuracy develop. To quantify this, he states that only 28 million people (4.4%) on the planet are in the 500-599 range (i.e., spiritually oriented people who have begun to transcend a linear way of being and are at different stages on the path of love and devotion). However, Hawkins specifies that even in the 500-599 range, accuracy in Truth Testing is not a guarantee.

In *The Eye of the I: From Which Nothing is Hidden* (p.57, 2001) he states that the process of Truth Testing itself calibrates at 600. This is reemphasized in his other books and is a significant distinction. While perhaps commonly interpreted to imply that using Truth Testing places the user in the 600s, I would suggest that it is more advisable to interpret this to mean that the user would need to be in the 600s (i.e., be Enlightened) to use it accurately.

In *Transcending the Levels of Consciousness* (p.275, 2006) he wrote that there were six people on the planet who were above consciousness level 600 at the time of writing, and since Hawkins has died subsequent to making this observation, presumably there are now only five people worldwide at that level, assuming none have been born. It stands to reason that if there is a need for complete, consistent accuracy in Truth Testing, the tester should be one of these five people. Statistically, you're not likely to be one of them.

Anyone who has experimented with Truth Testing will admit to sharing in a common hope that their results are accurate. Otherwise, why do it? But the obvious concern is that if consistent accuracy requires a minimum consciousness level of 600, the non-enlightened experimenter (i.e., everybody except for five people) will need to settle for inconsistent accuracy at best.

How inconsistent? How do we know which of the responses are correct and which are incorrect? Do we just plough through and hope for the best? But what if accuracy is important? What if we can't afford for the Truth Test to be wrong? Very simply then, don't do it.

For some people, perhaps partial accuracy in Truth Testing is sufficient. For example, someone might decide to Truth Test whether they had a past lifetime in medieval Europe, and the testing may indicate that they did (e.g., is this statement true? MT result is strong, therefore yes, this statement is true.). The person may then decide to believe they had a past lifetime in medieval Europe. This might put them in a great mood and explain to their satisfaction why they can't resist collecting suits of chain mail and have a dread of the bubonic plague. Maybe this really is true or maybe it isn't. Either way, the information isn't going to harm anybody and might even boost antique sales. This is an example of the idea that spiritual exploration is benign.

It is apparent, however, that even within the subjective, nonlinear, intuitive, consciousness-based, spiritual realm that lies beyond the vanishing point of the canvas referred to above, there are unexpected limitations to who can use Truth Testing, and further limits to how much accuracy, and therefore benefit those who do use it can expect.

Where Science and Spirituality Meet

When we step back onto the canvas and become anchored in **the linear domain** that is objective, logical, concrete and scientific there arises the reasonable concern that the unverifiable nature of Truth Testing data hinders rather than helps scientific and medical exploration by introducing constant doubt about the accuracy of the results and therefore the validity of the MT technique.

From the perspective of reason, the dilemma of perspective that culminates in the Truth Testing paradox has no solution, since the concern that the observer can influence the results of the test cannot be assuaged by more observation. Expressed differently, a circular argument will never get us out of a circle. This logical impasse arises from an inability to distinguish content from context, which entails a lack of understanding that the quality of perception can change. Einstein recognized this when he observed that we cannot solve the great problems of our age from the conceptual level we created them at.

Hawkins uses the example of trying to measure the beauty of a symphony with a thermometer. The thermometer is representative of linear, measurable science. Beauty is a quality of the nonlinear, subjective realm. Certainly there is temperature in the room where the symphony is being played and certainly it can be measured, but conflating the temperature that has been measured with the beauty of the composition misses the point of the performance.

While the linear field is quantitative, the nonlinear is qualitative. Differentiating between these two layers of awareness is not always simple since only in the nonlinear field of awareness can one truly understand (by experiencing) nonlinear reality. From a linear perspective, the nonlinear appears not to exist, or to be invalid, unprovable, subjective and inaccessible. This is probably at the root of the classic division between science and spirituality, where spirituality recognizes itself and science, but science is only capable of recognizing itself and feels out of its element with spirituality.

Understanding now that we exist in a progressive spectrum of consciousness that is divided metaphorically in half, where one half is oriented toward linear awareness and the other is inclusive of both linear and nonlinear awareness but only populated by about 28 million people, the core problem of interpreting MT becomes apparent. If someone's agenda is to explore the nonlinear domain, the unverifiability of Truth Testing may not deter them because non-linear information is filtered through intuition, not logic. However, if their desire is to explore the linear domain only, and if they are a scientifically-minded or even just a logical person, they will be rightly unwilling to use a technique like MT which is thought to derive information that is intrinsically subjective and unprovable. They may even be vehemently opposed to MT, and from their perspective, rightly so.

This is because they are failing to distinguish that MT can be applied to both the linear and the nonlinear. While MT and Truth Testing entail the same biomechanical process, they presuppose completely different energetic processes and are used to explore two different layers of reality. It is important to recognize this.

The scientific, linear world has until now been prejudiced against MT because MT has predominantly been associated with Truth Testing. The disadvantage of an anti-MT bias is that science then loses the significant opportunity to take advantage of MT and its applications in the scientific, and particularly medical worlds. We have been lost in the desert of health long enough. MT can get us out.

Hawkins made it clear that 85% of the planet can't expect to use Truth Testing at all. Perhaps he should have made it clearer that the other 15% can't expect to use it with anything approaching accuracy. Then, what he didn't make clear enough was that while 85% of the planet cannot use Truth Testing at all, they certainly can use MT. When MT is kept within the linear domain everyone can use it. To Hawkins' credit, if this had been posed to him as a question, I believe he would have agreed with the truth of it.

The advantage of the scientific MT methodology outlined in this book is that it can be used by everyone. When the testing is restricted to physical stimuli and not used to evaluate truth, there are no restrictions concerning who can MT. Level of consciousness has no impact on the results, only the three variables listed above: accuracy, repeatability and logic, which are all within the control of the tester.

All of the experiments in MT outlined in the chapters that follow have the essential quality of repeatability. Linear MT is free, immediate, simple, verifiable, logical, reliable and scientific. By contrast, as soon as the truth of a thought is MT, the limits of Truth Testing apply: we're off the canvas and into the nonlinear domain.

In this sense, we can view MT as spanning a great continental divide: in one direction, it carries the explorer toward spirituality; in the other, toward scientific and biomedical exploration. The spiritual direction is fundamentally subjective and nonlinear; the scientific direction is objective and linear. But while Hawkins has used Truth Testing to explore the nonlinear realm with such perfection that his written works should stand as one of history's greatest literary and spiritual accomplishments, only a few attempts have been made to elucidate the scientific and biomedical aspects of MT and none of them has been thorough. Decades after its discovery, we have not even scratched the surface of the linear applications.

Perhaps if the spiritual and scientific paths were followed to their ends, they would each lead to an Ultimate Reality where science and spirituality meet in one unified field. Until then, it will be helpful to differentiate this current body of work from the spiritual focus of Hawkins' works by specifying that while he covered the entire field of awareness from 1 to 1000, and did so using Truth Testing, this work is focused on the range from 1 to 599 (including reason, science and basic nonlinear awareness). There is a deep respect for the range of 600-1000 (The Field of Enlightenment) but an acknowledgement that the intrinsically unprovable (e.g., the Reality of Divinity) cannot be proved by science, it must be realized by experience. Thus, the use of Truth Testing has been strictly avoided in drawing any of the conclusions that follow. Only linear MT has been used.

We can now revisit the question posed at the beginning of this chapter: To what extent does the variable of perspective in MT render it unrepeatable and therefore unreliable?

The answer to this question is that as long as a physical stimulus is being MT (including the physiological effect of a thought per se on the nervous system), we remain rooted in science and perspective is irrelevant; as soon as a MT is used as Truth Testing to evaluate the truth of the energy field that a thought creates, we move beyond the vanishing point and are fundamentally in the realm of spirituality.

Every experiment in MT that is to follow is crafted to be linear so that the whole world, regardless of perspective or consciousness level, can join in and benefit from this methodology.

3

The Physics
of How Muscle Testing Works

Taraka timiram dipo	Stars, shadows, a lamp
Maya-avasyaya budbudam	Illusions, dewdrops, bubbles
Supinam vidyud abhram ca	A dream, lightning and a cloud
Evam drastavyam samskrtam.	In these is perceived the
	ultimate reality

—Buddha
The Diamond Sutra

(English translation from the Sanskrit by Leonard Carter)

In the mid 20th century, an awareness of the body's bioelectric field coalesced among what can most easily be termed the New Age crowd. Certain individuals who had the aptitude were able to notice a constant, fluctuating emanation of color that surrounded the body. Over time this phenomenon became more widely known as the aura.

Although it was and is quantifiable with Kirlian photography, a technique used to capture the electric coronal discharges of objects, in the 1970s when I was growing up the term aura was thrown in with strange meditation practices from the East, tarot card readings, Ouija boards, seances, crystal balls and darkened rooms with hanging bead doorways that you'd be lucky to escape from without meeting a deceased relative, paying a $20 fee or both.

By contrast, the real work in physics was being done in cosmology, the science of quantifying space, time and matter. The two major opposing schools were the unified field theory of Albert Einstein (1879-1955) and the quantum theory of Niels Bohr (1885-1962) and whether it was related or not, the term God particle seemed to hang in the balance. Nobody at the time was able to satisfactorily explain what a God particle was, just that it was the fundamental question to be answered, and people at my childhood church took the preposterous suggestion that God could be reduced to a particle as proof that science and spirituality would never meet.

The only thing that seemed to derail physicists from answering this essential question was that periodically they died an unexpected death from some medical condition: Einstein from an abdominal aneurism at 76 and Bohr from a heart attack at 77. Even at that young age I was left with the impression that the truly fundamental questions were not those of time and space but of what health is and why it inevitably fails us.

The fact is that the information about why health fails us has been rooted in the aura the whole time. This was probably overlooked and disregarded by scientists because the aura was called an aura and no serious scientist wanted to touch the topic with a 10-foot pole. Talking about an aura is a great way to lose a research grant. What it should have been called from the outset was what it is: the bioelectric field.

The Bioelectric Field

An understanding of the body's bioelectric field requires a basic familiarity with the physics of cell biology.

All cells have a membrane that is to them as our skin is to us. Each membrane is embedded with many different proteins which, because they carry things across the membrane are called trans-membrane proteins. Some of these trans-membrane proteins are pumps that give a cell its electric charge by moving ions (charged atoms) of sodium (Na#11), potassium (K#19) and calcium (Ca#20) in and out of the cell. Some of these pumps are called sodium-potassium (NaK) pumps, and because they pump ions, the core concept is that of **ion cycling**.

Here is an image for visual reference but an internet image search will bring up animated examples of NaK pump ion cycling that are more informative than a static picture.

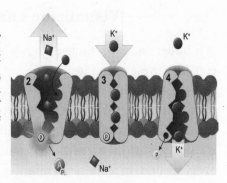

Sodium-Potassium Pump Math

One way to analyze the strength of the bioelectric field is to estimate its volume from the number of NaK ions cycling through the NaK pumps every second. Here is the raw data:

1. Each pump cycles sodium and potassium ions at a rate of 150 to 300 times per second. For this calculation, I've use the bottom end of the range: 150 cycles per second per pump. I have not factored in the number of sodium and potassium ion channels in each cell membrane, just the pumps, and this overlooks calcium ions as well.

2. Each individual cell membrane has anywhere from 80,000 to 30 million sodium potassium pumps. Let's take a low average of 10 million pumps per cell.

3. The Smithsonian Institute released a statement in 2015 that they calculate that the average human body has 37.2 trillion cells. I've used that number.

37.2 trillion cells x 10 million NaK pumps x 150 cycles/second = a number that you would have to look up to know how to express in language: 55,800,000,000,000,000,000,000, or 55.8 sextillion (e.g., million, billion, trillion, quadrillion, quintillion, sextillion).

That is how many times per second NaK ions cycle to produce our bioelectric field and this is a deliberately low estimate. I invite the Smithsonian Institute to arrive at a better, more accurate number once this book popularizes ion cycling in the bioelectric field.

Visualizing Large Numbers

It is understandably difficult to relate to numbers in the sextillions, so consider these examples:

According to the UK news periodical *The Telegraph* (article from Jan 24, 2016) the total property value of the planet earth at that time was $217 trillion. If 55.8 sextillion were translated into dollars, it could buy up all the real estate on 257 million earth sized planets... every second. In a matter of minutes that would buy the whole galaxy.

A more down to earth example is that our planet is thought to house roughly 7 quintillion grains of sand, so using that figure, if you took all the grains of sand on 7971 earth-sized planets, that would give you the number 55.8 sextillion, but again, 1 second later you would need another 7971 planets worth of sand, and then where would you put it all?

Simply put, it's enough cycles per second to create an electromagnetic field that surrounds and emanates from the body.

Description of the Bioelectric Field

This volume of ion cycling represents a significant enough movement of charged particles to produce an electromagnetic field that extends 3 to 5 inches beyond the body. For ease of reference this is termed a bioelectric field. Its size varies from one person to the next based on internal factors that influence electrical conductivity, such as hydration, sodium, potassium and calcium levels, circulatory capacity, bone density, nutrition, sleep, stress, mood, parasites, bacterial, fungal and viral interference, age, body composition, diet and genetic traits.

As an electromagnetic emanation it is probably only slightly stronger than brain waves, which are measured from 100 femtoteslas to 1 picotesla (e.g., 500,000 times less electromagnetism than a toaster).

There is a passive quality to the field such that it can conduct static electric charges inward, which renders people susceptible to picking up electric shocks from surfaces like a carpet despite the skin and fat layers being insulators. However, consistent with the nature of electricity, the bioelectric field also has the capacity to conduct inward charges outward, so that internal bioelectric information like organ functionality or nutrient levels for example can be measured at the outer surface of the body. Thus, the field serves the dual purpose of conducting information inward and outward, making it an ideal basis upon which to found a system of medical diagnostic inquiry.

The bioelectric field itself is invisible to the human eye, being in the near infrared spectrum (850nm to 1100nm). If you place your hand next to your cheek without touching it you may feel a slightly warm radiance. This is the result of the bioelectric feedback between two near infrared wavelength sources. What you are feeling in this experiment is your own bioelectric field or if you like, your own aura.

The field is pooled more densely in the core areas where the body, and therefore the ion cycling, is thicker, and is found more thinly in the extremities. This is why a MT of the field is more accurate when localized in the core, and why we place substances that are being MT against the abdomen or chest, as opposed to simply holding them in the hand, which by virtue of its distance from the core produces the least accurate bioelectric field response.

Since you carry this field with you wherever you go, it is a simple, immediate and free means of analyzing your internal and external environments, if you can learn how to interpret it accurately.

Summary of the Bioelectric Field

The bioelectric field is the cumulative electromagnetic field produced by the rapid cycling of 55.8 sextillion charged NaK atoms per second across cell membranes throughout the body.

It has a magnetic field strength in the low picotesla range and vibrates in the near infrared spectrum at 850-1100 nanometers. It conducts information both inward and outward. Though invisible to the average human eye, it emanates to a distance of 3 to 5 inches from the surface of the skin and is pooled most densely in the core. This field can be used as a simple internal and external diagnostic tool and is the scientific basis upon which MT is founded.

Interpreting the Bioelectric Field

Once we understand the presence of the field around the body, we are led to the practical concern of how we are supposed to interpret this information. There are different ways to do this.

These are summarized in chart form for ease of recognition:

	Ways to Interpret the Bioelectric Field	
1	**Mathematical** Understanding the bioelectric field using math and physics.	This chapter, below.
2	**Biological** The matter of how the MT response expresses itself physically. This has to do with neurology and muscle anatomy.	Pt1-Ch4: **The Biology of How MT Works**
3	**Biomechanical** The details about how to accurately perform a MT at home or in a clinical setting.	Pt2-Ch1:**The Motor Skills of MT**
4	**Logical** How to use reason to interpret and build on MT data.	Pt2-Ch2: **How to Interpret a MT**

While mathematical and logical interpretations might seem to be two sides of the same coin, they are different sides in that the math can stand alone, but logic depends on all the underlying interpretations. Without taking this multilayered approach to the logic, the data will lack meaning, utility or both.

For example, a physicist will agree with the binary nature of MT, a neurologist will understand the biological implications, and a clinical practitioner will grasp the motor skills, but only logic allows us to merge math, biology and biomechanics to see the big picture.

The bioelectric field cannot be taken at face value. If we don't understand its mathematical, biological and biomechanical implications, any attempt at interpretation will only get us more lost. For MT to be a sixth sense, to fulfill the promise at the beginning of this book and lead us out of the desert of poor health, we need to be able to comprehend what we are interpreting. This ends with logic but it starts with binary mathematics.

The Binary Bioelectric Field

The bioelectric field registers functional responses that are consistent with the rules of binary mathematics.

Binary is a mathematical system of 1 and 0, yes and not-yes. In the same manner, the bioelectric field carries a positive charge, expressed as a 1, or a negative charge, expressed as a 0. You don't need to write this expression out but you do need to constantly have it in mind: 1, 0, 1, 0. That's all you're looking for, a 1 or a 0.

Being able to interpret a MT requires that we start in the positive, otherwise we have nothing to build on. Imagine asking someone where they want to go out for dinner. Do they want to go to this place? No. That place? No. How about this place? No. We could ask for hours until finally, we discover that they didn't want to go out for dinner to begin with and we were asking the wrong question. We need to start with the right question. Do they want to go out for dinner at all? Yes. Okay, how about this place? No? Now at least we know that we have a legitimate negative response, a legitimate 0.

In the context of MT, this translates into the need to find a positive response to begin with. This is called a **baseline**. If we don't have a positive baseline as a starting point (or in binary thinking, a 1), there is no basis upon which to found any subsequent conclusions.

The whole point of doing a MT is to pursue a thought process: a diagnostic inquiry with a desired outcome that can be reduced mathematically to a 1 or a 0. We want to understand something. Keeping with the example above, although it has nothing to do with MT, we want to know where we can go out for dinner. But if we can only get yes or no responses, and nothing more sophisticated, yes and no are better than no answer at all. There are only a finite number of restaurants so eventually we will find one to go to.

The simplicity of this approach is necessary because we are dealing with our autonomic nervous system (ANS). What we need to grasp at this stage is that the ANS is completely incapable of expressing complex answers. It cannot so much as string two words together. We're lucky that it can express itself in yes and no, 1 and 0.

Comparison to the Baseline

At face value a positive MT baseline only tells us that the nervous system is functioning normally. Beyond that fact, there is nothing further we can learn from a baseline alone. To take the consideration process further, we need to compare something to it.

A positive baseline is assigned a value of 1. If the stimulus we are comparing shows no difference, that also gets a 1, which means nothing has happened and we still have nothing to go on. If instead the stimulus produces a negative response, this is indicated by a 0 and it tells us that something has happened. In binary, something has turned a 1 to a 0. Expressed in language, something has turned a positive baseline to a negative. We don't know why yet. At this binary stage of interpretation we are simply looking for the fact of a shift.

This consideration process is called making a **comparison to a baseline**. There is an implicit judgment that if a stimulus has turned a positive baseline to a negative MT response, a 1 to a 0, it must have some actual negative value for the body. In very simplistic language, it must be bad for the body in some way. But we don't know what form that badness is taking: it could be a lethal negative stimulus like radioactivity; there could be deadly parasite eggs in the thing being tested; there could be a virus; or it could have a simpler negative form like the presence of a heavy metal in a food that might feed a bad bacteria in the body but not do any major long-term harm.

The challenging thing about interpreting the body's binary response to negative stimuli is that we must contend with the whole range of negativity from barely negative to actually lethal. At the face-value level of using a MT to compare a stimulus to a baseline we don't have access to such qualitative information, so it is important to bear in mind that all we have identified is a negative response. Binary mathematics is perfect for this: we quantify the negative as a 0.

It is fair at this stage to articulate that we have identified a negative value but it is also essential to reiterate that the negative, or 0, is an unknown quantity. We don't know why it is negative, we just know that it is negative. For now, this is enough. It is a starting point.

Positive Versus Not-negative

If a **negative stimulus** can at some level be interpreted as bad, can we also interpret a positive stimulus as good? This brings up an interesting question: How exactly is a **positive stimulus** identified?

A stimulus is not positive simply because it fails to provoke a negative response. It may be positive but it may also be neutral. In a comparison to a baseline, all we can really conclude when a stimulus fails to turn a positive baseline to a negative is that it is not negative. Both a positive and a **neutral stimulus** will allow a positive baseline to remain positive and this has repercussions on how we interpret positivity. There is a big risk of mistakenly assuming that a stimulus is positive when in fact it is merely not-negative or neutral.

A common example of such misinterpretation is to see someone in a supplement store getting a product MT on their bioelectric field. They start with a positive baseline (1), then introduce the supplement and redo the MT in a comparison to the baseline. If the supplement MT negative (0) they correctly conclude that some factor in the product is a negative stimulus, and that it should be avoided. But if instead the supplement simply fails to turn the positive baseline (1) to a negative (i.e., it is still 1), can they conclude that it is a positive stimulus? They cannot. But they do anyway because they don't understand basic binary logic. This is the most common error of interpretation that a beginner in MT will make.

While a stimulus that is negative is indisputably negative, something that is not negative is not necessarily positive, it could simply be neutral. An example of something neutral is a brick. If you MT a brick on your bioelectric field it will fail to provoke a weak MT response. That doesn't mean you should eat the brick.

At this early level of consideration, which is still quite superficial, it is important to keep our conclusions narrow, precise and binary. There isn't enough information to draw any conclusion except the obvious: something that MT negative is negative, and we don't know why; something that fails to MT negative is either positive or neutral and we don't know why that is either. It is simply a binary fact.

Building on a Negative Baseline

When a stimulus MT negative in comparison to a baseline we have confirmed that it is a negative stimulus, but only at face value. We still don't know why it is negative. To begin to build on this fact and draw conclusions about it, we need more information. Specifically, we need to identify what stimulus cancels it out. This is expressed as **building on a negative baseline.**

First, we need to start with a positive baseline as outlined above. Then we need to find a stimulus that provokes a negative response. A beginner should repeat that MT a couple of times to be sure that their negative stimulus has the quality of repeatability.

When we have found something that provokes a negative MT response, we have found a void. If we can fill this void, then and only then can we begin to draw conclusions about why the stimulus MT weak.

The question is what additional stimulus can we introduce that will cancel out the negative response we have found?

Phrased in binary, we are looking for the stimulus that

> **MT Protocol: Building on a Negative Baseline**
>
> 1. Start with a (+) baseline.
> 2. Find something that MT (-).
> 3. Start introducing stimuli until you find which one cancels out the (-).
>
> **A:** If it fails to turn the (-) back to a (+), i.e., if the new stimulus is still only (-), there is no causal relationship.
>
> **B:** If it turns the (-) back to a (+) you have found a causal relationship.

turns the negative back to a positive. If we find one that does this, we can logically infer a causal relationship between the negative stimulus and the thing that cancelled it out (turned it back to a positive).

If instead the new stimulus fails to turn the negative back to a positive, so that the negative baseline we are trying to build on remains a negative baseline, then we have failed to find any causal relationship between those two stimuli.

The Holy Grail we are looking for is a **causal relationship**.

Binary Muscle Testing Process in Sequence

To link these concepts together let us consider them in sequence:

Baseline: this is simply a deltoid MT. For it to be a positive baseline, the arm must MT positive. This is to ensure that the muscle is working at all, otherwise we have no basis for a comparison.

Comparison to a baseline: we can now introduce a stimulus by holding it against the body's bioelectric field and MT it while using the original positive baseline as a comparison. A simple thing to MT would be a supplement bottle such as vitamin C. It should fail to MT negative, since vitamin C is generally good for us. From this we can conclude that it is either neutral or positive but not negative. However, once this is established, we don't have anything further to explore. The consideration process is over because it was quite superficial. Ideally, we want to find a negative.

A more intermediate application of MT is to evaluate the stomach. Press a few inches into your abdomen, localized around the stomach (under your bottom left rib). If you push deep enough this should provoke a negative MT. We can confirm that there is something going on in the stomach since it MT negative in comparison to the original baseline. We don't know why it is negative yet, only that it is.

Building on a negative baseline: Now, while maintaining the pressure that provoked the negative MT, we can introduce other stimuli simultaneously to see if any of them cancels out the negative stomach MT by turning it back to a positive.

For example, we might introduce the original vitamin C. If the process of placing it inside the body's bioelectric field alters the field in such a way that the negative MT of the stomach is turned back to a positive then we can infer that vitamin C is playing some role in why the stomach is MT negative. In this way we have built on a negative baseline and established a **causal relationship**. We appear to need the C.

This presents a solution to the supplement store problem outlined above. The person should have found a negative baseline, such as a stomach MT, and then built on it by MT different products to see which one turned the negative back to a positive.

Thinking in Binary

In the previous example, the binary thought process is that we start with a positive or a 1, find the stimulus that produces a negative or 0 and then build on the negative baseline to see which secondary stimulus cancels the negative out, turning it back to a positive or 1.

So, positive [baseline], negative [stimulus], positive [secondary stimulus] (1, 0, 1) leads us to a causal relationship while positive, negative, negative (1, 0, 0) does not provide the necessary information.

If instead we start with a negative or 0, it may be possible to introduce a stimulus that turns the negative back to a positive, or 1, but with 0 as our starting point the body wasn't expressing a normal response to begin with, so trying to build on that and draw more complex conclusions is going to be difficult and inaccurate.

This process is consistent with the nature of electricity which has either a positive or negative charge. What we are looking for in the binary responses of the MT is its correspondence with the behavior of electricity so that we can draw scientifically accurate and logically predictable conclusions.

Remember that at face value, the only valid conclusion is that the response is what it is—positive or negative. For this data to be interpreted relative to our health and wellness, we require the addition of a logical thought process (Pt2-Ch2: How to Interpret a MT) that is in turn dependent upon a knowledge of the products or stimuli being MT. This knowledge is based on the fields of pharmacology, molecular nutrition, organic chemistry, bacteriology, virology, organ physiology, waveform physics, electromagnetism, nonlinear math and parasite microbiology, and encompasses modern scientific theory.

The observation of a MT response is a matter of gathering binary data, covered in this section, while an interpretation of a MT response requires superimposing logic on the binary data.

This is a summary of the levels of complexity involved in correctly interpreting a MT response using a mathematical (binary) thought process and taking into account the diverse scientific disciplines this can be applied to.

Linear Versus Nonlinear Interpretation

While MT is scientific, repeatable, accessible to all, subject to simple binary interpretation and therefore based in the linear domain, Truth Testing is fundamentally nonlinear and accessible not as a repeatable process but only as a function of the subjectivity of consciousness itself.

It is relevant here to present the explanation that Hawkins gives of the non-dualistic nature of reality:

"In contrast, via the Heisenberg principle in quantum mechanics, the details of the evolutionary change can be contextualized in mathematical formulas. Intention (consciousness) collapses the wave function from the potential to the actual, from the potential state of the universe (the Schrödinger equations) to the collapsed wave state (the Dirac equation). The new state then becomes the new potential state that then "collapses" into the next defined state." (Hawkins, *Discovery of the Presence of God*, p. 107, 2006).

The Truth Test "is a general response of consciousness itself to the energy of a substance or a statement...that stems from the impersonal field of consciousness which is present in everyone living" (Hawkins, *Transcending the Levels of Consciousness*, p. 373, 2006).

As we can see, the math, science and contextualization of the nonlinear Truth Testing is radically different from the simple binary analysis that is suitable for standard, linear MT.

There is no comparison between these two modes of evaluation. The only thing they share in common is pressure on an indicator muscle.

To paraphrase Hawkins, he stated that the purpose of Truth Testing was consciousness research, not simple MT. (Hawkins, *Transcending the Levels of Consciousness*, p. 380, 2006).

Why Only Now?

The content in this chapter is monumental. Far from being a simple summary of existing knowledge, it provides a window on information that the average person hasn't encountered before. Why haven't they?

In the Information Age this is so rare an event that it deserves pause. How could something so immediate, technology-independent, accurate, important and relevant, and with such a strong scientific basis have been overlooked in the modern scientific era? Why is it only now coming to light? Why were we not all taught this in school?

Surely not due to complexity, as the principles are relatively simple: they are so simple, so obvious that they seem too good to be true. And that's the issue.

That the question of truth should arise so quickly here probes to the core of the matter. Scientific truth is concerned with admissible information. Bioelectricity, which MT is rooted in, should fall under the umbrella of modern scientific theory, so why is its truth so easily called into question?

The issue is most likely one of paradigm. The prevailing scientific paradigm must acknowledge the reality of bioelectricity, but isn't calibrated to consider any conclusions based on it to be admissible. Perhaps we are the inheritors of one too many centuries of the idea that seeing is believing to be comfortable delving into a thought process based on a science that is fundamentally unseeable.

Another possibility is that the intrinsic bias of the current paradigm is one of the supremacy of opinion, although it swears not to be, and the process of drawing conclusions from the bioelectric field via MT renders opinion obsolete. I'm sure nobody will deny that there are big egos in the scientific and medical worlds who hold their opinions very dear and may even have reputations staked on them.

We are left with one of these two interpretations: either modern scientific theory, with all its sacrosanctity is very biased indeed or it has been remiss in overlooking this information for the last six decades. The reader can decide for themselves, but let's take a quick look at history and see how this might have come about.

Paradigms in History

The best illustration of the dual problems of intellectual bias and genuine oversight in the history of science is the Copernican Revolution. In the two millennia prior to Copernicus (1473-1543), scholars interpreted the Sun's movement overhead to mean that it revolved around the Earth, placing the Earth at the center not only of our solar system but of the known universe. This was called geocentrism, though in retrospect it could also be called egocentrism.

Then over a 250 year period a number of astronomers, most notably Copernicus, Galileo, Kepler and finally Isaac Newton (1642-1727), published a series of works that provided the scientific basis for scholars to agree that the Sun belonged at the center of the solar system (heliocentrism). This is called the Copernican Revolution because it fomented a transformation in thought that paved the way for an understanding of universal gravitation, modern cosmology and modern scientific theory as we now know it.

That single shift in perception from the Earth at the center to the Sun at the center allowed all of this to happen. It is called a paradigm shift because it entailed not just new information but also a transformation of how we interpreted old information. This paradigm shift is thought to have made possible the level of scientific awareness we now use to think about the known universe.

When Europe still used the geocentric model of the universe, the father of physics was Aristotle (384-322 BC). He lived almost 2400 years before us and can be forgiven for lacking an adequate understanding of physics and cosmology. It was a credit to the Europeans that they finally recognized his limitations and replaced him as the father of physics with Isaac Newton, whom we rightly regard as the father of the modern scientific age. If we still clung to Aristotle today, knowing what we know now, that would reflect poorly upon us, not upon Aristotle, who had less information than we do.

I stated at the beginning of this chapter that I felt the fundamental questions of life were not those of time and space but of what health is and why it inevitably fails us.

Perhaps the most important question about health is that of how we came to think this way in the first place. Well, who is the father of modern medicine? The answer is Hippocrates of Cos (460-370 BC), an ancient Greek who lived even earlier than Aristotle. How does it reflect upon us that still today we choose as the father of modern medicine someone that lived almost 2400 years ago?

Is it possible that this attachment to such an antiquated view of health carries with it an unconscious bias or some oversight? For the moment, let's forget about Hippocrates and consider the state of modern health: Does it really make sense that the human race needs to live with illness? Is it logical to assume that the name of an illness is also somehow causing it (e.g., diabetes is causing diabetes)? Is it troubling to anyone that after 100 years of using modern technology to try to come up with cures to medical conditions, we haven't cured a single one and have instead found thousands of new ones? Could there be a historical blind spot in here somewhere?

The blind spot of geocentrism was the assumption that the Earth was at the center of the cosmos. By positioning the Sun at the center it became possible to realize that we were living in a universe.

The fact is that when it comes to medicine, as with everything else, there is an absolute truth; there is a way out of the desert. But how can we find it when we are buried in the sand of opinions?

It could be said that the blind spot of diagnosis lies in the assumption that the opinion is at the center of the truth. The truth, of course, is not determined by opinion. That is the essence of the error in a relativistic approach to reality. Absolute truth exists whether it is our opinion that it exists or not.

The fundamental truth about health is rooted in and expressed through bioelectricity. By placing the bioelectric field at the center of our understanding and **orbiting our opinions** around it we place ourselves in the best position to come to an awareness of information that the opinion alone, and our senses alone cannot.

Thus a practical solution to the dilemma of perspective is to understand that our perspective is not relevant to the truth.

Spirituality, Physics and Chaos

The questions in physics that apply to you and me have to do not with relativity (which deals with galaxy-sized problems) or quantum mechanics (which deals with subatomic-sized problems) but with chaos.

Chaos deals with human-sized problems like the question of what health is and why it periodically fails us. The answer to this question is to be found in the bioelectric field but bioelectricity, being electrical, is nonlinear, appears chaotic and needs to be analyzed using unprecedented mathematical sophistication.

Nonlinear reality has traditionally been so sophisticated that it was interpreted not through the lens of science but through spiritual study. We find an example of this in the *Diamond Sutra*, outlined at the top of this chapter, where the Buddha suggests a contemplation of fundamentally nonlinear forms like dreams, lightning and clouds for the purpose of giving nonlinearity a tangible quality that we can relate to using linear thinking.

In modern physics, chaos theory has arguably outpaced relativity and quantum mechanics in importance. In later chapters we will explore one of the problems in chaos as it relates to health (Pt3-Ch6, 7, 34). This has to do with calibrating an electromagnetic waveform to do the impossible: reach a terminal state of resonant frequency with a nonlinear system, something that has radical implications in the fields of physics, math, healthcare and parasitology.

However, in this chapter we are primarily interested in evaluating nonlinearity (chaos, if you prefer) using binary math to analyze the bioelectric field. We find that if we combine MT, binary mathematics and logic we can accurately interpret information from the bioelectric field that is not otherwise accessible to our five senses.

The act of doing so not only quantifies what is uncertain and begins to get us out of the desert but also represents a significant advancement in consciousness when compared to the standard, historical, linear method of cognition used in opinion-based diagnosis.

To apply MT we now need an understanding of biology that is consistent with the physics outlined above. We will explore this next.

4

The Biology
of How Muscle Testing Works

infirmos curate	**Heal the sick,**
mortuos suscitate	**cleanse the lepers,**
leprosos mundate	**raise the dead,**
daemones eicite	**cast out devils;**
gratis accepistis gratis date	**freely ye have received, freely give.**

—Jesus
The Gospel of St. Matthew. **10:8**

(English translation from the *King James Bible*)

O nce we understand that the bioelectric field functions according to the laws of physics, it remains to be identified how the field is able to express itself in the skeletal muscles. Manual MT wouldn't be necessary at all if there were a device that could read the bioelectric field, such as a Star Trek tricorder. Some Captain Kirk or Commander Spock of the future could scan you with it, look down at their device, frown, and announce elevated bacterial levels, a foreign parasite or biological contamination from a recent away-team mission on an alien world. All of that information is logged in the bioelectric field but we lack the interpretive senses and for that matter the tricorder to decode any of it.

Until then, at least, with a basic understanding of neurology and biomechanics, we can use a MT to access that information. This is the beginning of the pathway to healing.

53

The Turtle Response

Anyone who has been MT correctly will be familiar with the surprising, impossible-to-resist weak neurological response that occurs when something is MT on them. This response is what makes MT possible but how does it work?

It is simplest to think of the weak MT response as a recoil of the nervous system. If you have ever tapped on the glass of a fish tank (despite a sign saying not to), you will have noticed the fish dart away as the shockwave hits them. This darting-away recoil response is hardwired into all animal life.

We can see this demonstrated in turtles. When a turtle feels threatened, it retracts its legs and head. Our nervous systems respond in a similar fashion but when we experience physiological 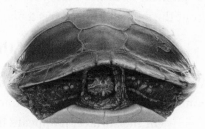 stress of some sort, we can't simply retract our limbs. They aren't retractable. Instead, the intensity of the outgoing motor signal itself is retracted, and this can be measured in pounds of force.

This reduction in outgoing signal is not visible to the eye but we can quantify that it has happened with a MT. This is done by performing a MT to establish a baseline of strength and then introducing a stimulus for comparison to the baseline.

If the perceived strength in the comparison is the same as the original, then logically there must be no change in the outgoing signal and we can conclude the stimulus we evaluated in the MT was positive or neutral since it failed to cause a motor signal retraction.

If instead the perceived strength is less than the baseline, the reduction in strength tells us that the motor signal was retracted.

This **Turtle Response**, or relative weakness, indicates whether or not the nervous system has experienced a negative stimulus or stressor. This is what we are looking for in a MT.

Positive/Negative Versus Strong/Weak

In the previous chapter, neurological responses were characterized as positive or negative as this is consistent with the binary nature of MT (i.e., 1, 0). In this chapter those same binary responses will instead be described as strong and weak (1, positive = strong; 0, negative = weak).

They are two sides of the same coin or different ways of looking at the same thing. The fact is that in the world, most people look at MT from the perspective of biology, particularly in a clinical setting, and use strong/weak as their frame of reference. It is best to be fluent in both the biological and mathematical ways of thinking about the subject as each has a place in the MT lexicon.

The Physiology of the Turtle Response

What region of our nervous system does the Turtle Response originate from? And is this even the right question?

On the surface, it appears that we can ascribe it to the brain. After all, in clinical terminology it is called a weak neurological response. There are multiple brain structures that respond to stress, such as the well-known HPA axis (hypothalamic/adrenal/pituitary) or the thalamus itself. But as we will see in the following chapter, the Turtle Response can be provoked simply by performing a two-handed MT against the arm. And then of course it is central to MT science that a stimulus held near the bioelectric field can provoke a weak response without any direct physical contact.

We might assign the response to the muscle itself, and this is possible based on the electrical nature of neurological communication but also seems limited. The most comprehensive explanation is that the bioelectric field as a whole undergoes a shift in response to internal or external stimuli. When the field is resonating with a positive charge, the MT response is strong; when a stressful stimulus causes it to switch to a negative charge, the MT response is weak.

It is most accurate to interpret the Turtle Response as an expression of the resonation of the bioelectric field as a whole.

The Neurology of Muscle Activation

Understanding that the weak MT response, or Turtle Response, is a quality of the bioelectric field itself, we can now examine how shifts in the field's electric charge translate into muscle activation.

Simply put, **a muscle is like a light switch**: it is interpreted to be on or off. However, muscles rarely tend to be fully off, so perhaps a dimmer switch is the more exact simile. The degree to which a muscle is on or off is its level of activation.

It is helpful to think of muscle activation in percentages. A muscle may be 100% activated, 80%, 50%, etc. If it is 80% activated, it is 20% inhibited. Activation and inhibition are two sides of the same coin. The degree of inhibition can vary from partial to full—this doesn't concern us here. It is simplest to overlook the technicality of partial activation and analyze the muscle comparatively. If it was activated in the strong baseline, and some stimulus inhibits it (renders it weak or negative) then comparatively, we have found a problem. We must now analyze the stimulus that caused the weakness: this is what MT is focused on.

A MT, then, seeks to identify any inhibition. As a reminder from the last chapter, we are looking for a stimulus that inhibits a positive baseline, creating a negative MT response so that we can begin to analyze the stimulus (build on a negative baseline).

The thing that determines muscle activation is the electric charge in the axon. This should recall your knowledge of muscle anatomy: the axon is like an electric wire that transmits the electric charge along the motor neuron from the brain (the motor cortex) to the muscle (the axon terminal). Similar to an actual wire, the axon is wrapped in a rubbery coating called the

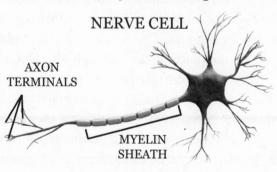

NERVE CELL

AXON TERMINALS

MYELIN SHEATH

myelin sheath. In cases of Multiple sclerosis, for example, the myelin sheath has deteriorated to the point that electric signal communication along the axon becomes progressively difficult.

It is this same reduction in electric charge that we are identifying in a MT except that when a negative stimulus is introduced to the bioelectric field, the reduction in activation is immediate but only temporary. In binary, this is a negative MT, clinically it is articulated as a weak MT and we can now quantify the stimulus that did this.

This provides an electrical perspective on the primary objection to MT since its introduction in the 1960s: that there is no obvious pathway for a negative stimulus to inhibit a muscle. That the identification of a pathway is even the desired outcome demonstrates the questioner's lack of understanding of the neurology of muscle activation. A muscle is like a light switch: it is on, off or at least dimmed as a result of the fluctuating electric charges in the axon. These fluctuations can originate directionally from the brain down to the muscle or from the muscle up to the brain; but they don't need to. They can also originate mid-way along the axon itself.

The electric charge can be influenced passively by various stimuli along the length of the axon. A positive electric charge originating from the brain might be interrupted by a negative stimulus somewhere along the axon, such that the muscle could fail to receive the intended activation signal, and fail to fully activate. This reduction in activation is interpreted clinically as a weak MT.

Any fluctuation in our bioelectric field as a whole will influence the electric charge along all axons, which depend on positive charges to fire the muscles. This is why something placed in the bioelectric field but not touching the body can still inhibit muscle activation.

This also explains how placing a strong magnet near the bioelectric field can enhance muscle activation. Based on Maxwell's equations (see p. 161), introducing a magnetic field near an electric charge will increase the electric charge. By increasing the amplitude of the electric charge along the axon, a magnet strengthens, albeit temporarily, the perceived MT response (it MT stronger).

The Awareness Threshold

Any stimulus that negatively affects the bioelectric field is a stressor. Obvious examples would be dropping a hammer on your foot or getting bitten by a snake, but we don't need a MT to tell us these things have happened because they register above our awareness threshold, that is, we are consciously aware of them.

The problem with the human nervous system is that many stimuli that can harm us fall below **the awareness threshold**, meaning that we are not able to perceive them with our senses.

Imagine looking at water. The human eye can't perceive the temperature of the water so we can't know if it is warm, cold or just above freezing. Only when we see the water crystallize can we know the temperature has dropped below 0°C/32°F.

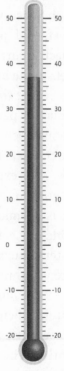

In a similar way, our nervous systems only register a stimulus as a harmful stressor when it reaches a sufficiently high level in our awareness threshold. Below this level, the stimulus is still harmful, just as the water can be very cold, but it doesn't register as harmful to us.

For something to register as a stressor, it needs to meet a set of requirements: it has to be above or below a certain temperature, or to be sharp or loud or have a bad taste or smell.

Anything outside of these requirements fails to register as a stressor: chemicals, poisons, radiation, toxic elements, parasite eggs and viruses, as well as internal stressors such as bad bacteria from parasites, infections, growths, tumors, deficiencies in vitamins, minerals, fat and protein, organ tissue deterioration and circulatory problems. Fortunately, these things will register negatively in our bioelectric field so they can be MT.

A MT shows us what our senses cannot by evaluating how our bioelectric field responds to stressors below the awareness threshold.

Pathways from the Physical to the Electrical

The role of the various sensory pathways in the body is to convert stimuli into electricity so the brain can interpret them.

Sight The eye perceives photons of light and converts them into an electric charge that is sent along the optic nerve to the brain.

Smell Chemoreceptors in the nose translate the physical contact with airborne molecules into an electric signal that is sent along the olfactory nerve to the brain.

Taste Taste buds in the tongue and throat translate chemical contact into an electric message that is sent along the gustatory nerve to the brain.

Hearing Cilia in the ear translate sound waves into an electric impulse that is sent along the auditory nerve to the brain.

Touch Sensory nerves throughout the body register physical contact as heat, cold, pressure, density and friction, which is converted into an electric current that both diffuses into the surrounding tissue and travels to the brain.

That the brain is the terminus for these signals strengthens the bias of perception, and is probably the main reason that our opinions about reality are more real to us than actual reality (i.e., more concrete than The Field that our perceptions interpret).

We exist in an extraordinarily narrow range of pressure, temperature, gravitation and radiation, and have intolerances to various chemicals, proteins and other stimuli. Many of the stimuli outside our comfort zone are in fact harmful to us, and these will register as such in the bioelectric field despite their falling below the awareness threshold.

The non-sensory nature of our physical reality becomes more apparent when we consider the effect that internal stimuli have on the bioelectric field as they are projected outward:

Emotion The manufacture of neuropeptides in a negative emotion will result in a shift in our bioelectric field, causing a weak MT.

Thought Engaging in a mental stimulus that is technically stressful (e.g., something you might be poor at, like math or logic) or that is physically stressful (e.g., making requirements of a brain structure that is inflamed due to bad bacteria in the cerebrospinal fluid) will result in a shift in our bioelectric field, causing a weak MT.

Organs An ongoing organ imbalance will exhibit a weak MT when the area is provoked (clinically, it is said to therapy-localize weak).

Nutrient Levels The fluctuating levels of vitamins, minerals, fats and amino acids in our bodies, as well as factors like dissolved salts and sugars, contribute to our cumulative electric charge. There are ways of isolating these factors which will register as strong or weak responses in a MT. Also, a strong baseline is dependent upon them.

Truth Our subjective perception of objective, absolute Reality tends to be inaccurate. At a minimum level of consciousness (calibrated by Hawkins as cal. 605) it is possible for absolute truth, which is The Substrate of Reality, to register as positive or negative shifts in bioelectric charge. This is dependent upon karmic inheritance as well as the amount of electricity our nervous systems can physically handle, since a particularly high capacity is required to be able to consistently, accurately respond to truth as a stimulus. For us non-enlightened persons this is not an option and should not be trusted.

The Bioelectric Field Our bioelectric fields are the sum total of our NaK ion cycling. The cumulative electric charge of this process acts as a connecting mechanism between our inner and outer fields. It both conducts external stimuli inward, such as information perceived (and for that matter, not perceived) by sight, smell, taste, hearing and touch, and projects our internal stimuli outward, such as our emotions, thoughts, organ information, nutrient levels and bacterial and viral load. Some of these stimuli register above the awareness threshold in our conscious minds but most of them fall below the awareness threshold. When such stimuli are stressors, they provoke a shift in bioelectric field functionality that is expressed as a weak MT response. On a more ethereal level, the bioelectric field also connects us with the nonlinear reality of Truth that, like Divinity, is both transcendent and immanent.

The Nervous System Disconnect

A more practical way of expressing the problem of the awareness threshold outlined above is to call it a **nervous system disconnect.** Plainly put, our bodies don't communicate well with our brains, there is a wiring problem. The bioelectric field registers internal and external stressors but we can't perceive that this is happening.

Homing pigeons, for example, have magnetoreceptors in their beaks that allow them to sense the geomagnetic field of the Earth. This enables them to navigate across great distances using a sense that we can only imagine. We do not have magnetoreceptors in our beaks.

A lack of awareness of our internal bodies could be blamed on inadequate wiring between the autonomic nervous system (that regulates our organs, circulation, nutrient levels and cellular repair) and our central nervous system (that we think with). In a similar way, a lack of awareness of our external environments can be blamed on our five senses for only being adapted to perceive a small slice of the infinity we live in.

However, our bioelectric field registers anything in our internal or external environments that is good or bad for us, making it a functioning sixth sense, so the real question is that of why we are so unaware of our bioelectric fields? This leads back to not having magnetoreceptors in our beaks: it becomes a circular argument.

This dissonance between our senses and our reality has resulted in a uniquely human disconnect between our understanding of our own health and the reality of our own health. We cannot bridge that gap by consciously accessing the missing information but it is registered in our bioelectric fields. It is literally at our fingertips, but a lifetime of thinking about it will not force it into the mind.

The truth at the root of our health is what we all search for. This is why we find ourselves lost in a desert of uncertainty, stuck following Somebody, Everybody, Anybody and Nobody. Paradoxically, thinking only drives us deeper into the problem, getting us more lost.

This is the problem that MT solves.

Health Philosophies in History

The irony of MT is that the thought process it makes possible is more sophisticated than our most advanced medical technologies or supercomputers and yet a Neanderthal could have used it. In fact, there is no way to prove that Neanderthals didn't use it. I have often wondered how so many ancient tribal societies were reputed to have achieved such an advanced knowledge of medicinal plants. It would be interesting to scour the old hieroglyphs for images indicative of MT in ancient societies. It is quite possible that MT is a skill that has faded in and out of human awareness over the millennia.

One thing is certain, and that is that the Ancient Greeks make no reference to it. When we consider that MT is essentially a new health philosophy, it is a valid question to ask what philosophy it is replacing. It was mentioned in the last chapter that as a thought process, placing the bioelectric field at the center of our understanding of health represents a shift from the historical way of thinking. Historically, we have always placed the opinion at the center of our understanding, and orbited various facts around our opinions to justify our perspectives.

An opinion-centric view of health has been the prevailing belief system since the age of Hippocrates (460-370 BC). This is where we inherited it from. It is worthwhile to explore the history of Ancient Greek health philosophy to see how this came about.

Before we do so, however, it will be revealing to go a little further back in time to the few centuries before Hippocrates, so that we can see what belief system Hippocratic diagnosis replaced.

In 900 BC, Bronze Age Greece was steeped in the belief in illness as a mystical event, sent by the gods or fate. Anyone who fell ill believed themselves to have been cursed and their only option was an obligatory visit to a temple where they would pay a fee, sacrifice a goat or some other poor unsuspecting animal and hope for the best. We find a reference in Homer's *Odyssey* to singing incantations over a bleeding wound (Homer, *Odyssey*, XIX, lines 455-458).

This is the level of ignorance that diagnosis came to replace.

Ancient Greek Diagnosis

The flowering of reason in Ancient Greek society is one of the pivotal periods in human history. An example of this is the emergence of **the philosophy of diagnosis** which represented a major upgrade over believing that illness was a curse from the gods. This new idea was based on the belief that illnesses were the result of biology and lifestyle.

It became apparent that there were a finite group of illnesses, each with their own sets of symptoms, and that anyone who fell sick could be placed into one of these categories. We now call such naming a diagnosis, which is derived from an Ancient Greek verb but there is no evidence that Hippocrates used the word.

Since there was no obvious reason for one person to get sick instead of another, Hippocrates proposed that the human body was governed by the four humors (blood, phlegm, vomit and diarrhea). It was assumed that imbalances in these humors caused the diverse diseases that afflicted the ancient world. The humors were thought to phase in and out of balance based on dietary and lifestyle behaviors. The supposed effect of weather and the seasons on the humors also figured prominently in his work (Hippocrates, *Airs, Waters, Places*; *Epidemics*).

At the core of any medical condition are three questions: What is wrong? Why is it wrong? How do we fix it? Hippocrates' answer to the first question was the name of the condition; to the second was the humors, the weather and lifestyle; and to the third was the prognosis.

A general Hippocratic prognosis was to do nothing in excess, drink clean water, eat good food, rest and go for a walk. More specific prognoses are to be found but might curdle our modern sensibilities. Many of them were herbal rubs or enemas, often boiled in wine, but we do periodically encounter ingredients like de-winged blister beetles and cow manure (Hippocrates, *Nature of Women*). One can certainly see where witches in the Middle Ages got the ideas for their brewing cauldrons made famous in Shakespeare's *Macbeth*.

Many works of Hippocrates have survived in their original form and were an inspiration for a later writer, Galen (129-c.210 AD).

What has also survived is the Hippocratic perspective on illness. We can see this most clearly when we look for cures. There aren't any. There isn't even the practical concept of a cure and this is perhaps why the use of the word cure is such a legally weighted issue.

Diagnosis is the medical version of geocentrism. The opinion about illness is at the center of the condition and facts are recruited accordingly. Understanding the history, we can appreciate that it represented an upgrade from being cursed, but the disadvantage of the diagnostic perspective was and is that it places so much emphasis on the opinion of the physician that the root causes of the symptoms are lost in the shuffle. The name of the diagnosis itself takes on so much importance that it not only summarizes the symptoms, it is basically presumed to cause them as well.

This is only a trick of language, of course. Everyone knows that the name itself is not also the cause of what it names, but when the cause of the name is another name, and the cause of that name is a third name, you stop asking questions, particularly when all the names are in Ancient Greek.

I had an experience like this when I was diagnosed at 16 years old with a medical condition called ulcerative colitis. When I asked my gastroenterologist, a modern day representative of the Hippocratic philosophy, what caused it, his answer was idiopathic proctitis. When I asked what the heck that was, he said inflammation of the rectum with an unknown cause. But saying that he didn't know the cause of it in Ancient Greek made it a real thing to him and 2400 years after Hippocrates, I was also expected to take that seriously.

"And it leads to colon cancer!" he added, tacking another name onto the roster.

It wasn't a conspiracy, he just didn't understand root causes. He had learned in medical school to have such an unquestioning belief in the supremacy of the name that it didn't make sense to him to invest any extra thought in identifying what was at the root of the inflammation. It might as well have been one of the four humors or the weather. It might as well have been 400 BC.

Diagnosis in Perspective

Compliments paid to the paradigm of diagnosis are that it can catch a preventable disease in time for a life-saving treatment, particularly when surgery is needed or when the immune system needs to be suppressed in a crisis. Also, it does indeed offer a better option than dying with the belief that the gods are angry with you. This observation is not intended as sarcasm: freedom from a belief in the anger of the gods was the original innovation of diagnosis and bearing this in mind may help to understand its odd lack of accountability to actual wellness.

Concerns about diagnosis are that it is frequently inaccurate; it places opinion at the center of the health cosmos; shifts emphasis from what caused the condition onto managing it; and paves the way for a reactive healthcare system based on surgery and pharmacology. Also, at 72.6 years of age, the average worldwide life expectancy today is not justifiably higher than it was in Ancient Greece, where many of the philosophers and historians lived into their 70s and beyond: Epicurus till 71, Plato till 81, Hippocrates till between 83-90.

An obvious criticism of diagnosis is that its obsession with naming illnesses is an end in itself. The preoccupation with giving symptoms a name removes any accountability to finding a cure for the condition. After all, a name cannot be cured. Since no actual cures are known for any medical conditions, the recourse of diagnosis is to give the sufferer a name so that they can feel at peace while they suffer. It may have been helpful 2400 years ago to know that we were dying from an actual illness rather than a curse but at this stage, few would dispute that it would be more helpful to know how to get healthy again. The assumption tacit in diagnosis is that ultimately there aren't any cures. The fact is that for millions of people every year in every country around the world, diagnosis is a death sentence.

Ultimately the inadequacy of diagnosis becomes apparent if we levy upon it the expectation that every single diagnosed patient should heal. This philosophy, so invested in naming conditions, has a poor track record with actual healing.

Recontextualizing Diagnosis

Heliocentrism didn't destroy the Earth by positioning the Sun at the center of our solar system. In fact, orbiting the Earth around the Sun was a more accurate model and we still got to keep the Moon.

In the same way, placing the bioelectric field at the center of our understanding and orbiting our opinions around it isn't going to destroy diagnosis. It will, however, reorient our perception so that we can arrive at a more accurate model of health that includes a cure. And we still get to keep the name of the medical condition. It's win-win and it's in our own best interest that this happens.

A cure is the thing that the philosophy of diagnosis obviously lacks, since originally the only expectation was that diagnosis should shift the burden away from the fear of having been cursed. When we look at the architecture of medical knowledge in this way, we can see now why there is such an odd lack of accountability to an actual cure. The cure was an afterthought: originally, naming the condition was an end in itself.

We can gain further perspective on this if we compare diagnosis to other ideas prevalent in 2400 BC. Physics at the time was rooted in the idea that there were not 118+ elements, as our modern periodic table demonstrates, but just four: earth, air, fire and water. Can you imagine where modern physics would be if we were still using the four elements? Philosophically, that is where modern medicine still is.

Like the four elements, diagnosis as a thought process is too unsophisticated to be able to address the root causes of illness, which are multidimensional. It is further impeded by the nervous system disconnect outlined above, where our conscious minds are unable to access information in the fluctuations of our own bioelectric fields.

In the gospel of Matthew (10:8), written 400 years after Hippocrates and reprinted at the top of this chapter, we encounter in the words of Christ such a powerful perspective on reality that it gives us cause to reconsider our basic assumptions about what is possible in healing. Certainly it is valid to wonder if there is anything scientific that we can do to bring that kind of healing into the world.

A Guide to Symptoms and Their Root Causes

To understand illness, we need to move beyond naming symptoms and ask—and find answers to—questions about root causes. We need to begin where diagnosis ends.

What is missing from the naming process is an understanding of the information that is contained in the bioelectric field. The answers are there but we're not asking the right questions.

We can take a journey together down the thought process and identify the questions very simply. In reverse order, let's consider as an example a well-known medical condition like diabetes.

7. At the level of naming the condition:
Q: What is the name? A: Diabetes (this is where diagnosis shines).

6. At the level of describing the symptom:
Q: What is the symptom? A: Inability to regulate sugar metabolism.

5. At the level of analyzing the location:
Q: What is the location? A: The pancreas.

4. At the level of a fungal or viral contributor:
Q: Is a fungus or virus involved? A: There's no evidence of this.

3. At the level of metal toxicity?
Q: Do we find any metal toxicity? A: Yes. Chromium (Cr#24).

2. At the level of bacteriology:
Q: Is there a bacteria involved? A: Yes, chromium-loving bacteria.

1. At the level of a parasitic contributor:
Q: Is there a parasite involved? A: It may or may not be a coincidence that every diabetic's pancreas MT for ivermectin (filaria medicine).

0. At the level of the parasite vector:
Q: Where did it come from? A: Filaria can be transmitted in utero but also come from diverse external sources like insect bites and manure.

Taken out of context like this, the questions above seem unrelated, abstract or irrelevant. However, when we consider them in the correct order, they make a lot more sense. A diabetic appears to have:

0. VECTOR: Lived in a world where parasites exist.
1. PARASITE: Picked up a parasite, possibly from the filarial family.
2. BACTERIA: Accumulated toxic, chromium-loving bacteria of the type that are excreted in the waste of some parasites.
3. METAL TOXICITY: Had their nutritional chromium converted into toxic chromium by bad bacteria, resulting in chromium toxicity.
4. FUNGUS/VIRUS: No evidence of a fungus or virus.
5. LOCATION: Experienced the accumulation of the above stressors in the pancreas which when starved of nutritional chromium and polluted by toxic, elemental chromium, stops functioning normally. Specifically, there is an insulin problem.
6. SYMPTOM: Prolonged pancreatic dysfunction that leads to spikes in blood sugar levels after eating. This can be life-threatening.
7. NAME: A syndrome that we use the word "diabetes" to describe.

This is a very different perspective on diabetes than the one we would expect from the health philosophy of diagnosis, which simply states that diabetes has happened, that it can be measured by monitoring blood sugar levels, and treated with insulin. When pressed as to why diabetes has happened, we get another name: autoimmune. And why does autoimmune happen? Diagnosis runs out of names.

This is where a MT analysis of the multilayered factors of a fungus, virus, metal, bacteria and parasite becomes highly relevant and none of this information is implicit in the diagnosis itself. Instead, we can only gather such detailed, specific information, and disambiguate it from all the other specific but irrelevant information in the body by performing a targeted MT analysis of the pancreas via the bioelectric field. We need to know what we're looking for.

When we do so, the conclusion is clear: diabetes hasn't simply happened because it happens. It appears to have happened because the patient has picked up a particular parasite. Understanding this opens the door to developing a strategy for a cure and is an illustration of how and why diagnosis is incapable of arriving at cures: not only does it not have enough information to create a context in which a cure is possible, it isn't even asking the right questions.

The point isn't to refrain from diagnosing diabetes, or to refrain from treating that condition with life-saving drugs. Rather, the point is to understand that diagnosis is not an end in itself. In fact, it should only be the beginning of a much deeper questioning process.

The desired outcome should be clear and practical: Healing. Healing in a way that hasn't been thought possible since biblical times.

When we understand this, we can ask questions about the root causes of symptoms that are not only calibrated to quantify them medically but are also focused on identifying and potentially resolving their true root causes.

This is where MT comes in. There is no simple medical test to evaluate whether there is a metal toxicity, bad bacteria or parasite in the pancreas. It would require a rather invasive tissue biopsy, which probably isn't the best idea for someone who already has pancreatic issues. Even with a biopsy, which lab would we send the tissue sample to that wouldn't simply report that it wasn't cancerous?

The factor that limits the thought process of diagnosis isn't the initial step of naming the condition, it is the lack of information about all of the subsequent steps: Is there a nutrient deficiency? We don't know. Is there a fungus or virus? We don't know. Is there a metal toxicity? We don't know. Is there a bad bacteria? We don't know. Is there a parasite? We don't know. Well, if we don't know anything, why are we so confident that we know what we're talking about?

Speaking of Ancient Greece, we read in Plato that Socrates posed a similar question to the citizens of Athens. Maybe it is time that we in the 21st century came up with some better answers.

One of the answers proposed here is the 8-step thought process outlined above. It is called The Health Ladder: A Guide to Symptoms and their Root Causes. By using The Health Ladder as a conceptual model and MT to gather information from our bioelectric fields, we may be able to find a way out of the desert of our symptoms.

Part 3 of this book explores this idea extensively and includes 36 chapters on specific Health Ladder applications. Part 2 which follows now, contains two quick chapters on how to MT correctly.

Part 2: Practicum

Contents of Part 2:

1

The Motor Skills of Muscle Testing

_____

O nly when we can perform a MT correctly is there the confidence to use it and more important, the ability to confirm (or the basis to contradict) the assertions made in this book.

It is simple enough to derive accurate information from a MT as long as it is done correctly, but for some people that's like saying it's simple enough to make money on the stock market as long as they buy low and sell high. Getting it right isn't a guarantee. MT requires instruction and some practice.

In this section we will explore the motor skills necessary to ensure that you can perform a MT correctly:

1. The anatomy of a strong MT
2. Correct form for a MT
3. Instructions for a MT
4. How to accurately identify a weak MT response
5. Common MT errors
6. Surrogate Testing
7. Self Testing
8. Before and after strength
9. Suggestions on how to practice

1. The Anatomy of a Strong Muscle Test

Before we explore the actual motor skills of a MT, we need to understand what aspect of muscle anatomy we are testing. It is not muscle strength we are looking for as everyone has a different level of strength. In a MT we are looking for a contraction of the fascia.

Fascia is a bit like plastic wrap on food in the grocery store. Every muscle and organ in your body is surrounded by fascia. Fascia separates your tissues, attaches them, stabilizes them and encloses them. Most important, fascia is an electrical conductor.

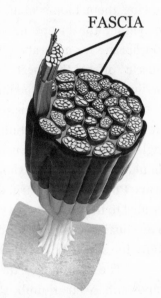

FASCIA

When the fascia grips the muscle there is an electrical response that allows the muscle to contract. A strong MT identifies this. If you poke your biceps muscle while it is flexed, it is the contraction of the facia that makes it feel firm.

When we perform a MT, we are evaluating the extent to which the fascia is contracting. This contraction can be very strong. If you put your elbow at a 90° angle and flex your biceps, someone pushing on your hand (thus performing a MT of the biceps short head in its mid-range of motion) would be hard-pressed to move it.

To bypass this strength issue so that we don't have to push so hard in a MT and risk injuring the person being tested, we place the muscle in what is called its **shortest range of motion**. This ensures that the fascial contraction is weakest and easiest to MT.

Each muscle has its own position for shortest range of motion and these can easily be learned. For the purpose of a basic MT, we are only interested in the deltoid muscle because it is relatively weak and your arm is a long lever, making it easy to MT without risk of injury.

2. Correct Form for a Muscle Test

The ideal muscle for testing purposes is the medial deltoid (shoulder). Remember, something like the biceps muscle is physically too strong and the finger muscles have too short of a lever length, making them biomechanically too strong, so neither the biceps nor the fingers are appropriate for accurate MT. The shoulder muscle offers the best combination of medium strength and medium lever length.

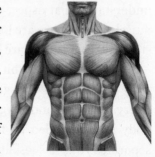

When your arm is straight down at your side, the deltoid is in the longest range of motion (ROM). When it is straight out at a 90° angle to your body, that is its shortest ROM. All MT of the shoulder should take place in the shortest ROM. This is the start position.

Start Position Your arm should be parallel to the ground with your hand at an equal level to your shoulder (not above the shoulder and not below).

The rotation of the wrist is important. Your thumb should be pointing straight forward (not up in the air or down at the ground). This ensures that you're isolating the medial deltoid only.

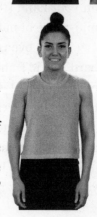

Vector of Force When testing, the arm is moved downward through its natural range of motion toward the same-side hip.

End Position The arm doesn't need to travel all the way to the hip, as seen in the adjacent image, just one foot or so in that direction. The purpose of the end position is to conclusively establish that the arm has moved away from its initial strong/positive baseline. Any movement is interpreted as a weak MT response. Lack of movement is a strong MT.

Testing Hand Position The hand of the person performing the MT is placed on the top of the wrist of the person being tested. Make sure you use a hand and not only the fingers: they aren't strong enough. And don't squeeze, just place your hand there. Squeezing will MT weak.

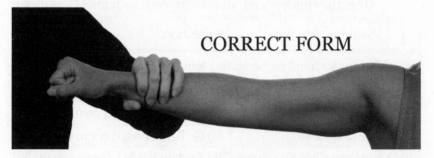

CORRECT FORM

It is vital not to place the hand on the wrist joint itself. This introduces a negative neurological signal which always provokes a weak MT response. Try it and see if you can reproduce that result.

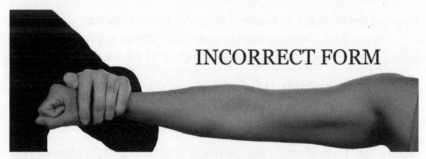

INCORRECT FORM

It is also important not to place the testing hand too close to the elbow. This reduces the lever length so much that the tester will have to push too hard for the MT to be accurate. It will generally always result in a strong response, even when the MT should test weak.

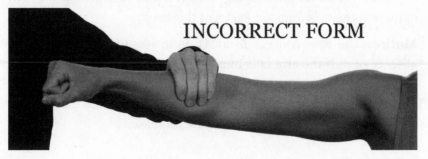

INCORRECT FORM

3. Instructions for a Muscle Test

If need be, explain to the person being MT what is going to happen and demonstrate the range of motion you'll be moving them through.

Once they understand, you can proceed with the MT as usual:

1	Move the arm into the start position.	
2	Place your hand in the testing hand position.	
3	Do the MT (i.e., try to move the arm through the normal range of motion). Make sure the MT has the following 4 components:	
i) Ease into it slowly		iii) Go light enough not to tire them
ii) Don't force their arm down		iv) Sustain the MT for 2-3 seconds
IF +	If the strength is the same compared to the baseline, it is a strong MT. MT for 2-3 sec., then cease pressure gently so that the process of ending the test is smooth and controlled.	
IF -	If the strength is weaker compared to the baseline, it is a weak MT. Gently move the arm through the appropriate range of motion until it reaches the end position.	

Baseline In a **baseline MT**, you should only be pressing as much as the person can resist. There should be no movement. The point of the baseline is to see how much pressure they can sustain without movement.

Stimulus To evaluate a **stimulus**, perform the MT either during the stimulus (as in the case of pressing an organ MT) or immediately after (as in the case of MT the effect of an exercise on the CNS).

A variety of stimuli are admissible for MT purposes. There is a specific format for introducing each stimulus. Instructions for each of these formats is found in Part 3 of this book.

Motion The core concept in a MT is to identify **motion** or the absence of it. If the arm fails to move, there is no evidence of a weak MT. If it has moved after being exposed to a stimulus, that is a weak MT. We can now build on this data and draw inferences about the stimulus being MT. That is how MT can act as a sixth sense.

4. How to Accurately Identify a Weak MT Response

The challenge in identifying a weak MT response lies in knowing what weak should feel like. It is legitimate to wonder if you are simply forcing the arm down as that is a constant potential problem.

The motor skill referenced on this page provides a way to provoke a weak MT response at will. Once there is certainty about what a genuine weak test should feel like, there can be confidence in differentiating weak from strong in each case.

This is called a **2-Handed MT**. The scientific basis for it is that each hand has its own electric charge. A single hand with a single electric charge works in the binary manner that we have come to expect.

However, when we place a second hand on top of the first, the overlapping of electric charges reverses the normal polarity in any muscle being tested. This is due to electricity, not the extra weight.

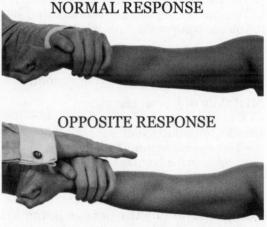

NORMAL RESPONSE

OPPOSITE RESPONSE

The result is that if a muscle is tested in the 2-Handed MT fashion, it will give exactly the opposite response from its normal functionality. A weak muscle will test strong and conversely, any strong muscle will test weak. This has limited clinical application but it is an invaluable technique for beginners when learning what a weak MT response should feel like. This is the best way to make sure you're not forcing the arm down and drawing the wrong conclusion.

As you fine-tune your MT motor skills, you are encouraged to use the process of the 2-Handed MT as a feedback loop until you are sure what a weak MT should feel like and the process becomes intuitive. Getting it right takes some effort but like riding a bicycle, once you learn the motor skill you won't forget it.

5. Common Muscle Testing Errors

The following is a systematic outline of the most common MT errors.

Mistakes of speed:
1. You can push with too much speed so that your momentum carries the arm down even if it is a strong MT.

Mistakes of timing:
2. You can push for too long (4+ seconds) and force the arm down.
3. You can fail to push long enough (-1 second) and stop before the arm has had a chance to express a weak response to the stimulus.
4. You can push too soon and catch the person off guard.

Mistakes of pressure:
5. You can push too hard and force the arm down.
6. You can fail to push hard enough and get a false positive.
7. You can squeeze the wrist while MT. That will cause a weak response.

Mistakes of control:
8. You can fail to meet the person's resistance smoothly, so their arm bobs up and down against your uncontrolled pressure.

Mistakes of biomechanics:
9. You can push in the wrong vector of force and test the wrong muscle, or nothing at all.
10. You can place your testing hand in the wrong position and lose biomechanical advantage.
11. Collapsed arches, bad shoes, compression socks, using an injured indicator muscle or a joint with hyper-flexible ligaments will MT weak.

Compensation by the person being MT:
12. The person can recruit another muscle to gain biomechanical advantage, such as shrugging the shoulder. It is your job to catch this.

Medical oversights:
13. The neurological strength of the person being tested can be reduced by a parasite, bacteria, virus or fungus, an extreme vitamin or mineral deficiency, dehydration, drugs, excessive alcohol, pronounced fatigue or hunger, low blood sugar or emotional stress.
14. The muscle might MT weak if the person rests their other hand on an organ that has an underlying imbalance, such as their stomach.
15. Electromagnetic interference from a strong power source.
16. Eyes closed will often MT weak as do bright lights in the eyes.

Note 1: Someone who has delicate health may need to be sitting down for the MT to be accurate. Standing up is sometimes contraindicated.
Note 2: Make sure the person's nervous system is behaving normally with a 2-Handed MT to rule out some of the above problems.

6. Surrogate Testing

Surrogate Testing requires three participants: the patient, the tester and the helper. It is necessary in cases where we need to MT someone who cannot produce their own muscular resistance. This applies to infants, children, seniors, the injured, the sick and pets. The person or pet who needs to be surrogate tested gets to sit there and watch, they don't have to do anything. Let's call them the patient.

Ordinarily, the person doing the MT, let's call them the tester, would use their testing hand to test the patient's muscle and their free hand to localize the area of the patient being tested (or hold a substance in the patient's bioelectric field, etc.). However, in the case of Surrogate Testing, instead of their testing hand doing the MT, this hand (or rather, arm) is being MT by a third party: the helper.

The helper doesn't need to know what's going on with the patient or the tester, they simply need to push. The helper doesn't even need to know how to MT, they just need to be told how to push.

As long as the tester is in physical contact with the patient, their bioelectric field will temporarily register the strong and weak charges of the patient in the same way you might pick up an electrostatic shock from another person. Electricity passes by touch.

Note: An important technicality is that many photographs of a tester Surrogate Testing a patient (or a pet) will show both the helper and the tester touching the patient. This doesn't line up with the functionality of bioelectricity. When all three participants touch, it creates a closed circuit electric charge 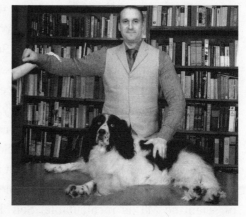 and the test is not accurate. The tester both touches the patient and is tested by the helper, but the helper and the patient cannot touch each other. That is correct Surrogate Testing form.

7. Self Testing

Self Testing isn't accurate for a number of reasons.

1. It involves the complicated motor skill of differentiating your own resistance from your own pressure. Since your own brain is producing both, there is no reality check. Error is almost guaranteed.

2. If the self-test is done on the fingers, the lever length is so short that the perceived strength difference, even during a Turtle Response, is far too small to be identifiable. The fingers shouldn't even be used as indicator muscles during two-party clinical MT.

3. Self Testing of the fingers (pulling apart interlocking circles) requires momentum as you would need to force the fingers apart from each other. This is a recipe for inaccuracy.

4. If Self Testing is done with one hand pushing on the wrist of the opposing arm, so that the anterior deltoid is being MT, then in the same way that a 2-Handed MT produces a negative charge during nervous system verification, your own two hands are likely to cancel each other out, making that test highly inaccurate.

5. With your two hands occupied in a Self Test, where is the third hand to introduce the stimulus being MT?

Presumably, a third hand isn't needed because the same people who Self Test combine this modality with Truth Testing. And they wonder why MT has a bad reputation? Why people think they're crazy?

Whole books are dedicated to Self Testing, there are pictures of fingers making circles on the covers. Goodness gracious me. How are we to untangle this web of misconceptions?

The margin of error in a binary guess is 50% (e.g., yes or no, you have a 50% chance of guessing correctly). By contrast, in my experience, the margin of error with Self Testing is about 95%. You would be statistically more likely to get it right if you simply guessed.

But beyond the accuracy problem, the cost to the reputation of scientific MT is incalculable. Self Testing is charlatanry and it causes scientific MT to be painted with that same brush. If you love the world enough to want truth to unfold to support the highest good, please understand that Self Testing is contradictory to that end.

8. Before and After Strength

Everyone's nervous system has its own unique before strength and after strength.

Yourself

Before | After

The **before strength** is the amount of resistance a person can exert in a baseline MT. This typically ranges from 1 to 10 lbs of resistance and can be thought of on a scale from 1 to 10. It is necessary to quantify the before strength as precisely as possible since this is the basis for identifying whether subsequent MT are strong (the same as the baseline) or weak (less than the baseline).

The **after strength** is the amount of resistance a person can exert during a 2-Handed MT. This will always produce a negative response in the muscle being tested but the degree of muscular inhibition will vary from one person to the next. It can also be assigned a value from 1 to 10.

Variance In addition to everyone's before and after strength being unique, the ratio between the before and after will vary in each case. The examples on the opposing chart represent the range of variance you will encounter throughout the population:

Examples

Before | After

Example A: This person has a perceived before strength of 10 and an after strength of 9. They will be very difficult to MT because it is an advanced motor skill to be able to recognize a variance as small as 1 lb.
Example B: This person has a before strength of 8 and an after strength of 1. They are ideal to MT since you and they will easily notice the difference in a variance of 7 lbs.
Example C: This person has a perceived before strength of 2 and an after strength of 0. They will be difficult to MT because they can't produce enough resistance to be tested. This is typical of someone who is unwell or full of parasites. They will need surrogate MT.
Yourself: You should establish your own variance as a frame of reference.

9. Suggestions on How to Practice

Since everyone that you MT will have their own unique before and after strength, it is suggested that you approach each new person with the mentality of quantifying this variance before proceeding.

To create the habit of doing this, you are encouraged to find at least four people that you can try it on right away.

For each person, see what their before strength is (with a baseline MT) and then compare it with their after strength (a 2-Handed MT). Assign a numeric value in each case and observe the differences. If it helps, you can fill in the values on the page below.

Person 1:   **Person 2:**   **Person 3:**   **Person 4:**

Before	After		Before	After		Before	After		Before	After
10	10		10	10		10	10		10	10
9	9		9	9		9	9		9	9
8	8		8	8		8	8		8	8
7	7		7	7		7	7		7	7
6	6		6	6		6	6		6	6
5	5		5	5		5	5		5	5
4	4		4	4		4	4		4	4
3	3		3	3		3	3		3	3
2	2		2	2		2	2		2	2
1	1		1	1		1	1		1	1
0	0		0	0		0	0		0	0

Fatigue You will find in every case that after a certain number of MT, the person being tested reaches a stage of **fatigue** where everything MT weak. Sometimes a short rest will suffice, sometimes rubbing or gently pinching the medial deltoid muscle will reset it enough to proceed, but other times you will need to stop for the day.

If you don't catch this, you might mistakenly throw out half the food in your kitchen thinking it all MT weak, so be aware of it.

MT Myths That you can't be MT while wearing a leather belt, or with a cell phone in your pocket, with a jacket on, or sunglasses, or if you've had alcohol or not until you say your name. The biggest nonsense in the field is that you have to grant the practitioner silent, energetic permission to MT you. And we wonder why MT wasn't taken seriously.

2

How to Interpret a Muscle Test

If health were as simple as accurately differentiating a strong MT from a weak one, there would be little need for a book of this nature.

The complexity of health is related to how we interpret the data and that interpretation is the result of what questions we base our consideration process on.

Is there a logic to MT? What are we MT, where are we MT it, and why are we drawing that particular conclusion? How should we interpret quantity testing, Truth Testing, Surrogate Testing and nonlocal testing?

Is there a unified theory of health that we can use to guide our thought process or is MT just a glorified diagnostic screen that ultimately reinforces our preexisting biases? These might sound like casual questions but when applied to medical matters the right answer can be the difference between life and death.

What is needed is an understanding of how to interpret information about these issues, how to be right and how to be certain that we're right. In short, we need to know how to interpret a MT.

The Logic of Muscle Testing

The essence of MT is that we are interpreting the body's binary responses to stimuli in an attempt to draw logical conclusions about information that is not otherwise available to sensory awareness.

However, logic is limited by what information is available. We can see this clearly in the example of Aristotle who more or less invented logic. Using the best information at his disposal, he logically concluded that the universe was made up of 4 elements: Earth, Air, Fire and Water. European alchemists followed his example for almost 2000 years. We now know that lacking an understanding of atomic physics, this conclusion, though logical, was neither complete nor accurate.

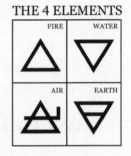

THE 4 ELEMENTS

In the same way, MT only contains the binary information of yes/positive/strong and no/negative/weak. It is not enough to use logic to sort out that something has happened, the onus is also on the person drawing the conclusion to educate themselves on what the variables are (i.e., what premises they choose as the basis for their logic).

For this reason, it is overly simplistic to interpret strong/positive MT responses as intrinsically good and weak/negative responses as bad. All that is intrinsic to a MT is that it has happened.

Drawing Basic Conclusions from a Muscle Test		
IF	AND	THEN
Baseline is positive	Comparison is positive	Stimulus is not negative
Baseline is positive	Comparison is negative	Stimulus is negative
Baseline is weak		You have no basis for a MT

What do positive and negative mean? In the following sections we will explore basic, intermediate and advanced MT applications to see how the available information determines what kind of conclusions we can draw. We will then explore how to think about quantity testing, Truth Testing, Surrogate Testing and nonlocal MT.

Basic Muscle Testing Applications

In a basic MT we are focused on identifying **What**.

Because our nervous systems do not allow us to consciously perceive most electromagnetic stimuli, knowing what stimuli are harmful effectively allows us to use MT as a sixth sense.

There are numerous applications of basic MT but it is important to hesitate to draw too broad of a conclusion. A MT will identify whether a stimulus appears likely to cause a harmful effect and you are encouraged to put **The Golden Rule of MT** into effect: If it MT weak, avoid it.

But beyond this rule, a basic MT won't give you enough data to draw a more advanced conclusion.

> ### Basic MT Protocol: What
>
> 1. Start with a baseline.
> 2. Introduce a stimulus.
> 3. Redo the MT: ideally during, if not possible, immediately afterwards (as in an exercise).
>
> **A:** If the MT is still strong, there is no evidence that the stimulus was harmful.
>
> **B:** If the MT is now weak, there is evidence that the stimulus was harmful but we still don't know where or why.

It is wise to remind yourself that you don't know what you don't know, and just because a MT has produced a weak response, that doesn't mean that you suddenly do know what you don't know. All you really know is that a stimulus you were curious about is MT weak, but you still don't know why.

If understanding is desired, it is necessary to progress from basic MT to intermediate and advanced MT (outlined below).

Note 1: A common misinterpretation is that if something MT strong, that means it is good for you. This is not the case. With basic MT, a strong response is merely the absence of a weak response.

Note 2: Probably the most common error at this level is for the student to lapse into Truth Testing and ask the universe if a strong MT means they need the product. Do this at your own peril but don't pretend that it is MT. Unless you're Enlightened, Truth Testing won't provide you with accurate or repeatable responses.

Intermediate Muscle Testing Applications

An intermediate use of MT is to establish **Where**.

This presupposes that you are identifying a location somewhere in the body of the person being MT (yourself, a pet, a child, etc.). It bridges the nervous system disconnect.

The process of MT a location requires being able to **provoke the location** for MT purposes. If you think of a church bell, it has within it the potential to ring but only does so when something strikes it. It rings when it has been provoked.

In the same manner, a body location may contain an imbalance (parasite, bacteria, virus, nutritional deficiency) but it must be provoked so that the imbalance can express itself as the electromagnetic plume that shows up in a MT. If imbalances couldn't phase in and out in this way, how would it be possible to ever find a strong baseline? And interestingly enough, with severe medical pathologies this is exactly what we see: it is impossible to ever find a strong baseline, everything MT weak. That's why certain people need Surrogate Testing.

> **Intermediate MT Protocol: Where**
>
> 1. Start with a baseline.
> 2. Touch an indicator point on the person being MT.
> 3. While touching, redo the MT.
>
> **A:** If the MT is still strong, there is no evidence of an imbalance at that location.
>
> **B:** If the MT is now weak, there is evidence of an imbalance at that location but we still don't know why, only where it is.

There are different techniques to provoke a location. These are often specific to the location being MT and are covered extensively in Part 3 of this book.

Here, our interest is restricted to interpreting where the imbalance is and this is very simple: we know we have found an imbalance—a where—when we can touch or provoke any location that results in a weak MT response. The eye cannot see this negative electromagnetic plume happening but the MT identifies it.

Advanced Muscle Testing Applications

It is our goal with advanced MT to understand **Why**.

While a basic MT looks for a stimulus that can produce a negative response and an intermediate MT tries to provoke a negative response from a location, an advanced MT looks for the stimulus that turns those negatives back to a positive.

This is where the fun begins and where logic takes a dominant role. By identifying which stimulus turns a negative baseline back to the original positive, we can try to logically conclude why there is a causal relationship between them.

This is the basis for the why we are looking for. However, extrapolating causality from a logical relationship is not as simple as it might sound. It depends upon an advanced understanding of the field of knowledge that the MT pertains to.

Whether we are MT something having to do with vector biology, parasite microbiology, pharmacology, bacteriology, organic chemistry, fungal biology, virology, medical physiology, internal and diagnostic medicines, biomechanics, molecular nutrition, biophysics, waveform physics or electromagnetism, we should recognize that simply having access to information about bioelectric field fluctuations (i.e., MT) does not mean that we are excused from mastering these areas of study.

For any conclusion to be logical it must also be scientifically coherent, so it is best to understand our expertise and our limitations.

MT — MT

Advanced MT Protocol: Why

1. Start with a baseline.
2. Identify an indicator that produces a negative MT. This indicator becomes the negative baseline.
3. Build on the negative baseline. Identify which stimulus turns the negative MT back to a positive.

A: If a stimulus fails to turn the negative back to a positive, there is no relationship.

B: If a stimulus succeeds in turning the negative back to a positive, we can logically conclude that there is some relationship between it and the negative baseline.

The nature of our conclusion depends upon what is being MT.

MT — MT

Interpreting Quantitative Responses

Quantity Testing is one of the advanced applications of MT. The dimension of quantity adds a new layer of understanding to evaluating the MT result.

Imagine MT someone for how much water they needed (though water is one of the few things we don't need to MT for). If the quantity testing indicated that they were dehydrated to the verge of death, that would tell us something very different about what they had been doing in the previous few days than if they only needed a small sip. By contrast, the more basic binary interpretation of water=yes/no fails to convey this nuance.

The best simile to describe quantity testing is that it is like putting **weights on a scale**.

On the reference side of the scale we have the quantity that the body needs. This is the passive consequence of various internal biochemical and electromagnetic fluctuations.

On the variable side of the scale we have the quantity being added. The scale will balance when the necessary minimum quantity is placed in the body's bioelectric field and this balancing is expressed as a strong MT response.

MT Protocol For Quantity Testing

1. Start with a baseline.
2. Identify an indicator that produces a negative MT. This indicator becomes the negative baseline.
3. Identify which stimulus turns the negative MT back to a positive.

Then,

4. In cases where this stimulus is divisible into quantities, MT the lowest increment and then increase by one quantity at a time until the negative turns back to a positive. Make note of the exact quantity.

We can logically conclude that there is some relationship between that exact quantity and the negative baseline.

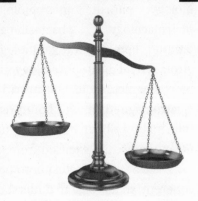

Interpreting Bioelectric Field Fluctuations

The functioning of the body's bioelectric field, which a MT allows us to interpret, is based on positive (+) and negative (-) charges that behave in accordance with Coulomb's Law (like charges repel, opposite attract).

The interior of most cells is thought to have a net (-) charge. This seems most conducive to the continued functioning of the sodium/potassium pumps that maintain cellular electricity and that cumulatively are the basis for the bioelectric field.

Nerves, by contrast, rapidly cycle between (+) and (-) charges. This **polarity switching** seems most conducive to conveying information inward and outward along the axon. It is this neural electric charge that we are interested in, since its presence allows for fascial innervation or deinnervation that we identify in strong and weak MT responses. This is the essence of bioelectricity.

It is understood that a single electron (-) is sufficient to create a shift in the electric charge of the nerve. This was referenced in the textbook *Applied Kinesiology,* (Frost, p.55, 2002) and explains how a substance held near the bioelectric field is able to produce a weak response in the muscles.

This also explains how thoughts are able to produce a weak MT response. The human brain generates an electromagnetic field measurable in femtoteslas (100-1000 fT) which is fainter than the picotesla range of the bioelectric field itself but capable of affecting it by adding 1 electron (-) to the mix. That shift of 1 electron temporarily switches the fascia (and muscle) on or off.

This is the scientific basis for how Truth Testing works. A fabricated thought propels a real electron. The thought thereby temporarily echoes in reality. The question isn't whether Truth is possible or whether our thoughts can provoke (+) and (-) charges in a Truth Test, it is whether our thoughts can access Absolute Truth at all and that is a deeper matter having to do with levels of consciousness.

Interpreting Other Phenomenon

Surrogate MT: As we explored, a helper pushes on the arm of the tester who is thereby both being MT and evaluating the patient.

Surrogate MT is fully as accurate as standard MT and in some cases more so, because the tester knows their own arm best, assuming that they have a stably functioning bioelectric field. When the tester is in physical contact with the patient, so that this contact is the only new stimulus for the tester, it is understood that the tester picks up the fluctuating electric charges from the patient. If some new stimulus is introduced to the patient, it will temporarily also affect the tester. This is what the helper identifies when MT the tester.

The (+) and (-) charges of the patient have an innervating and deinnervating effect on the tester's fascia, which results in the tester's medial deltoid (or any other indicator muscle) temporarily expressing the same strong or weak MT responses that the patient would have.

Nonlocal MT (also called Remote MT): This happens when the person doing the MT has no physical contact with the person being MT. They may still MT a surrogate (who is also not in contact with the person being MT) but more frequently they are self-testing.

This is neither scientific, accurate nor ethical. There is too great of a margin of error and no accountability.

The person doing the **nonlocal MT** will elicit strong and weak responses (in themselves or the person they're using as a surrogate) but these are the result of the random cycling of (+) and (-) charges in their own nervous system. What they are doing is recognizing this natural phenomenon and imposing upon it the imaginary interpretation that the strong or weak responses correspond with the nervous system of the person they're talking to or thinking about.

It should be understood that there is no actual causal relationship between nonlocal test responses and the test subject.

Such practitioners reinforce preexisting negative impressions of MT. Their adoption of nonlocal MT is one of the primary reasons (along with Self Testing and Truth Testing) that MT has remained largely unaccepted since George Goodheart developed it in the 1960s.

Interpretation Matrix: The Health Ladder

As we move deeper into interpreting health matters, we encounter more questions than answers:

Is there a society-wide solution to viruses other than economically devastating lockdowns? Why are some people more deficient in nutrients than others, or have more bacterial infections? Why do toxic metals stick to one person and not the next? Why do some people get parasites and not others? Or if everyone has parasites, why do they not affect everyone the same? Why do some people develop medical conditions? What is the "auto" in autoimmune?

Eventually these questions expand to society as a whole:

Can natural and alternative practitioners agree on how to interpret health and come up with better solutions to illness? Can we work with the body instead of against it but still be scientific? Can we do anything to incorporate energy medicine into modern healthcare? Do we have to wait hundreds of years for nanotechnology to save us all or is there something we can do right now? Is there no way for medical specialists to put their heads together and find some new solutions?

We all need to be healthy, we all share the same concerns and eventually we all start to wonder:

Is it possible to start getting some answers instead of only more questions? Is it time for a paradigm shift in how we look at health? Is it time that healthcare had its scientific revolution?

The binary information contained in a MT is not in itself sufficient to tell us how we should be interpreting the data we identify. What is needed is a better way of interpreting all of this information: a way to synthesize the data from every field and make it coherent by using a more accurate interpretation matrix than our current outdated diagnostic model. What is needed to get out of the desert of uncertainty is a unified theory of health.

This theory is called The Health Ladder. In Part 3 that follows, we will explore The Health Ladder applications in detail.

Part 3:
Applications

Contents of Part 3:

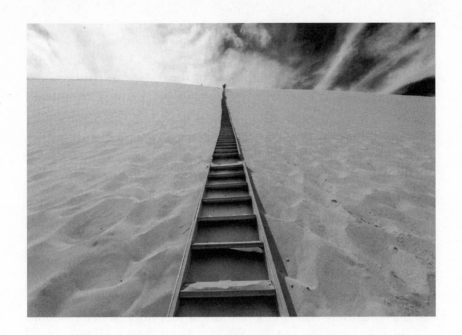

1

The Health Ladder:
A Guide to Symptoms and Their Root Causes

C ontent often appears arbitrary until it is placed in its context. David Hawkins illustrated this with his *Map of Consciousness*, a conceptual device that takes the content of the human experience—fear, desire, anger, pride, courage, reason, lovingness and Enlightenment—and organizes it within the context of The Field of awareness, which spans from the lowest levels (apathy and guilt) to the highest (Salvation and Enlightenment).

The challenge arises when we try to fit health into Hawkins' *Map of Consciousness*. There is no easy way to do this since good health and illness can equally manifest throughout the levels. A saint at Hawkins calibration (cal.) 575 may be spasmed with arthritis, while a sinner at cal. 100 may have vibrant health and live to be 100, pain-free. Hawkins ascribes this variance to karma and suggests the letting go technique (Hawkins, *Letting Go*, 2012) to minimize suffering. This is spiritually valid but not the physical solution that most people are looking for.

The process of justifying poor health by blaming it on karma is exaggerated in much of the spiritual-based health literature of the late 20th century, which takes karma a step further and proposes that psychosomatic processes are at the root of illness such as emotional blockages, memories being manifested in physical tissue, poor strategies for coping with stress and energetic negativity.

The unavoidable result of this interpretation agenda is guilt. The implication is that you are sick because it is your fault: whether you did something wrong in a past life or just can't handle this one, you must deserve to be sick because you had it coming to you.

This perspective leaves us in a prison of sorts: the prison of our own health. What person in chronic pain hasn't felt the toll of a life sentence? What loving parent has seen the suffering of their child (or child the suffering of their parent) and not been reminded of their 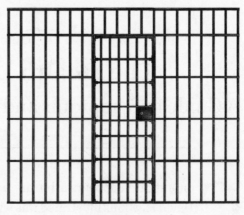 powerlessness in the face of the prison of health? Who has not felt lost in a desert?

The health philosophy of diagnosis strengthens the bars of this prison. We are taught that a location in the body develops a symptom; that the symptom has a name; and the name describes what is happening in the location. We could call this a health wheel. It might as well be a hamster wheel because once on it there's no way off. It is a prison of the mind to go with the body's prison of health.

A prison in a prison in a desert: now that is a life sentence.

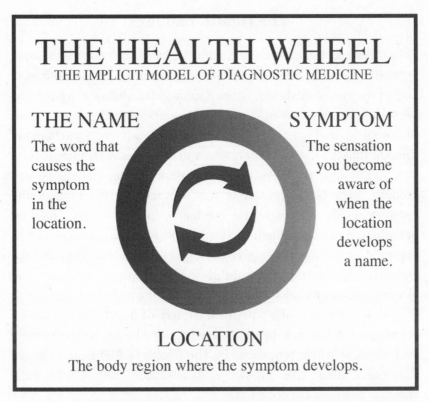

THE HEALTH WHEEL
THE IMPLICIT MODEL OF DIAGNOSTIC MEDICINE

THE NAME

The word that causes the symptom in the location.

SYMPTOM

The sensation you become aware of when the location develops a name.

LOCATION

The body region where the symptom develops.

It is certainly recommended that you use your illness to find peace, to develop patience, humility, compassion and lovingness; to learn to cherish life, to be gentle, respectful of others and kind. In fact, it is ideal if we can all learn to radiate joy into the world and for some people, illness is a teacher on this pathway.

But surely we don't all have to be sick to learn these valuable spiritual lessons? Wouldn't it be nice if there were a way out of illness? To understand how to get out of the prison of health, first we need to get out of the prison of the mind and on a very practical level, this is a consequence of our understanding of health.

As long as the health wheel is our theoretical model, we will never escape this prison. To get out of an actual prison we might be able to use a ladder to climb over the wall. Perhaps we can also use a theoretical ladder to get out of a theoretical prison.

We can think of this as a Health Ladder.

The Health Ladder

To understand the content of health, we need to see it in its larger context. Historical attempts at this have included the disciplines of Indian Ayurvedic medicine, Greek diagnostic medicine, acupuncture, Western botanical medicine, naturopathic and homeopathic philosophies and a host of body-mind and body-energy schools of thought that the 21st century reader will be basically familiar with.

But how do these fit into modern Western medicine and modern scientific theory? How can we reconcile the various and complex fields of diagnostic medicine, pharmacology, medical pathology, molecular nutrition, fungal biology, virology, bacteriology, organic chemistry, parasite microbiology, epidemiology, immunology, endocrinology and the more subtle branches of waveform physics and electromagnetism that seem to have something to do with health?

What is needed is a **unified theory of health**. What follows is a proposal for such a theory. Extensive consultation with experts in each applicable field referenced by The Health Ladder has confirmed that the content that follows is scientifically valid, biologically accurate and logically coherent.

The Health Ladder is divided into two sides: The A-side describes the condition, the B-side its resolution. For example, at Rung 2A the condition is Bad Bacteria, while its resolution at Rung 2B is taking Antibiotics (to eliminate the bad bacteria) or Probiotics (to repopulate the good bacteria). Even when a condition doesn't appear to have any resolution, there is still an implicit resolution. At Rung 7A, The Name of a condition is resolved at Rung 7B by getting Social Support. This equilibrium between the condition and resolution is present at each rung.

The **rungs** of The Health Ladder provide a context that gives us perspective on the content of the symptom we are concerned with. It becomes clear that there is a causal relationship moving from the bottom of the ladder to the top. Rung 0 leads to Rung 1, and so on. This awareness of context allows us to recontextualize the various factors of health and helps to prioritize which solution to pursue.

THE HEALTH LADDER
A GUIDE TO SYMPTOMS AND THEIR ROOT CAUSES

CONDITION

RESOLUTION

7A. THE NAME

Rung 7

The word agreed upon to summarize the Symptom (6A), that historically was also presumed to cause it.

7B. SOCIAL SUPPORT

At RUNG 7B, everyone can support you better when they know The Name (7A) that summarizes your symptoms.

6A. SYMPTOM

Rung 6

The expression of RUNGS 1A–5A at a level that can be perceived or measured.

6B. TREATMENT

RUNG 6B Treatment is symptom-focused: surgery, drugs and some manual modalities are all designed to suppress the Symptom (6A).

5A. LOCATION

Rung 5

The regions of the body that manifest the stress from RUNGS 1A–4A, often below the awareness threshold.

5B. THERAPY

RUNG 5B Therapy is support-focused: vitamins, supplements, herbs and some manual modalities attempt to heal the Location (5A).

4A. FUNGUS / VIRUS

Rung 4

Fungus: your best friend, helps you break down Bad Bacteria (2A).
Virus: your worst enemy, thrives in an environment of Metal Toxicity (3A).

4B. ANTIFUNGAL / VIRAL

Anti-fungals: overlook the fact that fungi play a vital role in health.

Anti-virals: don't generally provide a long-term solution.

3A. METAL TOXICITY

Rung 3

Elements in their non-bioavailable form adhere to you when Bad Bacteria (2A) absorb them for cellular metabolism.

3B. METAL DETOX

RUNG 3B Metal Detox can minimize the Symptom (6A) by starving Bad Bacteria (2A) of the Metals (3A) that they metabolize.

2A. BAD BACTERIA

Rung 2

At some stage all Bad Bacteria (2A) come from a Parasite (1A). Once excreted into your body they circulate everywhere, causing inflammation and tissue damage.

2B. BAD BACTERIA

Probiotics: temporarily replace good bacteria but don't eliminate Bad Bacteria (2A) from Parasites (1A).

Antibiotics: kill off Bad Bacteria (2A) but never Parasites (1A).

1A. PARASITES

Rung 1

Various Parasites (1A) inhabit your body. They deplete nutrients, damage tissue and excrete Bad Bacteria (2A). Best eliminated by Frequency Therapy (1B).

1B. FREQUENCY THERAPY

Eliminates all species of Parasites (1A) from all locations. Clean, quick, comprehensive and free of side effects, it is **the future of human healthcare.**

0A. THE VECTOR

Rung 0

All animals in nature are the primary or intermediate hosts to various species of Parasites (1A), many of which can infect humans.

0B. AWARENESS

Educate yourself. Start by reading *Experiments in Muscle Testing* by Leonard Carter. Then, apply what you learn.

Start Here

www.TheHealthLadder.com

Start Here

At the bottom left corner of The Health Ladder you will see the words "Start Here." This is the conceptual beginning. You can either read the rungs horizontally from left (Side A) to right (Side B) or vertically from bottom (Rung 0A) to top (Rung 7A). It works both ways.

A sentence form summary of side A of The Health Ladder is that parasites exist in nature (0A), they infect our bodies (1A), excrete bad bacteria into us (2A), which leads to metal toxicity (3A) and a susceptibility to fungi and viruses (4A). Eventually a location (5A) develops a symptom (6A) and we name it (7A) to understand it better.

Discussion

The primary message of The Health Ladder is that 1A Parasites cause 6A Symptoms that are generally known as 7A Names. These include every known medical condition. The secondary message is that parasites can be eliminated using applications of advanced physics at Rung 1B. This concept will be explored in later chapters.

However, there is an implication of The Health Ladder that is even more valuable than knowing what the answers to a problem are: the implication is that now we **know what the questions are**.

When we're dealing with something like a life-long, potentially fatal medical condition, it is vital that we understand it, and invariably there will be something about it that we won't know. A central question is: Why did I get this condition?

How can we understand a problem when we don't know what the problem really is? To find out what we don't know, it isn't enough to simply ask questions. Our uncertainty lies in not knowing what questions to ask. More often than not, we're not even aware that we're not asking the right questions.

The Health Ladder resolves this challenge by breaking down the questions we should be asking into Rungs 0-7. Let's take a walk together through the rungs to see how we can find out what questions we should be asking. For this purpose, we can use the example of the well-known medical condition of diabetes.

Diabetes: Health Ladder Analysis (fill in the blanks)

Rung 7: The Name   Diabetes
Rung 6: Symptom   Poor insulin regulation
Rung 5: Location   Pancreas
Rung 4: Fungus/Virus
Rung 3: Metal Toxicity
Rung 2: Bad Bacteria
Rung 1: Parasites
Rung 0: The Vector

At first glance it appears that Rungs 0-4 are all unknowns but we have gained a valuable insight: Now we know what questions to ask.

As a predictive model, The Health Ladder tells us that every Name (Rung 7A), Symptom (Rung 6A) and Location (Rung 5A) will have corresponding information at the lower rungs.

Did you know that diabetes had a 3A Metal Toxicity component? Or that all diabetics appear to have the same 1A Parasite in common? Are these questions that anyone is asking about diabetes? If not, why not? The answer is probably because adding in these extra dimensions appears to make a condition like diabetes seem more complicated than it needs to be. Paradoxically, The Health Ladder model demonstrates that by missing these rungs of information we are making conditions more complicated than they really are because now we need to explain the spontaneous manifestation of a 6A Symptom in a 5A Location in the absence of an obvious causal agent.

Perhaps this is why diabetes is classified as an autoimmune disorder. And just what is the "auto" in autoimmune? We don't know, the answer goes. Maybe stress, maybe genetics, maybe bacteria, maybe environment but really, we don't know.

The Health Ladder is a better interpretation model. It provides us with direction as to what further avenues we can explore and what we should be asking questions about.

We can do the following:

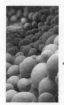

Rung 4A: Fungus/Virus MT the pancreas for anti-fungal and anti-viral medications to see if we can find evidence of the presence of a fungus or virus. While it would be unusual to find either one in diabetics, it helps us to rule out some possibilities and eliminates the fear of the unknown.

Rung 3A: Metal Toxicity MT the pancreas for metal toxicity. A laboratory blood analysis will show various metal toxicities but only a MT will isolate which ones coincide with the pancreas. The most common in diabetics is chromium. This is medically relevant to the disease because chromium in its nutritional form 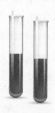 (chromium picolinate) is a major cofactor in blood sugar metabolism. Could it be significant that the very mineral involved in regulating healthy blood sugar levels is consistently found in its toxic, elemental form in the pancreas of someone with diabetes?

The Health Ladder predicted this because it tells us that elements in their non-bioavailable form adhere to us when Bad Bacteria (2A) absorb them for cellular metabolism. Could a Bad Bacteria be eating up the available nutritional chromium picolinate and spitting out elemental chromium #24? Is that what we're finding at Rung 3A? Is anyone asking this question? Can we partially confirm this by establishing the presence of 2A Bad Bacteria in the pancreas?

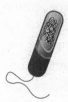

Rung 2A: Bad Bacteria MT the pancreas for various antibiotics to confirm the presence of bad bacteria. Azithromycin and clarithromycin tend to indicate as being needed in diabetics. Does taking a 2B Antibiotic cure diabetes? Certainly not. At this level of understanding we're not even looking at cures, just quantifying the rungs. The Health Ladder tells us that at some stage all Bad Bacteria (2A) come from a Parasite (1A). It predicts that we will find a 1A Parasite if we look for it: Various parasites inhabit your body. They deplete nutrients, damage tissue and excrete Bad Bacteria (2A). Can we find the parasite?

Rung 1A: Parasites A MT analysis of roughly 50 diabetics shows that their pancreases all test for one parasite medicine in common: ivermectin. Ivermectin treats filarial parasites.

Filaria are complex organisms capable of living in the pancreas or elsewhere. Furthermore, some filaria are able to autopopulate, meaning that depending on the subspecies (serotype) in question, there is a chance that unless it is fully eliminated, a diabetic might never be rid of it. Is anyone else finding this? Is anybody else looking for it?

Rung 0A: The Vector It is well understood by parasite biologists that filarial larvae and their eggs are widely distributed throughout nature. One such 0A Vector is a mosquito bite. All mosquitoes bite and everyone has been bitten at some time.

Understanding all of this, we arrive at a set of questions that we can now ask: Could a diabetic have been bitten by just the wrong mosquito? Could a filarial parasite be the "auto" in "autoimmune" for this condition? Could the spontaneous acquisition of the parasite explain the sudden onset of diabetes? Could a higher load of filaria explain more severe forms of diabetes (e.g., Type 1 or insulin-dependent diabetes)? Is there any evidence that diabetic symptoms have improved or resolved when filaria have been eliminated? Can all filaria be eliminated? Have autopsies of diabetics revealed filaria in the pancreas some or all of the time? Is anyone checking this?

These are all valid questions and relevant to someone with diabetes. But do we even know that we should be asking them? Could the obsolete Health Wheel model outlined above, the remnant of our Western diagnostic medical philosophy, explain why we have such a blind spot in this area?

The point of The Health Ladder model isn't to get caught up in the analysis of any one condition. It is intended as a universal model for all conditions: a unified theory of health, a guide to symptoms and their root causes.

Summary of The Health Ladder

Once we have adopted The Health Ladder as an interpretation model to understand the 8 layers of every health condition, we find ourselves in a better position to navigate our way out of the desert we're lost in.

We may not immediately be free from suffering, but we can at least be free from the prison of believing that illness causes itself; free from the guilt of believing that we caused it; free from needing to use metaphors like autoimmune as placeholders to represent what we don't understand; and in a much better place scientifically to arrive at a functional understanding of how to bring about permanent change with any condition.

This understanding is facilitated when we can use The Health Ladder as a guide to symptoms and their root causes.

You can download a Health Ladder image for your phone or computer at: **www.TheHealthLadder.com**.

Or, if you find The Health Ladder to be a helpful learning and teaching tool, and would like to own it in a high-resolution 24"x 36" poster format for your home, school, office, clinic or hospital, you can order one at:

www.MuscleTesting.com

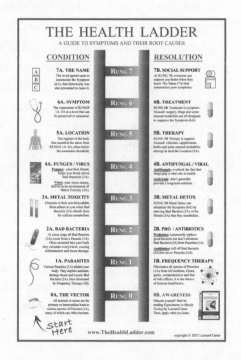

5A. LOCATION

The regions of the body that manifest the stress from RUNGS 1A–4A, often below the awareness threshold.

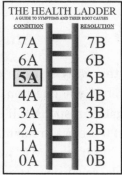

THE HEALTH LADDER
A GUIDE TO SYMPTOMS AND THEIR ROOT CAUSES

CONDITION		RESOLUTION
7A		7B
6A		6B
5A		5B
4A		4B
3A		3B
2A		2B
1A		1B
0A		0B

2

Muscle Testing
The Organ Systems

We need MT because of the nervous system disconnect outlined in Pt1-Ch4. If our minds knew the inner workings of 5A Locations like our liver, heart, kidneys and intestines as well as they could interpret basic urges like hunger and thirst, we wouldn't be lost in a desert of health. We would instead be extraordinarily healthy or at least understand exactly why we weren't.

Instead, we are unaware of these inner processes, and modern testing protocols, though they might quantify the presence of a major imbalance or medical condition, cannot qualify what we really need to know: Is the organ fundamentally healthy and if not why not?

This qualitative question is explored when we MT the organ systems. A MT will indicate what a medical test will not: the state of balance or imbalance that the organ is in. When there is a negative baseline, we can build on this to answer the life or death questions of what is wrong, how to quantify it and how to fix it.

MT the organs allows us to build a bridge between the mind and the body.

Muscle Testing an Organ

At this early stage in our analysis, we are MT an organ to answer a very basic question. Can we provoke a 5A Location to exhibit a negative response? If so, we won't know what the problem is, just that there is a problem.

If the MT we perform while localizing (touching) the organ reference point is weaker than the original baseline MT, we have found a problem area. If instead the examination fails to produce a weak response, we have failed to find a problem area. Failing to find a problem doesn't guarantee that the organ or region is balanced, but it is a step in that direction.

> ### MT Protocol
> ### For An Organ Location
> 1. Start with a baseline.
> 2. Place your 4 fingertips over one of the organ locations outlined below.
> 3. While holding this pressure, redo the baseline MT.
>
> **A:** If the MT is the same, there is no evidence of a problem.
>
> **B:** If the MT is weaker, you have identified an imbalance. You can now build on this negative baseline to draw inferences.

At this level of enquiry we are only examining 5A Locations to identify whether there is a problem in any of them. There is not yet enough information to build on the negative baseline to identify specific factors of the problem, such as nutrient deficiencies, metal toxicities or the presence of parasites. Those are for later chapters. We are focused here only on mastering the manual skill of MT the location for the purpose of seeing whether it produces a strong or weak MT.

Once we have identified where a **problem area** is, the question becomes: What stimulus can we introduce into the bioelectric field to cancel out the weak response elicited by the MT? This surprisingly simple question leads in a number of different directions, depending on the MT agenda. If it is your agenda to MT for a 5B Therapy such as a vitamin or supplement, see Pt3-Ch3. If you are looking for a 3A Metal Toxicity, see Pt3-Ch4. If instead you wish to identify a 1A Parasite in the location, see Pt3-Ch5. All of these applications build on the 5A Location.

Organ Muscle Testing Locations

The testing locations for the organs and glands are straightforward: once you have identified the 5A Location you want to MT, simply place your four fingertips onto that area. Remember that we need to provoke an electromagnetic response similar to striking a bell with a hammer, so beware of touching a deep organ too lightly. Often, pressure is needed.

It is a misconception inherited from the field of acupuncture that we need to find a precise spot the size of a pin to accurately MT an organ. Each organ produces its own miniature version of the body's bioelectric field. These mini organ fields emanate around the tissue, leading to two interesting phenomena:

1. No single point There is **no single point** that is indicative of an organ. A MT anywhere in the lung region, for example, will indicate the lungs. Also, look for variance from one lung to the other as single-side pathologies can be an issue.

2. Depth is a factor A shallow MT pressure will evaluate shallow tissue; a deeper pressure, deeper tissue. **Depth is a factor.** For insulated organs like the heart, lungs, kidneys, liver and brain, there is no means of accurately localizing the deep areas with touch, only shallow tests are possible. This is one of the main limitations in MT organ locations: after a certain depth the MT is general, not specific.

For these reasons, in the organ location section that follows, there are no landmarking circles placed over the images to clarify the exact testing positions. Practically speaking, there are no exact locations, just general guidelines that for better or for worse, are open to interpretation.

It is the responsibility of the serious student and the practitioner to familiarize themselves with these locations and endeavor to draw conclusions that are as precise, binary and scientific as possible.

One technique that helps to be more precise when MT adjacent organs or glands is to use the tip of a single finger instead of four fingertips when localizing a particular region.

Organ Locations

Note: left = LT   right = RT

1. STOMACH (GASTRIC) **Where** Under the LT ribs. **Function** Produces acid, begins digestion, timed release of food into the small intestine. **Dysfunctions** Acid reflux, stomach ache, cramps, ulcers, initial allergic responses to foods.	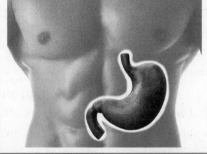
2. SMALL INTESTINE (ENTERIC) **Where** All around belly button. **Function** Breakdown of food and nutrient extraction. **Dysfunctions** Pain, ulcers, mucous, bloating, gassiness, back pain, neck pain, abdominal sensitivity, most digestive-related medical conditions.	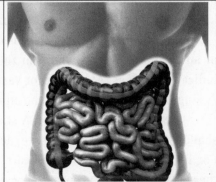
3. LARGE INTESTINE (COLONIC) **Where** 1) **Ascending colon** RT-side abdomen above pelvis. 2) **Transverse colon** Center abdomen below ribs. 3) **Descending colon** LT-side abdomen above pelvis. **Function** Further breakdown of foods, good bacteria produce vitamin B, absorption of water, formation and storage of feces. **Dysfunctions** Constipation, bloating, colitis, gassiness, cramping, pelvic and back pain.	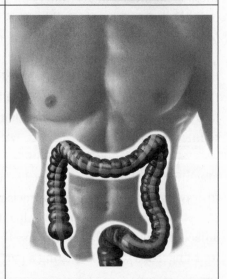

4. LUNGS (PULMONARY)

Where Behind RT and LT pecs.

Function Oxygen absorption, excretion of C02 and some lymphatic waste.

Dysfunctions Shortness of breath, cough, lung conditions like asthma and COPD, proneness to viruses. Pain in the upper back, shoulder, neck.

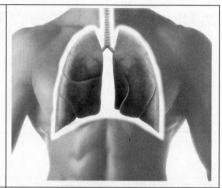

5. LIVER (HEPATIC)

Where Under RT side and rear RT rib cage (wraps around back).

Function Filters blood from the digestive tract, produces bile and over 500 enzymes and specialized proteins.

Dysfunctions Cholesterol and bile issues, reduced enzyme production, general inflammation, RT side rib and back pain, jaundice, cirrhosis.

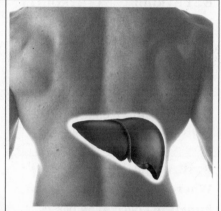

6. KIDNEYS (RENAL)

Where Underneath the back LT and RT 12th (bottom) ribs, push into the soft tissue.

Function Filter urea and bacteria out of the blood, controls blood pressure and levels of water, acids, bases and electrolytes.

Dysfunctions Fluid retention, anemia, decreased sex drive, changes in appetite, urine output, potassium levels. Also kidney stones, cyst formation, mid-back pain and some adrenal disorders.

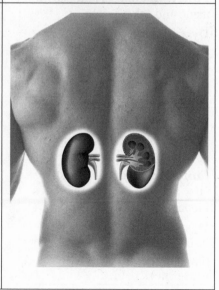

7. HEART (CARDIAC)

Where Direct center of chest. It's only off to the left in the movies.

Function Circulates blood.

Dysfunctions Irregular heart beat, narrowing of the arteries, heart attack, heart failure.

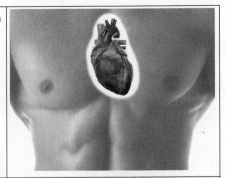

8. THYROID (THYROID)

Where In the throat below the jaw, both sides of the trachea.

Function Produces hormones that regulate metabolic rate, muscle control, mood, bones.

Dysfunctions Weight gain, depression, skeletal issues.

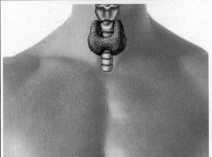

9. BLADDER (CYSTIC)

Where Above pelvic bone.

Function Collects and passes urine and other waste.

Dysfunctions UTIs (urinary tract infections), cysts, urine leakage, loss of sphincter control, bed wetting.

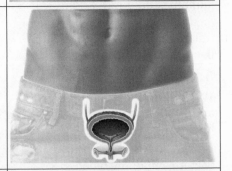

10. PANCREAS (PANCREATIC)

Where Behind the LT ribs that are below the LT pectoral.

Function Produces digestive enzymes and insulin, regulates blood sugar.

Dysfunctions Blood sugar issues including diabetes, digestive imbalances. Often causes neck pain.

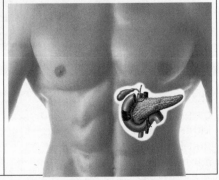

Building on a Negative Organ Muscle Test

As with every MT, if the area tests strong you have failed to find a problem. That doesn't guarantee there isn't one, but it's a good start.

Your goal, however, is to find a weak MT and then, as a reminder from earlier sections, build on a negative baseline. There are numerous Health Ladder applications for this, depending on your testing agenda, expertise and what kind of MT Kits you have access to.

Here are some examples, based on a weak MT of the stomach:

Rung 6B Treatment MT medications such as those for acid reflux against a negative stomach test. Do they turn the (-) back to a (+)?

Rung 5B Therapy MT the stomach for various supplements.

Rung 4B Antifungal MT various antifungal medications to infer the presence of a fungus. Be cautious about taking the antifungal, though.

Rung 4B Antiviral MT antiviral medications to identify a virus.

Rung 3A Metal Toxicity MT various element samples to determine local metal toxicity. This will often be specific to each organ.

Rung 3B Metal Detox Check which metal binders or chelators are needed as a way of minimizing symptoms of metal toxicity.

Rung 2B Probiotics Check which probiotic the stomach needs.

Rung 2B Antibiotics Determine which antibiotic the stomach needs.

Rung 1A Parasites MT various antiparasitic medicines against the stomach. Make sure you quantity test the dosage, this is essential.

Rung 1B Frequency Therapy Perform a MT to determine whether the particular stimulus of your frequency is relevant to the stomach.

Summary of Organ Muscle Testing

If you have no idea what is going on with your organs, you have no power over them. Knowledge is power.

Since you depend upon your organ and endocrine systems for survival, developing the skill of MT these areas is arguably the most important health action you can or will ever take.

Once you have learned how to MT the 5A Location, you are empowered to take further action at your own discretion.

Further Reading on the Organ Systems

The factor that limits exploration into MT the organ systems is a lack of information about applications in this area. That is addressed in The Complete Muscle Testing Series: *Book 2 Muscle Testing the Organ Systems*, where information about each organ and gland is expanded upon:

Part 1 concerns the organ systems. An individual chapter is devoted to each organ, including the stomach, small intestine, large intestine, kidneys, bladder, lungs, heart, liver, gall bladder and brain.

Part 2 covers the endocrine system including pancreas, adrenals, thymus, thyroid, ovaries, testes, pineal, pituitary and hypothalamus.

Part 3 deals with how to MT other body regions such as the skin, bones, hair, teeth, eyes, sinuses, ears, muscles, joints and circulatory system.

With an emphasis on functional MT of each location, Book 2 is addressed to the lay person but is intended to convey clinical-level understanding of the subject matter that can be used in practical MT scenarios by professionals and amateurs alike.

As a thorough explication of all 5A Locations in the body, this book is the foundation upon which the science of MT is based.

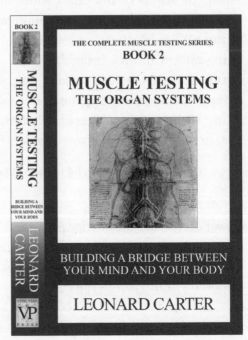

BOOK 2

THE COMPLETE MUSCLE TESTING SERIES:
BOOK 2

MUSCLE TESTING
THE ORGAN SYSTEMS

BUILDING A BRIDGE BETWEEN YOUR MIND AND YOUR BODY

LEONARD CARTER

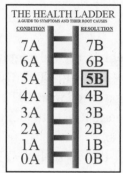

THE HEALTH LADDER		
A GUIDE TO SYMPTOMS AND THEIR ROOT CAUSES		
CONDITION		RESOLUTION
7A		7B
6A		6B
5A		5B
4A		4B
3A		3B
2A		2B
1A		1B
0A		0B

5B. THERAPY

RUNG 5B Therapy is support-focused: vitamins, supplements, herbs and some manual treatments attempt to heal the Location (5A).

3

Muscle Testing
Nutrients and Supplements

There are hundreds of supplements we could take, and if we looked into what each of them did it might sound like we needed them all. DNA synthesis? Check. Tissue repair? Check. Mucosal lining support? Check. Protein metabolism, digestion, sleep? Check. But we can't just eat a bowl of pills for breakfast, we need real food.

From all of those that sound good, which supplements do we actually need? Identifying this is a major application of MT. A 5A Location will often MT weak because there is a local nutrient deficiency. Supplements are positioned at Rung 5B on The Health Ladder because nutrition is a 5B Therapy.

At this level of thinking we are not focused on the root cause, just on how to support the body in a state of crisis and for this purpose, supplementation can be highly effective. People who for whatever reason need to supplement will have the best experience if they use MT to confirm the right product, its quantity and frequency.

The Process

The process of determining which supplement is needed requires that we build on a negative MT for a 5A Location (Pt3-Ch2). Once we have found a location that provokes a negative or weak MT, we can introduce various supplements to the bioelectric field to identify which of them cancels out the negative response.

For clarification, it is best to think of this as seeing which supplement turns the negative MT back to a positive. When we isolate one such product, we can infer that there is a positive (beneficial) bioelectromagnetic relationship between the 5A Location and the 5B Therapy, or in simple English: that's the one we need.

Factors to be aware of are:

1. MT a supplement against the correct 5B Location.
2. Variance in product quality.
3. Quantity testing to get the dosage right.
4. Understanding the number of times per day needed.
5. Understanding the number of days it is needed for.
6. Understanding what these supplements do.

We will cover each of these details below.

1. MT a supplement against the correct 5B Location

As a reminder from Pt1-Ch4 The Biology of MT, it is not enough to MT a product against the bioelectric field as a whole. This is far too general to indicate anything useful. We need to **MT against a location**.

The methodology needed to draw an effective conclusion requires starting with a specific negative MT of a 5A Location and introducing single-ingredient supplements one at a time to determine which if any of them cancels out the negative. When you find one, you can draw the single conclusion that this supplement is deficient in this location. If it is the stomach, for example, you might have narrowed down that the stomach needs vitamin C, specifically.

When this becomes an ingrained thought process it will help to make sense of overlapping symptoms from different locations.

2. Variance in product quality

It should be understood that not all products are created equal. The label is seldom accurate. **Variance in quality** can be due to bioavailability, concentration or the presence of additional toxins in the form of binders, fillers, flavors and sweeteners. You can't know this from reading the label or necessarily the product reviews and price is not a guaranteed indicator of quality although there is a correlation. The product needs to be MT. There are two ways to do this:

i. Bad for you? MT it on your own bioelectric field in the clear, to determine if it provokes a negative response. You are not testing it against a particular organ, just against yourself, and the information you are looking for in this test isn't whether you need the product or whether it will help you. You are only determining here whether it will hurt you.

> **MT Protocol:**
> **Is It Bad For You?**
>
> 1. Start with a baseline.
> 2. MT the product against your bioelectric field; remember you can't MT through metal.
>
> **A:** If the product MT weak, it is not good for you.
> **B:** If the product fails to MT weak, it is not bad for you.

ii. Good for you? Once you have confirmed that it won't hurt you, the next concern is whether it will actually help you. This is a technicality because a product will fail to provoke a positive MT against a location for 2 reasons: 1) It may not be the right product, but there is always the chance that 2) it is the right product only it isn't concentrated or bioavailable enough to produce the MT response you are looking for.

Starting from scratch, it would be difficult and time consuming to correctly orient yourself in this area. To facilitate understanding, some charts are provided below that summarize which supplements tend to consistently MT against which locations at which dosages. This is your guideline. If there is a failure to replicate the findings below, you might assume that the problem is quality and try a different product.

3. Quantity testing to get the dosage right

Once you have established that you have the right product for the right location, you will need to tailor the quantity to your needs. This is called **quantity testing the dosage**. Since every bottle states "Take 1-2 capsules daily," we can't reasonably interpret this as personalized advice.

Refer to Pt2-Ch2 for a review of the protocol for quantity testing (p.87). As a quick summary, start with the whole bottle to confirm whether the product is needed. Then introduce 1 pill at a time and MT each increment to identify the minimum number of pills that are needed to turn the negative back to a positive.

Be careful not to consume an unsafe quantity of a product. A MT will often indicate a dosage far in excess of what it is safe to take. Such a deficiency cannot be solved at the level of 5B supplementation.

4. Understanding the number of times per day needed

There is no way to determine this at the time of the initial MT. Someone who doesn't recognize the difference between scientific MT and spiritual Truth Testing might feel tempted to use MT to ask a question of the universe, namely "Universe, do I need to take this product once a day or twice?" I hope it is clear by now that this is not likely to produce an accurate result. At best this methodology will undermine the science of MT and erode its public credibility. At worst a person can believe that a toxic dose is safe and make themselves or someone else very sick. And all for what? Because Truth Testing seemed like a shortcut? That's either laziness or ego but it's neither science nor medicine. It is essential that we differentiate scientific MT from Truth Testing, not confuse or intermingle them and not use Truth Testing with health issues.

The only process that clarifies the times per day needed is retesting the product against the location every 4 to 8 hours. As a guideline, every product MT for being needed 1-2 times per day. 1x/day is an ongoing support dose, 2x/day is more of a therapeutic dose and anything 3x/day or more is a clinical or medical-grade dose that is only appropriate for a serious, short-term deficiency. Supplementing with any vitamin or mineral 3x/day long term will cause toxicity and is strongly recommended against.

5. Understanding the number of days it is needed for

There are a few aspects to this variable. First, the quantity will lessen from a higher initial amount to a lower eventual amount. Don't continue taking the quantity you MT for at the outset for the duration, or very quickly you'll be taking too much. Retest every few days.

Second, watch for a toxicity reaction within the first week. The main reason you'll be deficient in something is that you have a 1A Parasite creating that deficiency. You are deficient in the parasite's favorite food. Be careful about supplementing long-term with the thing you're deficient in as it can switch, over time, from being something that you need (i.e., something that turns a negative 5A Location back to a positive MT), to being something that is toxic for you and provokes its own negative MT in a screen. This subsequent switching of your result isn't an issue of product quality, it is a function of how your system processes supplement toxicity over time.

Third and final, if you have found a product that continues to MT positive on you, and to help a negative 5A Location you're trying to support, the ultimate question you need to ask and answer is that of how long it is appropriate to take a supplement knowing that the reason you are deficient in it stems from a cause lower down on The Health Ladder. That decision will vary by case and is yours to make.

Summary So Far

If you can confirm that a supplement is needed against a particular location, verify its quality and tailor your dosage by MT for quantity, times per day and duration, you have identified the important variables.

It is advisable to think of this in mental slots as if you were filling in your own prescription pad. Everyone already informally does this with supplements. Here is a way to be scientific about it.

Personal Supplement Regimen				
Supplement Name	**Unit Size**	**Quantity**	**Times/Day**	**Duration**
Your Supplement				
Example: Vitamin C	1000mg	2 pills	Twice	Ongoing

6. Understanding what these supplements do

There isn't space here to list every supplement you could possibly use, so instead we will focus on the following combination of factors: the best for you, the safest and the ones that support the organs listed in the previous chapter. This information is below.

Muscle Testing Water-Soluble Vitamins

There are several water-soluble vitamins: about twenty Bs and one C. Vitamin C has about five main forms commercially but they all do the same thing. A MT will confirm this. We will touch on the five most common forms of vitamin B but eight of them are very important.

When MT vitamin B, be aware that different parasites will create different toxicities. If you've ever heard of someone having an allergy to a B vitamin, that's an example of this. When MT, always look for that paradoxical deficiency on day 1 and toxicity a week later. This will confirm you've found a parasite that likes a B vitamin.

Water-soluble Vitamins	Unit Quantity	Dosage Range	5A Location to MT it on	Function
Vitamin C (Ascorbic Acid)	1000 mg pills	1 - 5 pills	Stomach, Intestines, Lungs	Formation, repair and maintenance of all body tissues
Deficiency: Scurvy		**Toxicity:** Loose/watery stools		
Vitamin B3 (Niacin)	500 mg	1 - 5 pills	Small Intestine, Liver	Converts food into glucose
Vitamin B6 (Pyridoxine)	100 mg	1 - 5 pills	Liver, Intestines	Essential factor in amino acid metabolism
Vitamin B7 (Biotin)	1000 mcg (1mg)	1 - 5 pills	Large Intestine	Protein formation, especially hair and nails
Vitamin B9 (Folic Acid)	1000 mcg (1mg)	1 - 5 pills	Large Intestine	Helps iron metabolism, red blood cell formation
Vitamin B12 (methylcobalamin)	1000 mcg (1mg)	1 - 5 pills	Liver, Heart	Helps with DNA synthesis
Deficiency: B3 is pellagra. Other B deficiencies don't have special names.		**Toxicity:** Generally there is no toxicity, but excessive supplementation is unwise. Also, a day 2 or 3 toxicity reaction indicates a parasite.		

Muscle Testing Fat-Soluble Vitamins

There are four main fat-soluble vitamins (A, D, E, and K) and many sub-forms, particularly in the carotenoid group. Similar to the B vitamins, it is a standard pathology that certain parasites will cause a toxicity reaction to the fat-soluble vitamins.

Note: i.u. = international units, a term generally used for fat-soluble vitamins

Fat-soluble Vitamins	Unit Quantity	Dosage Range	5A Location to MT it on	Function
Vitamin A (Retinol)	10,000 i.u.	1 - 3 pills	Primarily the eyes	It is fuel to your eyes in the same way electricity is fuel to your phone
Deficiency: Nyctalopia (Night blindness)			**Toxicity:** Hypervitaminosis A. Beware: over-supplementation is very dangerous.	
Beta Carotene (compound vitamin A)	30,000 i.u.	1 - 10 pills, 2-3x/ day	Stomach, Intestines, Lungs, Liver, All mucosa	Up-regulates production of mucosal lining, allowing for digestion and breathing
Deficiency: Depletion of mucosal linings			**Toxicity:** Your skin will turn progressively brighter shades of orange until you look like a carrot.	
Vitamin D3 (Calcitriol)	1000 to 10,000 i.u. gel caps	5 - 10 pills	Thymus, Stomach, Intestines	Backbone of your immune system, kills 2A Bad Bacteria
Deficiency: Rickets, osteomalacia			**Toxicity:** Hypervitaminosis D. Beware: over-supplementation is dangerous.	

Vitamins E and K are more complex in terms of what 5A Location we would MT to identify a deficiency in them, and what conclusion we would draw from this information. We will not be exploring them yet.

A detailed analysis of fat-soluble vitamins in the carotenoid category (there are over 600 but the main ones are alpha carotene, beta carotene, lutein, lycopene, astaxanthin and zeaxanthin) has interesting longevity implications, not only on hair, nail and skin quality but also on organ tissue repair. However, this field is only illuminated once the underlying carotenoid drain—parasites—is fully eliminated. Remember, 1A Parasites want a mucosal lining, too, and they use our beta carotene and other carotenoids for this purpose.

Bacteria, Minerals and Amino Acids

Minerals that have a biological role are all drawn from the periodic table. In their elemental form they are poisonous to us but good for our 2A Bad Bacteria.

To render them bioavailable, a **nutritional molecule** is added onto them, usually by a plant. There is a basic group of these molecules and their role is to render the element capable of being absorbed and metabolized by us at the cellular level. The names of the molecules might be familiar from the supplement store: citrate, oxide, glycinate, picolinate, orotate and carbonate. Here is how it works:

Magnesium (Mg#12) + Citrate (C6H8O7) = Magnesium Citrate

It is important to understand that the action of the 2A Bad Bacteria involves separating these minerals from their nutritional molecule so they can be metabolized by the bacteria.

2A Bad Bacteria + Magnesium Citrate = Magnesium (Mg#12) + Citrate

2A Bad Bacteria transform our useful minerals back into a toxic molecule and are the reason that MT minerals generally leads to the paradoxical switch outlined above, where 2 to 7 days after supplementing, a mineral that MT strong will now MT weak.

It is vital to understand this principle about MT minerals or none of your data will make sense for more than a few days.

Regarding fats and amino acids, we will not have space to go into them here, partly because they are even more complex than the mineral example, but in concept the application is identical. If you have no parasites you should be able to derive your nutrients from your diet. If by contrast you're full of parasites, not only will you be chronically fat- and amino acid-deficient, but supplementing in concentrated forms of them will lead to the paradoxical switch where they will MT weak and be a source of negative dietary symptoms for you, up to and including food allergies and various other medical pathologies. This dramatically accelerates the aging process.

Muscle Testing Minerals

Understanding the danger of over-supplementing with minerals doesn't detract from an awareness of their importance in various metabolic functions. It is worth noting that mineral deficiency and toxicity becomes a major factor when we begin to explore their role in 6A Symptoms.

In medical pathologies, the action of the 2A Bad Bacteria in mineral deficiency takes on a whole new significance. All cases of diabetes have chromium deficiency in common. A bacteria is doing this. Multiple sclerosis involves selenium. Migraines are associated with manganese, selenium or molybdenum and psoriasis is associated with zinc. The minerals are not pivotal in themselves but by pointing to the 2A Bad Bacteria, they tell us what else might be going on.

The list below is not a complete outline of all the minerals we use for metabolic processes. It leaves out more complex minerals like copper, lithium, molybdenum, phosphorus, sodium and vanadium and a few others, but it provides a solid foundation from which to start thinking about this area and some useful things to MT for:

Muscle Testing Minerals				
Minerals	**Unit Quantity**	**Dosage Range**	**5A Location to MT it on**	**Function**
Boron	3 mg	1-5 pills	Intestines	Bones, muscles, hormones
Calcium	300 mg	1-2 pills	Muscles	Bones, muscles, electricity
Chromium	200 mcg	1-4 pills	Pancreas	Helps glucose metabolism
Fluoride	250 mcg	1-2 pills	Teeth	Hardens the teeth
Iodine	15 mg	1-2 pills	Thyroid	Makes thyroxin hormone
Iron	50 mg	1-2 pills	Veins	Helps blood hold oxygen
Magnesium	500 mg	1-2 pills	Stomach	Almost everything
Manganese	10 mg	1-2 pills	CNS	Protein and vitamin uptake
Potassium	99 mg	1-2 pills	Stomach	Maintains bioelectric field
Selenium	100 mcg	1-2 pills	CNS	Muscle function and energy
Silicon	8 mg	1-4 pills	Bones	Skin, bones and teeth
Strontium	250 mg	1-4 pills	Bones	Skin, bones and teeth
Zinc	30 mg	1 pill	Skin	Skin and immune system

Other Core Concepts with Supplementation

Deficiency It is wise to remember that if you need to supplement just to maintain basic health, something is siphoning off your nutrients. Rung 5B Therapies like supplementation solve a short-term deficiency but fail to change the larger context of what is creating the deficiency.

Indication of need There should always be a MT indication that you need a supplement. If you can't build on the negative baseline from a 5A Location with the 5B supplements from your regimen then why are you taking them? You will find that there are enough supplements you MT for needing without wasting time, effort and money taking things you're not testing for.

Toxicity Because your parasites are nourished by your supplements every time you take them, one way of looking at this is that you are deficient in your parasites' favorite foods. Be cautious of MT and then consuming high doses of supplements as you will reach a point where you are creating your own nutrient toxicity. The more you consume, the more the parasite consumes and the more it excretes bacteria into you. This snowballing toxicity can intensify the very symptoms you're taking supplements to minimize. This is particularly evident with minerals, amino acids and the B vitamins.

Application Start by applying what you have learned here. Go through your supplement cupboard and run the following MT screens:
1. Which supplements MT weak on you (stop using them).
2. Which supplements turn a negative baseline back to a positive.

Then make a dosage chart for yourself and do the MT to identify the right quantities of the right products at the right frequency. If you want to make this a fun project, do the same thing for your spouse, kids, parents and friends.

Supplement Name	Unit Size	Quantity	Times/Day	Duration
Your Supplement				

Priorities At some point, you will need to strategize which organs you should prioritize for long-term support. This is a conversation to be had with your doctor or naturopath.

Clarification

The rationale for MT your supplements is often expressed in misleading language. Common examples are that "your body is telling you what it needs," that "your body can talk"or that "your body doesn't lie." This way of putting it places emphasis on a face-value interpretation of the MT response and leads to confusion.

It can confuse you because the fact is, your interpretation of any MT is subject to your level of understanding of the rungs on The Health Ladder as well as your agenda in the matter.

It can also confuse other people who may not understand this content and may be wary of unscientific language. When teaching others, it is always advisable to refrain from speaking in esoteric terms, particularly when it is important that they believe you.

The body's MT response to a supplement should be phrased in the following way: **The body is expressing binary neurological responses** (positive/negative, strong/weak) **to physiological stimuli** (such as nutrients, supplements and organ test points). These responses are open to a wide range of interpretations based on your knowledge of The Health Ladder, your level of education in molecular nutrition and your interpretation agenda.

An interpretation of a MT that is based on an awareness of The Health Ladder and free from any overt agenda to consume or sell a product would lead to the following conclusions:

1. Short-term nutritional support is an appropriate 5B Therapy.
2. A supplement regimen will be most optimal if it is customized using the MT process outlined in this chapter.
3. Long-term nutritional support should only be a last resort when there is an inability to deal with Rungs 1-4 on The Health Ladder.
4. Over-supplementation should be avoided due to the danger of strengthening the 1A Parasites that caused the deficiency.

This clarifies how to think about, interpret and express the process of MT nutrients and supplements as a Rung 5B Therapy.

Further Reading on Nutrients and Supplements

An expanded form of this information is found in The Complete Muscle Testing Series: *Book 3 Muscle Testing Nutrients and Supplements*. It is divided into 4 parts:

Part 1 examines detailed information about water-soluble and fat-soluble vitamins

Part 2 looks at all the minerals, with an emphasis on their role in metabolic functions.

Part 3 covers proteins and the amino acids, detailing the metabolic processes they are responsible for, how and where to MT them and their role in various medical conditions.

Part 4 is devoted to MT which fats the body utilizes and where they are needed, a fascinating area full of misconceptions and oversights.

Part 5 explores the diverse and complex world of herbal supplementation, one with a rich history and interesting MT applications in modern pharmacology.

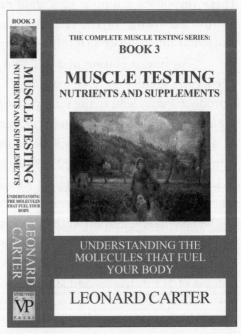

3A. METAL TOXICITY

Elements in their non-bioavailable form adhere to you when Bad Bacteria (2A) absorb them for cellular metabolism.

3B. METAL DETOX

RUNG 3B Metal Detox can minimize the Symptom (6A) by starving Bad Bacteria (2A) of the Metals (3A) that they metabolize.

THE HEALTH LADDER
A GUIDE TO SYMPTOMS AND THEIR ROOT CAUSES

CONDITION	RESOLUTION
7A	7B
6A	6B
5A	5B
4A	4B
3A	3B
2A	2B
1A	1B
0A	0B

4

Muscle Testing

For Metal Toxicity

The core questions at this level of thinking are 1) To what extent is metal toxicity involved with illness? 2) How can this be quantified? 3) What can be done about the findings?

Measuring specific metal toxicities in particular locations leads to further questions: Why do metals stick to one person more than another? What is the effect of high levels of toxicity versus low levels? What constitutes a toxic amount? What symptoms do the different metals cause? How do we get them out? When they are removed, will that translate into any difference in health? Is there anything we can do to avoid them in the future? Do we need to avoid them? Where do they come from? Is metal toxicity even the correct term for what is happening? Can MT help with these considerations?

It is appropriate to position these questions at Rung 3 on The Health Ladder. 3A Metal Toxicity adheres to us because of 2A Bad Bacteria and is the means by which 4A Fungi and Viruses express themselves.

Metal Toxicity Terminology

To start with, the word heavy in heavy metal is not accurate. The weight of an element refers to the number of protons in the nucleus of the atom. Heavier metals like mercury (Hg#80) and lead (Pb#82) are known to be very toxic but lighter metals like lithium (Li#3) or calcium (Ca#20) can be equally toxic in their own ways. An element doesn't need to be heavy to be toxic: Light elements are toxic too.

The metal in heavy metal is also a misnomer. Arsenic (As#33) is classified as a metalloid (not exactly a metal), while selenium (Se#34) is a non-metal and fluorine (F#9) is a halogen.

Last, the idea of toxicity in metal toxicity is misleading. Someone can appear to experience great suffering from arsenic while their arsenic levels are within a medically acceptable range. Disregarding obvious, industrial-level poisoning, the bulk of the negative physiological reactions to the elements have to do not with toxicity in them but with 2A Bad Bacteria on The Health Ladder.

So, if 2A Bad Bacteria are the things that cause 6A Symptoms in most cases, and we can neither describe this accurately by the terms heavy or metal or toxicity, then how should we describe it?

Element saturation is most accurate but we will proceed by using the more common term metal toxicity interchangeably with **element toxicity** so as to build understanding on an existing term.

There is a further distinction to be made regarding whether or not an element has a **biological role**. Arsenic (As#33) is not known to contribute to any biological function so it is perceived as exclusively toxic, whereas calcium (Ca#20) has numerous functions and is essential to life. But is calcium (Ca#20) bioavailable? This is a different concept.

The **bioavailability** of an element has to do with whether it can be used or metabolized for cellular functioning. In the same way that the tip of a screwdriver determines which screw it can work with, for an element to be bioavailable, it must be combined with an amino acid tag (e.g., calcium (Ca#20) + citrate = calcium citrate). Elemental calcium (Ca#20) without its amino acid tag can be almost as toxic as elemental arsenic. This distinction applies to all the elements.

Metal Toxicity Analysis

On the surface, metal toxicity sounds very dangerous. Mercury (Hg#80), thallium (Tl#81), lead (Pb#82) and bismuth (Bi#83) are known neurotoxins and arsenic (As#33) is a deadly poison. But how about the rest of the periodic table? If we subtract the 2 radioactive elements below bismuth and the 5 noble gases that don't stick to anything, there are 76 elements that it is possible to have toxicity in.

Anyone wanting to see which toxicities apply to them can have a hair metal analysis done. This looks wonderfully scientific, you even get your results printed in color, but there are problems with this approach:

1. It only covers 38 of 76 possible elements. What about the other 38?

2. It divides the elements into toxic and essential groups, which overlooks the fact that even essential elements with a biological role can be toxic if they are not made bioavailable by an amino acid.

3. It takes content out of context, assigning low importance to elements that show up low on the chart but that may still be causing serious symptoms in your case.

	Metal	Healthy Range	LOW	NORMAL	HIGH	TOXIC
				TRACE ELEMENT TESTING SCREEN		
1	Boron	B= LOW				
2	Calcium	Ca= LOW				
3	Chromium	Cr= LOW				
4	Cobalt	Co= LOW				
5	Copper	Cu= LOW				
6	Fluoride	F= LOW				
7	Iodine	I= LOW				
8	Iron	Fe= LOW				
9	Magnesium	Mg= LOW				
10	Manganese	Mn= LOW				
11	Potassium	K= LOW				
12	Selenium	Se= LOW				
13	Vanadium	V= LOW				
14	Zinc	Zn= LOW				
15	Aluminum	Al= LOW				
16	Antimony	Sb= LOW				
17	Arsenic	As= LOW				
18	Beryllium	Be= LOW				
19	Bismuth	Bi= LOW				
20	Cadmium	Cd= LOW				
21	Gadolinium	Gd= LOW				
22	Germanium	Ge= LOW				
23	Gold	Au= LOW				
24	Lead	Pb= LOW				
25	Mercury	Hg= LOW				
26	Molybdenum	Mo= LOW				
27	Nickel	Ni= LOW				
28	Palladium	Pd= LOW				
29	Platinum	Pt= LOW				
30	Silicon	Si= LOW				
31	Silver	Ag= LOW				
32	Strontium	Sr= LOW				
33	Sulphur	S= LOW				
34	Tellurium	Te= LOW				
35	Tin	Sn= LOW				
36	Titanium	Ti= LOW				
37	Tungsten	W= LOW				

4. It is not qualitative. When an element toxicity shows up high, the analysis won't tell you if it's doing you harm, or how, or why. You can only assume.

5. There is no explicit location. If you have a high arsenic level, is it high everywhere or just in your liver? Without understanding where the element is collecting, you can't draw any practical conclusions.

And then where are all these element toxicities coming from? A toxic environment, we are told. And how do we get them out? We can do oral or injectable chelation with DMSA, EDTA or DMPS or get our mercury fillings removed. But does that even work? More often than not, chelation is a lifestyle. And then what? It never ends.

Muscle Testing Metals

If you have toxicity in an element, a sample of that same element will MT weak on you when held within your bioelectric field.

When an element exists in the body at a toxic level, this information is incorporated into the bioelectric field. The presence of the element contributes to a net negative charge within the field such that if a further quantity of that element is held near the body, the resulting neurological reaction will be that a strong MT baseline will change to a weak response.

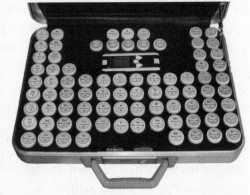

A Periodic Table MT Kit is needed for this purpose containing pure samples of all 76 testable elements. Even platinum (Pt#78) and gold (Au#79) can show up as toxicities.

Extensive cross-referencing with lab-based metal toxicity analyses has confirmed that a MT-based analysis of the elements produces consistent and accurate results.

A MT analysis improves on lab results in the following ways:
1. It makes it possible to test for all 76 elements, not just 38.
2. It bypasses the misconception of toxic versus essential elements.
3. It identifies elements that may be producing toxicity in your case even though they would register in a medically acceptable range.
4. It is by definition qualitative. Any element that MT weak is a problem.
5. It allows us to establish a location. When MT an element sample against an organ location we can isolate exactly where the toxicity rests. This has never been possible with a hair metal analysis.
6. Last, the results are immediate and you don't have to lose any hair.

It should be reiterated that Truth Testing won't work for this purpose, Self Testing isn't accurate and MT vials of water supposedly imprinted with an element is not a replacement for pure element samples.

Metal Toxicity Patterns

The average person who is MT for all 76 elements will exhibit a weak response to about 20 of them. People with a medical condition can MT weak to as many as 50. There is a correlation between the number of elements someone MT weak to and their degree of illness.

While MT an element per se is interesting, we can only draw inferences about causality (e.g., understanding what it is doing to us) when we MT it against a location. This is essential when analyzing a medical condition.

When a MT screen of the 76 elements is applied to medical conditions, some obvious patterns emerge: everyone who has Multiple sclerosis (MS) will MT for selenium toxicity; people with fibromyalgia MT for arsenic toxicity; Parkinson's cases always have thallium in the motor cortex; low iron is paradoxically often associated with iron toxicity; diabetics always MT for chromium toxicity in the pancreas; chronic vomiting MT for mercury in the stomach; bloody stools is usually cadmium in the large intestine and someone with hot flashes consistently MT for aluminum; with high blood pressure, circulatory points around the body MT for lead; with migraines we find manganese; with asthma, the lungs MT for a concoction of elements but always arsenic.

> ### MT Protocol For Metals In A Location
>
> 1. Start with a baseline.
> 2. Find an element that MT negative.
> 3. With the negative element sample resting on the stomach, MT various organ locations to see which one cancels out the negative element.
>
> A: If organ plus negative element still tests weak, no correlation.
>
> B: If organ plus negative element tests strong, then there is a correlation. We can then infer that the element is localized in this particular organ.

So, what are we seeing here? Patterns of element toxicity show up in many medical conditions. But are the elements the root cause? Can we get them out and keep them out? Will getting them out resolve the symptoms? On The Health Ladder, we treat a 3A Metal Toxicity with a 3B Metal Detox: chelation (pronounced key-lation).

Chelation

The term for drawing toxic elements out of the body is chelation. A **chelator** or binder is a compound that binds to an element.

We can quantify that chelation has worked if a MT analysis can identify the presence of an element before the binder is used, and then fail to identify the element in the days afterward (e.g., if you no longer MT for mercury, presumably the chelator worked).

A MT analysis of the chelators on the market reveals that no single product (DMSA, EDTA or DMPS) universally binds to all elements. For example, EDTA MT against arsenic, DMSA does not.

There are numerous nutritional products that have a chelating action on the elements: barley grass, chlorella, spirulina, wheat grass, activated charcoal, magnesium citrate, boron glycinate and MSM. There is in fact a science to this but there isn't space to go into it here.

What is needed at this introductory level is the knowledge

> **MT Protocol For Metal Chelators**
> 1. Start with a baseline.
> 2. MT the element sample.
> 3. MT the chelator at the same time as a weak-testing element sample.
>
> **A:** If the chelator cancels out the weak MT, it must bind to the weak sample.
> **B:** If the chelator does not cancel the weak element sample out, it does not bind to it.

of how to identify element toxicity by MT pure element samples from a Periodic Table MT Kit. Only then will it make sense to cross reference this with a given chelator to identify a binding relationship.

This paves the way for a process of getting the elements out. When we utilize the correct binder for a specific element toxicity we can reasonably answer the above questions: Will chelating an element in a symptomatic location resolve the symptom? Is element toxicity the root cause of illness?

When this is approached scientifically it becomes clear that a symptom may lessen during chelation but it will not resolve from chelation. In fact, the element toxicity quickly returns after chelation. This leads to the next question, From where does toxicity return?

Sources of Metal Toxicity

The problem with trying to use a binder to chelate element toxicity is that you will acquire more of the element from your environment, probably that same day.

To identify the sources of any metal toxicity, you will need a sample of the metal to MT against a product so as to quantify it. Without the element sample, there is little point in thinking about this because you'll have no more than common misconceptions to go on (e.g., fish and some dental fillings have trace amounts of mercury, but did you know that whipped cream and laundry detergent have just as much if not more?).

> ## MT Protocol For Metals In A Product
>
> 1. Start with a baseline.
> 2. MT the product, remember you can't MT through metal.
> 3. MT which element sample cancels out a weak product.
>
> **A:** If weak product plus element still tests weak, no correlation.
>
> **B:** If weak product plus element tests strong, then there is a correlation. We can infer that the element is in the product.

An analysis of thousands of household products indicates that there is metal toxicity in everything we use.

Foods: sauces, cream, dairy, fish, meats, cereal, grains, fruit, vegetables, oils, syrups, butter, ice cream, cheese and spices, not to mention alcohol and tobacco. So, you can't eat anything.

Household products: perfumes, makeup, floor cleaners, shampoo, soap, deodorant, tooth paste, laundry detergent, dish soap and room fresheners, essential oils and candles. So, you can't breathe anything.

The result is paranoia, and this isn't a healthy way to live your life. A shift in perspective illustrates why: There are just as many heavy metals in organic, raw and vegan foods and household products as there are in processed items. You can't avoid the periodic table because you're living in it, you're made of it, it is the universe. We need to move on from this mentality of avoidance by letting go of the idea that the environment is toxic. This leads to the original question:

To what extent is metal toxicity involved with illness?

Metal Toxicity on The Health Ladder

We can quantify metal toxicity with a hair metal analysis or more precisely with a MT analysis using a Periodic Table MT Kit. This information can be built upon to identify both the source of the elements in our environment, the location in the body where they are collecting and which chelator can best be used to extract them.

An analysis that cross-references the elements with various medical conditions indicates a relationship but the systematic removal of the elements using chelation fails to eliminate the symptom, so it is clear that element toxicity is not the root cause of illness. This is why metal toxicity is positioned at Rung 3 on The Health Ladder.

Moving conceptually down to Rung 2, it becomes apparent that Bad Bacteria are the agents that absorb the elements and utilize them for energy metabolism. This is why element toxicity appears to stick to us, particularly in its nonbioavailable forms; why everyone has their own toxicity profile; why people have differing amounts of the same element and in different locations; why toxicity appears to be related to illness; and why chelation doesn't resolve the 6A Symptom.

It is clear that the root cause of the symptom is the 1A Parasite that is excreting the 2A Bad Bacteria that is causing the 3A Metal Toxicity to adhere to us. When this is understood, it allows us to use the incidence of a metal toxicity as an indicator of the parasite. Frankly, there is no better way to find parasites than by MT element samples. There is even a pattern to this: mercury indicates roundworm, lead indicates whipworm, arsenic indicates flatworm. Because of this pattern of indication, an analysis of metal toxicity is highly relevant. Perhaps it is the most relevant thing you can MT. But only when the 1A Parasite is eliminated will we cease to find the 3A Metal Toxicity. Until then, there is little to be gained from chelation.

The end conclusion is quite empowering: You can live back on the grid, stop fearing food, stop fearing your environment and understand that the elements are your friends. They either help directly in your metabolic processes or they help indirectly by telling you which parasites you have. Focus then moves to the 1A Parasite.

Further Reading on Metal Toxicity

A thorough and systematic analysis of metal toxicity is found in The Complete Muscle Testing Series: *Book 4 Muscle Testing for Metal Toxicity.*

Part 1 outlines the science of metal toxicity, valence electrons, and the electrochemical nature of how chelators work to reduce metal toxicity in the body.

Part 2 explores how the elements are absorbed by bacteria and used for their cellular metabolism in a way that harms us.

Part 3 expands on the difference between toxic elements and nutritional minerals with a biological role, with more information on the amino acids that render the elements bioavailable.

Part 4 examines the architecture of how metal toxicities relate to common medical conditions, as well as how they can affect our mood and wellbeing.

Part 5 is an encyclopedic list of the elements from #1 to #83 (and also #84 to #101 for the sake of interest) with a profile for each that includes symptoms of toxicity, what sources they come from, what they are used for in society, what medical conditions they are associated with, what parasite they indicate and what binders are used on them.

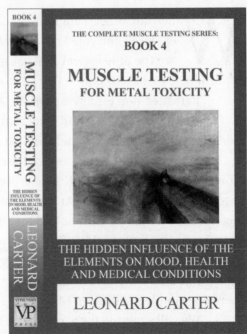

BOOK 4

THE COMPLETE MUSCLE TESTING SERIES:
BOOK 4

MUSCLE TESTING
FOR METAL TOXICITY

THE HIDDEN INFLUENCE OF THE
ELEMENTS ON MOOD, HEALTH
AND MEDICAL CONDITIONS

LEONARD CARTER

1A. PARASITES

Various Parasites (1A) inhabit your body. They deplete nutrients, damage tissue and excrete Bad Bacteria (2A). Best eliminated by Frequency Therapy (1B).

THE HEALTH LADDER	
A GUIDE TO SYMPTOMS AND THEIR ROOT CAUSES	
CONDITION	RESOLUTION
7A	7B
6A	6B
5A	5B
4A	4B
3A	3B
2A	2B
1A	1B
0A	0B

5

Muscle Testing

For Parasites

When all other rungs on The Health Ladder have been explored and ruled out, it becomes clear that 1A Parasites are the only logical root cause of illness. But how can we confirm that we have them?

Parasites don't show up on an X-ray or MRI because they don't have bones or a shell, and stool testing, generally assumed to be a definitive process, is extremely limited, subjective and inaccurate.

To what extent are parasites at the root of medical conditions? How can we quantify this? How can we differentiate between one species and the next? How can we isolate their presence in specific locations? How do we eliminate them? How do we know that they have been eliminated? How do we know there aren't more that haven't been eliminated? Aren't there only a few parasites to worry about? Shouldn't we have none? Are any of them good for us? Isn't there one simple medication that treats all organisms?

We will examine these questions below.

The Limitations of Stool Testing

Most stool tests focus exclusively on bacteria, particularly the highly pathogenic forms like those associated with cholera, bubonic plague, blood poisoning, bloody diarrhea and flesh eating disease. Bacteria, although detrimental and even fatal, are not parasites.

Stool testing results include a brief nod toward parasites with the statement "no ovum seen" at the bottom of the report. *Ovum* is Latin for egg, meaning parasite egg. But did the parasites you were searching for excrete eggs in that particular bowel movement? Did you happen to scoop those eggs into your sample for the lab? Did the lab tech chance to extract them in their pipette for the microscope slide? Then, did they see them? And if seen, were they recognized as such? How long do lab techs spend looking for parasite eggs? Did you know they are told not to look too hard because everybody has them, anyway?

And then if parasite eggs are found, are the right ones found? It is common to misidentify as the root problem dientamoeba fragilis, a harmless protozoan, or H.pylori which is a bacterium. If ovum from roundworm or flatworm eggs are seen, is the right medication prescribed at the right dosage for the right duration? And does it work?

Stool testing leaves us with more questions than answers.

The Parasite Problem

We are faced with an impasse. Parasites are clearly central to an understanding of health but there is no straightforward way of knowing which ones we have or where they are, let alone how to get them out. We might agree to label this **The Parasite Problem**.

There are 4 central questions to The Parasite Problem:

1. Which parasites do we have (and where in the body are they)?
2. How do we know?
3. How do we get rid of them?
4. How do we know they're gone?
5. Where do they come from? This question is almost a side-note since most of the species we think we need to avoid are already in us.

Top 10 Parasite Myths

Before we can address The Parasite Problem, it is important to clarify what is not the case. Throughout the world there are major blind spots in the understanding of parasites. The top 10 parasite myths are outlined below. It is a myth that...

1. Nobody in a Western country has parasites In fact, every single human in the world without exception hosts multiple species.

2. You have to travel to get parasites You get your first few species from your mother and the rest from unboiled dairy, deli meats, manure-based oils and syrups and insect bites. By the time you pick up an unusual parasite on a trip, it is a drop in the bucket of your lifelong collection, but every food poisoning instance is a new species.

3. Parasites lay eggs in you which hatch in you With the exception of pinworm and filaria, all parasites have a life cycle that requires the eggs to leave the body, and often involves one or more intermediate hosts. Many eggs, for example, can only hatch in a snail.

4. Parasites breed (or only die) based on the phases of the Moon There is no correlation between parasites and the Moon though some of them do feed on hormones. Parasites are not so complicated that we need to understand them using astrophysics.

5. Parasites are only in the intestines Different species are adapted to live in every cubic inch of your body, including all organs and the brain.

6. Regular deworming helps you stay parasite free Medications will never get you parasite free because of The Dosage Toxicity Problem.

7. There is a medication for every parasite out there Even if all the main medications exist, the problem is that there is not a single or even a safe dosage for every organism.

8. A single antiparasitic medication treats all parasites There is no single medication that treats all parasite species.

9. A single dosage will always work There are in fact thousands of potential dosages and most of them are too toxic to take.

10. Antiparasitic medication dosages are based on your body weight This is not the case. You are medicating the parasite, not yourself.

Types of Parasites

The world of parasites can be understood very simply if we divide it into two categories: single-celled and multi-celled.

Single-celled Plasmodium, the parasite that causes malaria, is single-celled. This category also includes the amoeba and giardia, sometimes called beaver fever. There is little benefit in displaying them on a life-sized chart because they are microscopic.

Multi-celled These are definitely macroscopic. They can be subdivided into three main groups: flatworms, roundworms and filaria.

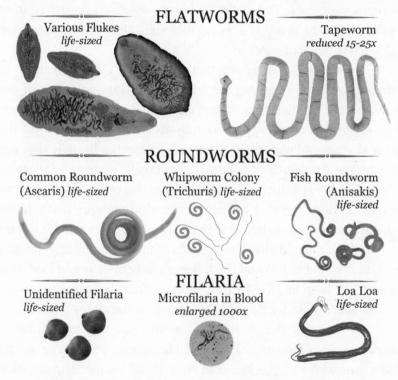

FLATWORMS

Various Flukes
life-sized

Tapeworm
reduced 15-25x

ROUNDWORMS

Common Roundworm
(Ascaris) *life-sized*

Whipworm Colony
(Trichuris) *life-sized*

Fish Roundworm
(Anisakis)
life-sized

FILARIA

Unidentified Filaria
life-sized

Microfilaria in Blood
enlarged 1000x

Loa Loa
life-sized

If you understand this, you understand basic parasitology.

The complexity arises when we consider which sub-species (serotype) we might be hosting. There are hundreds of thousands of possibilities, biologists don't even know them all. It doesn't matter how we classify them, it matters which ones we have. It is wisest to assume that we have multi-celled parasites from all three groups.

The Motel Room Concept

Since untold quantities of parasite eggs exist in nature, and since we have no natural defense to them, the question we should be asking isn't how could we get a parasite but rather, how could we possibly avoid it?

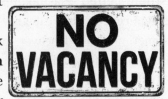

To clarify this idea, we can think of our bodies using **The Motel Room Concept**. With a roadside motel there are thousands of cars driving by but only 20 or so vacancies. The factor that stops every single driver from checking into the motel is a no vacancy sign. Once all the rooms are full, nobody new can check in.

It works the same way with parasites. Using flukes as an example, we have a vacancy for flukes in the various rooms of our health motel: the liver, lungs and different parts of the intestines. Since exposure to fluke eggs is continuous on the highway of life, the factor that stops flukes from continually hatching in us is that our fluke rooms are already full of flukes. Eventually we have no vacancy.

Physiologically, the probable process here is that the organism excretes a bacterium that contains a chemical message that inhibits same-species eggs from hatching in that location ever again. This is for the benefit of the parasite. If thousands of flukes continually hatched in us, that would kill us and the flukes already in us would lose their home. They keep us alive by protecting us from being overwhelmed by their species. Better the devil you know, as the saying goes.

Now take this idea and multiply it by roundworms, hookworms, whipworms, filaria and tapeworms and you've got an idea about who has checked into your motel rooms. The question isn't whether you have a parasite but which serotype you have that is protecting you from getting more of the same or something worse.

An example of why it would be beneficial to host the 4-foot long human tapeworm is that if you didn't have it, you would be at risk of picking up the 60-foot long fish tapeworm, and that would kill you. There is a certain, strange benefit, then, to hosting a parasite.

Medications as Parasite Placeholders

The Health Ladder and The Motel Room Concept both predict that we will find various parasite species throughout the body. It is possible to improve on the limitations of stool testing by using MT to find them.

However, what parasite indicator should we use in a MT? An herbal antiparasitic like black walnut shell or wormwood is so non-specific as to be futile and a watery vial claimed to indicate the parasites in a species group is based on a fraudulent claim.

What is needed is a specific quantity of a chemical that can be used as a concise, reproducible **placeholder** for the actual parasite. In this example we will consider praziquantel (biltricide), a well-known fluke medication.

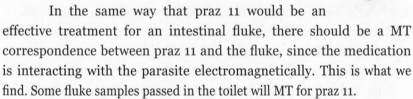

Praziquantel (abbr.: praz) pills come in 600mg doses. Therefore, praz 1=600mg and praz 11=6600mg. It is standard to administer a dosage of praz 11 to treat an intestinal fluke, seen at life-size in the adjacent image.

In the same way that praz 11 would be an effective treatment for an intestinal fluke, there should be a MT correspondence between praz 11 and the fluke, since the medication is interacting with the parasite electromagnetically. This is what we find. Some fluke samples passed in the toilet will MT for praz 11.

This correspondence between the amount of medication needed to kill the parasite and the amount that the parasite will MT for is the basis for the science that follows.

It leads us to a simple realization: If praz 11 is the effective treatment for the fluke and if the fluke MT for praz 11 when outside the body, might it also MT for praz 11 while still inside the body?

If so, it is a scientific revolution as it allows us to effectively bypass the limitation of stool testing and answer questions 1, 2 and 4 of The Parasite Problem (above). All that is needed is to learn basic antiparasitic pharmacology and then by MT a body location against an antiparasitic medication, we can reasonably infer the presence of every parasite species that we MT for needing the medication for.

There are only five main medications. This is relatively simple.

Antiparasitic Medications

To be able to MT for parasites, we need to understand which anti-parasitic medication works on which parasite. In this way we can use the medication as a conceptual placeholder to represent the organism we are looking for but cannot otherwise perceive with our senses.

The top 5 medications are presented below in chart form:

Antiparasitic Medications I: Brands and Targets			
	Medication	**Brand Name**	**Parasite it Targets**
1	Praziquantel	Biltricide	Flatworms (flukes and tapeworms)
2	Albendazole	Albenza	Hookworm, whipworm, others
3	Mebendazole	Vermox	Roundworms, possibly others
4	Ivermectin	Stromectol	Filaria, scabies
5	Metronidazole	Flagyl	Single-celled protozoans

Here is the logic that follows: If a 5A Location is MT for...

1. Praziquantel, then we probably have a fluke or tapeworm.

2. Albendazole, then we probably have a hookworm or whipworm.

3. Mebendazole, then we probably have a roundworm.

4. Ivermectin, then we probably have a filaria.

5. Metronidazole, then we probably have a single-celled parasite.

6. Other medications not listed here are subject to the same logic.

This largely demystifies the field of parasites. These five medications correspond nicely with the types of parasites listed above. There are thousands of details and some technicalities, exceptions and exclusions but they don't obscure the big picture: If we MT our organ locations for these medications, we can begin to develop an accurate profile of what parasites we have and where they are. Then focus can move to getting them out.

This bypasses the uncertainty of stool testing and of our own nervous system disconnect. All that is needed is a Parasite MT Kit with samples of the pills, and the know-how to use it.

Parasite Muscle Testing Kit

It is ideal to have samples of these medications in a Parasite MT Kit for home or clinical use.

A few challenges arise. In most Western countries they are sold by prescription only. In other countries most can be obtained over the counter. Then, cost is a factor. Mebendazole in Canada can cost $20/pill, whereas in India or Mexico it might only be 0.50¢/pill. Even though the point isn't to take the pills, only to MT them as placeholders, the costs can rack up. In a clinical setting people can MT for high doses.

Here are some other questions to think about: Where will you get these pills? Are they reliable? Do they expire? Do you have to declare them when you travel across borders? If you don't declare them, can the retail value of the pills get you arrested for smuggling a controlled substance? (e.g., mebendazole x 1000 pills might only have cost $200 but would retail for $20,000 in Canadian currency).

The simple solution is to get them at non-prescription costs from a reliable re-seller, remember never to travel with them and just get what you would basically need to MT for the most common parasites. This is presented in chart form below.

Antiparasitic Medications II: mg/pill and MT ranges				
	Medication	mg /pill	Pill # to MT for	Safe oral dose
1	Praziquantel	600 mg	33	11
2	Albendazole	200 mg	15	4
3	Mebendazole	100 mg	30	4
4	Ivermectin	12 mg	30	1
5	Metronidazole	200 mg	10	4

For simplicity, moving forward the medication names are abbreviated to praz, alb, meb, iver and metro. If we had 33 praz pills, 15 alb, 30 meb, 30 iver and 10 metro we could easily perform a broad range of basic MT for parasites against every organ location. For MT purposes, these pills don't expire.

Muscle Testing for Parasites

Once we understand which parasite species the medications are placeholders for, and have a Parasite MT Kit for practical use, the process is straightforward: we MT the medications against various weak organ indicator locations to find a correspondence. It usually makes sense to start with an area that is already symptomatic.

This is the same process as MT for a Rung 5B Therapy like a vitamin (Pt3-Ch3) but here we are MT antiparasitic medications.

The logic is as follows:

• If the MT is done accurately,
• If the medication is reliable,
• If we can agree that the medication is a placeholder for the parasite,
• Then:

Any indicator location that MT for any antiparasitic medication must contain whatever parasite the medication treats.

MT Protocol For Antiparasitic Medications

1. Start with a baseline.
2. Find a weak organ indicator.
3. Identify which antiparasitic medication cancels out the weak indicator.

A: If the medication fails to cancel out the weak indicator, there is no correspondence.
B: If the medication cancels out the weak indicator, there is a correspondence. The type of medication indicates the parasite species.

Phrased more practically, if your stomach is MT for whipworm medicine then you probably have whipworm in your stomach. If your lungs are MT for fluke medicine, chances are you have a lung fluke.

This level of simplicity helps us to understand and demystify 1A Parasites. Our cultural inheritance until now has led us to confuse, obscure and make impenetrable the language of medical conditions, partly by assigning disproportionate importance to the 6A Symptom and the 7A Name. We need to focus on and quantify the 1A Parasite.

When we have a simple means of finding a parasite, all that needs to happen to confirm that a treatment has been effective is to no longer find the organism 24 hours after the treatment.

Quantity Testing Antiparasitic Medications

When we use quantity testing with the pills from our Parasite MT Kit, we are able to quantify parasites in greater detail.

We find that meb 1 (1 x 100mg) may not MT against a location, but then meb 10 will. Or praz 15 might not, but praz 18 will. Remember that this is like adding weights onto a scale, we need to find the right number of pills before the medication will MT against the location.

There are different possible interpretations of these quantities. A unique quantity of pills (e.g., praz 11, meb 1) could represent:

1. A single organism.
2. A group of organisms

Certainly, multiple parasite samples that have passed out of the body will MT for a single quantity of pills.

The problem is that the body will frequently MT for doses in excess of the safe oral dose. In this sense we can use the doses to identify the parasite, but taking the pills is not always possible.

MT Protocol: Quantity Testing Medications

1. Start with a baseline.
2. Locate a weak indicator.
3. Identify which antiparasitic medication cancels out the weak indicator.
4. For more detail, try quantity testing the exact number of pills:

-Test with the whole bottle.
-When you have the right medication, test pill by pill until the MT is strongest.
-Take note of the exact number of pills.

Note: Annotate your findings using abbreviations and number codes: praz 11, meb 1, etc.

A medication may MT against different locations at the same dosage. Because of the process of blood circulation, it is difficult to be certain where the organism actually resides. It is common for the electromagnetic signature of an intestinal parasite to show up in the lungs (probably via its 2A Bad Bacteria), making accurate identification of the location of the organism quite difficult.

Either way, if some quantity of an antiparasitic medication is MT, a parasite from that species is definitely somewhere in the body.

Dosage Toxicity

Toxicity is the major limitation in antiparasitic pharmacology.

The maximum safe dose that these medications can be consumed at is praz 11 pills, alb 4, meb 4, iver 2 and metro 4. By contrast, the maximum quantity of pills that someone could MT for (i.e., thousands of pills) doesn't simply exceed the safe dose, it exceeds the imagination. We can see from the discrepancy between how many pills it is safe to take and how many pills someone will MT for that we can use the pills to find the parasite but not to treat it.

This is **The Dosage Toxicity Problem**. It may be that these astronomical dosages reflect some natural immunity that the parasite has built up while living in the host. There is some evidence to support that the dosage we MT for may increase over time.

The Parasite Problem

We can now revisit The Parasite Problem outlined above:

1. Which parasites do we have (and where in the body are they)?
Due to The Motel Room Concept and using a Parasite MT Kit, we host organisms from every species category. They are distributed throughout the body and often localized in symptomatic areas.

2. How do we know?
We can use antiparasitic medications as parasite placeholders and MT them against specific locations to draw conclusions about which species we host and make further distinctions using quantity testing.

3. How do we get rid of them?
At the lower doses we can take the medicines but at the higher doses above the safe limit (e.g., most doses), an electrical frequency is the only option. This will be explored in detail in the next chapter.

4. How do we know they're gone?
Simple logic: If the original location is no longer MT for the original antiparasitic medication at the original dosage (e.g., stomach no longer MT for praz 11) then we can infer that the treatment has worked and the organism is dead. Otherwise, we would still be finding it.

Conclusions

The general conclusion we can draw is that we can use antiparasitic medications to find parasites but not to treat them. This solves the problem of stool testing, bypasses the nervous system disconnect, confirms the predictions of The Health Ladder and to a large extent gets us out of the uncertainty of the desert of health.

Despite not being able to take most of the dosages of medications that we will MT for, it is still essential to understand what parasites we have. This information strengthens an awareness that every 6A Symptom is associated with some 1A Parasite.

By extension, knowing how to find parasites using this method gives us a means of confirming whether a treatment has worked (e.g., if we are treating praz 11, then praz 11 should no longer show up in a MT of the stomach after the treatment). This is how we know that herbal antiparasitic products, for example, are almost universally ineffective and why handheld parasite zappers and other antiparasitic frequency devices bought on the internet don't work.

In fact, MT the medications outlined above can act as the basis for a new science of MT for parasites. Science depends on data. Without this data we can see why the current science of parasites and antiparasitic pharmacology is still in its infancy.

The specific conclusion we can draw is that quantity testing makes us acutely aware of The Dosage Toxicity Problem. Because it is clear that medications can't work on most parasites due to toxicity, it is plain that it is time for a better alternative.

And now we can express this problem using a common language: How can we eliminate parasites that are identified in a MT at values of medications above the safe doses (e.g., anything above praz 11, alb 4, meb 4, iver 1, metro 4) that we know for certain are in the body?

This leads to a fundamental question that we will explore in detail in the next chapter: Is it possible to use an electrical frequency that mimics the action of antiparasitic medications to kill the parasites that medications cannot due to The Dosage Toxicity Problem?

Further Reading on Parasites

A detailed analysis of parasites is provided in The Complete Muscle Testing Series: *Book 5 Muscle Testing for Parasites*.

Part 1 covers parasite theory: what categories of organisms there are, how their life cycles vary and physical traits such as how they are adapted to live in different body regions and how their biochemistry interacts with ours, from infection to adaptation and feeding.

Part 2 outlines each of the antiparasitic medications from how they work to what dosages they can be MT at. Then, emphasis is placed on how we can use a logical analysis of this data to create a theoretical holographic parasite profile in the absence of formal visual evidence.

Part 3 is an encyclopedic list of all the main parasites that are a danger to humans. It can be read for entertainment or used as a reference.

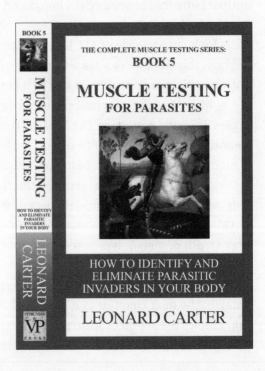

THE COMPLETE MUSCLE TESTING SERIES:
BOOK 5

MUSCLE TESTING
FOR PARASITES

HOW TO IDENTIFY AND
ELIMINATE PARASITIC
INVADERS IN YOUR BODY

LEONARD CARTER

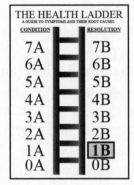

THE HEALTH LADDER
A GUIDE TO SYMPTOMS AND THEIR ROOT CAUSES

CONDITION	RESOLUTION
7A	7B
6A	6B
5A	5B
4A	4B
3A	3B
2A	2B
1A	**1B**
0A	0B

1B. FREQUENCY THERAPY

Eliminates all species of Parasites (1A) from all locations. Clean, quick, comprehensive and free of side effects, it is **the future of human healthcare.**

6

Muscle Testing
Healing Frequencies

A s we have explored, we can MT antiparasitic medications to confirm the presence of a parasite, but since most of the dosages we arrive at through quantity testing are too high (toxic) to be consumed, it is necessary to find an alternative to ingesting the pills. We will examine here whether a frequency can be used for this purpose.

This is thought of as a healing frequency, but to understand the variables, we need to define:

1. What a frequency is.
2. What constitutes healing.
3. Whether a frequency can replicate the action of an antiparasitic medication.
4. Whether it is possible to isolate that frequency in its root electrical form.

The first three points have simple answers, the fourth is a socially, politically and scientifically complex issue.

Frequencies

A frequency, measured in hertz, is the technical description for the number of times per second that something happens.

Once defined, the term can be applied to anything. A heart rate of 1 beat per second or 60 beats per minute would have a frequency (FQ) of 1 hertz (Hz). A heart rate of 72 bmp would have a FQ of 1.2 Hz.

FQs can be understood best if we divide them into 2 forms: audible and electrical. We will also examine chemical FQs.

Audible FQs are in the spectrum of sound, which spans from 20 Hz to 20,000 Hz. For example, low C on a piano vibrates at 32.7 Hz, middle C is 261.6 Hz and high C is 4186 Hz. For comparison, the range of human hearing covers the whole 20 to 20,000 Hz but adults tend to lose the high end of the range as their hearing deteriorates, and by age 60 can often only detect 10,000 Hz and below.

Electrical FQs are harder to conceptualize because we can't perceive most of them with our senses. An example is that the electric current in the wiring of a North American home cycles at 60 Hz (but at 120 volts, is lethal—voltage is its own variable). Even though 60 Hz falls within the spectrum of sound, it has not been translated into a sound wave so it is not an audible FQ. The entire spectrum of radiation can be thought of as electrical FQs, from audible sound to ultrasound, radio waves, microwaves, infrared, visible light, ultraviolet, X-rays and cosmic rays.

The best known example of a FQ destroying something is when an opera singer produces a pitch that shatters a wine glass. This is said to be the **resonant FQ** of the glass, the FQ at which a synchronization between the sound and the glass causes the glass to rupture.

Electrical FQs can also shatter something if the resonant FQ is reached.

It is understood that a FQ can shatter something but how can it heal?

Healing

Healing as a term is open to a wide range of subjective interpretations. To be able to scientifically evaluate a healing claim it is first necessary to clarify how healing is defined within the claim.

For example, the King's Chamber of the Great Pyramid in Egypt is asserted to resonate at 16 Hz, which is claimed to be a healing FQ. Or different sources will suggest 20 Hz or 460 Hz for the same room. The variance doesn't actually matter because these numbers are made up. A random FQ is proposed, the claim is tacked on that it is a healing FQ, and the reader is supposed to infer the rest. The more in need of healing they are, the more inferring they'll do. Sweeping statements like "healing is voltage" also prey upon a public that lacks a language of waveform physics and an understanding of how to define healing. This concern applies equally to all actual FQs, such as the Earth's Schumann resonance of 7.83 Hz, which is what it is, but cannot be demonstrated to be healing in any way.

Claims of this sort underscore the need for a clear definition of healing and a way to cross-reference it with a FQ.

In the context of The Health Ladder, healing is something that takes place at the 5A Location, but from this perspective we can see that a healthy state depends upon the absence of 3 underlying factors: the 4A Virus, the 2A Bad Bacteria and the 1A Parasite. Since the implication of The Health Ladder is that the 4A Virus and 2A Bad Bacteria are dependent upon 1A Parasites, we can safely define healing as: a state of wellness at 5A that is able to express itself when 1A Parasites are eliminated. **Healing is killing a parasite.**

When we revisit the claims about the King's Chamber in the Great Pyramid above, it is common sense that the room has no antiparasitic properties but if we wanted to take the claim seriously and evaluate it, we now have a means of doing so: do the proposed FQs of 16, 20 or 460 Hz MT against the same 5A Location that anti-parasitic medications (e.g., praz 11) MT against?

We are brought to the sudden awareness that we don't know anything about FQs or how to reproduce them to evaluate this idea.

How to Reproduce a Frequency

For an analysis of a FQ to be scientific we need to be able to accurately reproduce it. Here are some factors that need to be modified:

1. **FQ range** A tone generator phone APP ranges from 20 to 20,000 Hz but is not programmable in any useful way. Laboratory grade devices produce FQs into the microwave spectrum (300 GHz) but are restricted in who can buy them so that people don't microwave themselves.

A commercially available scientific function generator ranges from 0 Hz to 25 MHz. 2 MHz is at the high end of what is considered safe. Medical ultrasound by comparison ranges from 2.5 to 18 MHz.

2. **Decimal places** In technical scientific work, the more decimal places we can add, the more accurate the FQ is. A full six decimals are recommended (e.g., 0.123456). For this reason, an analog (non-digital) function generator is not suitable for work in FQs.

3. **Waveform** Sine, square, ramp and pulse waves all have different properties. Sine waves, for example, do not MT against any parasite indicator point at any FQ.

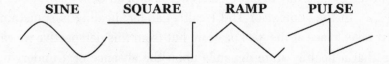

| SINE | SQUARE | RAMP | PULSE |

4. **Voltage balance** There is a positive and negative curve to every FQ wave. It can be +1v and -1V or some other combination (e.g., +2/-6v).

5. **Symmetry/Duty cycle** The percentage of the angle of the wave is programmable. This factor profoundly influences its behavior.

6. **Phase or Degree** The phases of a FQ, easiest to think of as the angle of rotation are measured in degrees from -180° to 0° to +180°.

If this sounds quite technical, it is. To be able to evaluate whether a FQ can match the claims made about it, we need to be able to reproduce its range, decimal places, waveform, voltage balance, symmetry and phase orientation using a scientific function generator.

There are further distinctions to be made in how that FQ, once generated, is conducted into the body. We will explore this below.

Delivering a Frequency to the Body

To MT a FQ we must be able to deliver it to the body in a form that can produce a measurable stimulus.

With an audible FQ, it might be simplest to run it through a speaker. The effect of a sound wave on the body can be MT.

However, the bulk of FQs are above the audible range, and must be MT in their root electrical form. This is the default output form of a function generator so nothing special needs to be done to the device, but to MT an electrical FQ, it will need to be wired up to the body.

At an amateur level this is often done by attaching the output wires to bits of copper pipe but this isn't recommended for scientific applications as many things can and do go wrong: there is extensive loss of signal (possibly full loss), the hands are not free for MT purposes and it isn't practical to hold copper pipes for more than a few minutes. What if the experiment requires a duration of hours?

The most scientific application is to adapt medical grade sticky electrode pads like the type used in TENS machines. Function generators have an output port that fits a type of wire called a BNC cable. To deliver the output FQ to the body, you will need a BNC to RCA adaptor and some electrode pads and wires, pictured below.

BNC to RCA   Electrode Wires   Electrode Pads

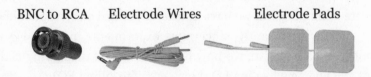

By connecting the electrode pads (via a wire) to the BNC/RCA adaptor there is no loss of signal. This keeps the hands free for MT and allows for extended FQ experimentation times. These items are not included with a function generator, which itself can cost between $500 and $5,000, but they can easily be ordered on the internet.

The typical electrode attachment points are the wrist and ankle. Note that voltage is a consideration. Any FQ above 10 volts will not only MT weak, it will shock or burn the skin and should be avoided.

Muscle Testing Frequencies

We can now apply a number of related principles to MT a FQ.

Once there is an understanding of how to:

1. MT an organ location

2. MT an antiparasitic medication against it (e.g., praz from a MT Kit)

3. Use quantity testing to isolate the specific dosage of medication (e.g., praz 11 MT against stomach)

And when we remember:

4. That healing is killing a parasite

5. The specifics of how to tune a FQ (waveform, symmetry, etc.)

6. How to set up a delivery system (cables, electrode placement)

7. How to MT a FQ against a location

Then finally:

8. We have a frame of reference by which to evaluate its effectiveness.

Once we can find a FQ that MT against a location, we don't have enough data to draw the major conclusion that we have found a parasite killing FQ, but we have at least identified a correspondence.

> **MT Protocol:**
> **How to MT a Frequency**
>
> 1. Start with a baseline.
> 2. Find a weak organ MT.
> 3. Identify the antiparasitic medication and dosage that cancels out the weak location (e.g., praz 11 cancels stomach).
> 4. Using that location, introduce a FQ using medical electrodes and a function generator.
>
> **A:** If the FQ cancels out the same location as the antiparasitic medication did, you have a correspondence.
>
> **B:** If it doesn't, you don't.
>
> Note: This doesn't guarantee it will kill the parasite, just that it looks like it will. Chances are, it won't.

More importantly, since most experiments in MT a FQ will demonstrate a negative, we now have a means of disproving claims about a FQ being a healing FQ (i.e., a parasite killing FQ).

This is because of the core **Principle of Negation**: while a FQ that MT positive may (but only may) kill the parasite, any FQ that fails to MT positive will definitely not kill the parasite. It is much easier to negate a FQ than it is to find one that works. But now at least we know what we didn't know before: how to identify a false claim.

Now that we have a definition of what does not work and a methodology to prove it, we can reexamine the King's Chamber.

Evaluating Frequencies

MT a FQ against a location provides the necessary data to evaluate claims made about the FQ and its healing (i.e., killing) properties.

Using the stomach and praz 11 as an example, we find that neither 16, 20 nor 460 Hz cancels out that reference point (or for that matter, any other point). There is no correspondence, so these are not healing FQs. We encounter the same failure with 7.83 Hz so there goes the Earth's Schumann resonance and your trip to Giza plateau.

We can now see why these are false claims: What dosage of antiparasitic medication are these FQ claimed to correspond with? None. What location? None. What are the decimal places? What is the waveform, the voltage, the symmetry, the phase? ...Crickets. Just a random number dangled in front of an audience desperate for the truth.

We finally have a shared frame of reference to evaluate the work of Royal Rife (1888-1971), an American researcher who invented a Beam Ray that he claimed could cure diseases and among other things, kill parasites. Whether his work has survived in its original form is unclear but as it stands now, his purported parasite killing FQs are typically presented in the following format:

Fluke: 6 Hz, 23, 133, 200, 475, 900, 1800
Roundworm: 5 Hz, 19, 125, 197, 475, 872, 2100

Well, we know what flukes are, that's what praz indicates and it would be rare for any person not to MT for praz 11. But can anyone find any MT correspondence between any of these fabled Rife FQ and their praz 11 indicator points? Of course not, and now we understand why: the numbers are in a form that is too simplistic.

A typical Rife manual will contain tens of thousands of FQ like those listed above, all supposedly tuned to specific microorganisms (e.g., fluke, roundworm, giardia, amoeba). One wonders if the poor guy was simply listing his failures as not a single FQ MT positive.

Unfortunately, Rife's work had a strong if corrupting influence on late 20th century alternative medicine and resulted in the widespread misconception that parasite zappers worked.

Evaluating Frequency Devices

When we combine a poorly understood topic like healing with a poorly understood field like waveform physics, a tragic hero like Rife and an industrious charlatan like Hulda Clark we find what we might expect: a thriving market of fraudulent devices called parasite zappers.

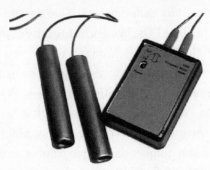

These are hand-held or desktop FQ generators sold on the pretext that they emit a FQ that can eliminate parasites. Often with confidence-inspiring names like the Spooky Plasma, the Spooky 2, the Miracle Rife, the Royal Rife Machine and the BCX Ultra Deluxe, these devices share a set of attributes in common: they all use the FQ delivery system of holding metal pipes that as we now understand isn't effective for a few reasons; they are all programmed with Rife numbers that we can use MT and the principle of negation to rule out as effective; and the usage instructions are based on Hulda Clark's inaccurate assertions that an effective treatment duration is 7 minutes, and that repeated treatments are needed to get the eggs, a rehashing of the misconception that parasites lay eggs in us that can hatch in us.

A feature of the more sophisticated devices is that they cycle between different FQs or run through a preset sequence. This means that even if they accidentally passed by an effective FQ, there wouldn't be enough duration of exposure to it to confer a therapeutic benefit.

Desperation. These devices cater to and fuel desperation. A simple MT of their output FQ rules them out as effective and this brings us to the core of the issue: the problem isn't that no device works, it is that we as a society don't have a simple frame of reference to use MT to evaluate whether any device works or not.

If we knew how to MT, we might encounter the startling fact that some FQs do test for a correspondence with a parasite indicator point.

The Nuclear Chemistry of Frequencies

We have now made enough distinctions to revisit the questions posed at the beginning of this chapter. It is now clear 1) What a FQ is and 2) What constitutes healing. We can finally examine 3) Whether a FQ can replicate the action of an antiparasitic medication.

It may surprise the reader to consider that antiparasitic medications are themselves positioned at Rung 1B on The Health Ladder: **Frequency Therapy**. This has to do with the principle from nuclear chemistry that at the atomic level, nothing touches anything else. Atoms don't touch other atoms. Instead, their electrons swirl around them and share electrostatic bonds with other electrons. In bonding together, electrons still don't touch each other. At the subatomic level they are nowhere near each other. Solidity is an illusion of the senses.

This means that an antiparasitic medication isn't touching you or your parasite, it is simply propagating temporary electrostatic bonds and delivering an electrical FQ based on a chemical form: a **chemical FQ**. When we take a medication we are consuming a chemical FQ. The question of whether a FQ can replicate a medication is redundant: the FQ is the medication. Medications are chemical FQs.

The practical question is 4) Whether it is possible to isolate that FQ in its root electrical form without depending upon pharmaceutical chemistry with its Dosage Toxicity Problem.

Within the parameters of physics, there is a way to replicate the electrical signal that underlies the action of an antiparasitic medication. A function generator can work for this purpose as long as the necessary FQ falls within the safe range (i.e., 0 to 2.3 MHz) and a MT can be used to confirm a correspondence.

This leads to 3 deceptively simple questions:
1. Does this FQ require any special math to mesh with the body?
2. Does this FQ require a special delivery system?
3. What is the FQ and what are the subordinate details?

Question 1 will be addressed in Pt3-Ch34: The New Science of MT. Question 2 is explored in Pt3-Ch7: MT Healing Compounds and question 3 is touched on in the remainder of this chapter.

Criteria of a Successful Frequency

For an electrical FQ to replace the action of a chemical FQ it must meet 2 criteria: 1) Correspondence and 2) Outcome.

A **correspondence** is what happens when a MT indicates a binary electromagnetic relationship between two factors. The recommended factors in this case are that an electrical FQ (factor 1) should turn a negative organ location (factor 2) back to a positive when a chemical FQ like praz 11 has also MT against that same location.

This doesn't confirm that the electrical FQ will work but it helps us to use the principle of negation, outlined above, to rule out when it definitely will not work. This saves some time. The term correspondence is used, instead of a more definitive term like causal relationship, as an admission that based on MT data alone, we can't yet be sure of explicit causality, only of an implicit relationship.

The desired **outcome** is that after introducing the FQ, an indicator location that formerly MT for a medication (e.g., praz 11) should now no longer MT for it. That would mean the FQ had worked.

No FQ could possibly be successful that didn't first demonstrate a correspondence, and no FQ (audible, electrical or chemical) could be said to have worked if it did not result in the outcome that the initial medication indicator was no longer apparent.

These are the two main criteria of a successful frequency.

The ultimate criterion of a successful FQ is not only that it demonstrates a correspondence and results in an outcome but also that it can be recognized as such. For this to be the case, there are a number of requirements of the person doing the recognizing:

Can they MT? Can they MT an organ location? Can they cross-reference this with antiparasitic medications? Can they quantify a dosage? Do they have a function generator? Do they have the right wires? Can they program the FQ, the decimals, the waveform, the voltage, symmetry and phase? Do they use the right programming? Are they familiar with the criteria of success: do they know how to identify a MT correspondence? Can they identify when the desired outcome has happened? Do they employ the FQ for the right duration?

Questions About Frequencies

If the ultimate answer to question 4) above is yes, this leads to a fifth question: What is the FQ? But is that the question we need an answer to?

What has been outlined so far is simple, or if not simple at least it is quantifiable using a MT. We can draw logical conclusions from these MT responses. They are starting points.

However, when we look for the correct FQ we find a nonlinear field, one that is filled with mathematics and within that space is the truth. But will anyone recognize it as such? In translating nonlinear mathematics back into linear language will we encounter more questions than answers?

What follows is a set of questions that do not have simple answers. It becomes apparent that for the truth to be articulated, the world needs to be at a conceptual, perhaps even a spiritual level where truth can be understood. Are we at that stage? Or are we as a society only ready for more questions? Here are some:

1. **Differentiation** How do we differentiate the desired outcome from mere MT correspondences when there are more correspondences than there are seconds in the history of the universe (i.e., more than 432 quadrillion)? Then, are there many correct FQ or only one?

2. **Identification** How is a successful FQ identified as such? Who understands the math (infinite nonlinear dynamics) needed to recognize what an effective FQ looks like? With no historical precedent, what is the basis for a mutually acceptable definition?

3. **Communication** How should a methodology that has not previously been perfected be introduced to the world? In a book? In an interview? A 2-page spread in a scientific journal? On the evening news? In a podcast? A social media post? Does it go viral? Does anyone believe it? Does anyone even get the memo?

4. **Side Effects** Is it safe? How do we find out? What are the long-term effects? How long should we take to evaluate this? Will we ever know if it's safe? What constitutes safe? What constitutes proof? Who does these experiments? Who believes them? Who decides?

5. **Accuracy** Who is in a technical position to be the arbiter of whether the proposed FQ is effective? Math professors? The institution? Health regulatory agencies? The old guard? The avant-garde? Energy healers? Eccentrics? Skeptics? The end-consumer?

6. **Admissibility** Since a FQ is an abstract mathematical construct, who is empirical proof assumed to be admissible to? Hospitals? Doctors? Clinics? Administrators of studies? Professors? Health ministers? Bureaucrats? Patients? Investors? The sick? The dying?

7. **Scientific** What constitutes an adequate scientific explanation? More studies? Decades of public digestion? A democratic vote? A totalitarian directive? A political endorsement? A documentary? A scientific award? A critical mass of exposure? A purchase by a major pharmaceutical corporation? A merger? An acquisition?

8. **Delivery Mechanism** How is the correct FQ to be delivered to the target location? Did you know that a FQ needed to be delivered to a target location? Did you know that wires and electrodes were too simple to work? That the voltage is too high and the amplitude is too low? That without a delivery system the FQ is useless? Who solves this problem? Is there a solution? Who can we ask?

9. **Intellectual Property** How is the IP to be handled? Is it patented by a developer only to be stolen around the world by governments that decide it is too important not to steal? Is it patented by an interest group and then buried in a basement for 20 years while they profit from a more lucrative alternative? Or besmirched with fake lawsuits so that no institution will touch it? Is it given away? To who? And what do they do with it when they get it?

10. **Regulatory Approval** How is approval granted? Years of paperwork? As a favor? A bribe? Part of an election platform? Country by country? Are the whole 20 years of patent protection wasted while governments sit in boardrooms debating in committees whether the public has a right to use the technology? Does it ever get approved? Can the economy handle the upheaval that the information represents? Will lobby groups approve or intervene? And then who implements it? Who regulates them?

11. **Public Reaction** How does the public respond to this information? With skepticism? Disbelief? Desperate attempts to contact the inventor, begging him to fly to their city and set up a FQ in their living rooms because a family member is dying and this is their last hope? Are there petitions? Protests? Riots? Does a stereotypical Edison torch a metaphorical Tesla's lab? Is it a favorite topic of conspiracy theorists? Is Monday's apothecary burned as Friday's witch? A target of the outrage mob? The victim of cancel culture? Is this the guy we love to hate or the hero we've all been waiting for?

12. **Economic Impact** How does the economy handle it? Will pension plan funds take a dive? Will insurance stocks soar? Will pharmaceutical valuations simmer while the analysts digest the information? Will hospital boards consider leasing the technology? Do venture capital firms try to swoop in and buy it up, ratchet up the price, get a good rate of return, post a great quarterly profit, line their pockets, pay their shareholders?

13. **Media Matters** How is it digested by the news media? Is it a partisan issue? A grass roots movement? Are hit pieces put out? Investigative journalism? Primetime showcases? Myth busters? Documentaries? Human interest pieces? A flurry of references by people in the know? A tour of the talk shows? Breakfast television? Those blessed 10 minutes of fame? The flavor of the week? Old news?

14. **Insurance** Who will insure such a technology? Against what? And what about the inevitable lawsuits? Can somebody get cancer from a frequency? Is it a lawsuit waiting to happen? Does someone else get lupus, shingles and myxomatosis simultaneously? Is that a class action suit? Do law firms advertise for participants on commercial breaks?

15. **Accessibility** What form will 1B Frequency Therapy eventually take? Where will you get it? What will it cost? Is it a 1-time thing? Are follow up treatments needed? Will it be affordable? Will there be a waiting list? Who goes first? How do the people that can't get an appointment react to the news? Who tells them?

These are not simple questions. The way out of the quandaries they represent is lovingness and ultimately that is a spiritual matter.

Further Reading on Frequencies

Further exploration of this subject is found in The Complete Muscle Testing Series: *Book 6 Muscle Testing Healing Frequencies*.

Part 1 is devoted to the physics of frequencies, from a detailed analysis of the electromagnetic spectrum to a new language of frequency involving numeric ranges, waveforms and other factors. This is a simple language but metaphorically speaking, like hieroglyphics, the pronunciation needs to be learned.

Part 2 explores the biology of resonant frequency with a structural analysis of how an electrical waveform can be terminal to a biological system. It follows this consideration process to the extent of what is possible using FQs alone, and then examines the intrinsic limitations of trying to use undeveloped electromagnetic waveforms in a treatment format.

This is a summary of the latest science of bioelectrodynamics.

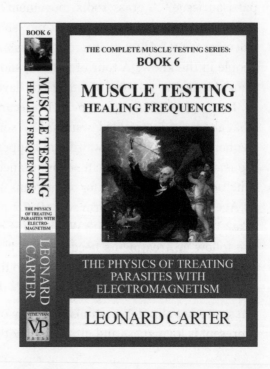

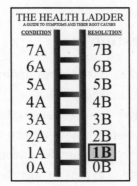

THE HEALTH LADDER
A GUIDE TO SYMPTOMS AND THEIR ROOT CAUSES

CONDITION		RESOLUTION
7A		7B
6A		6B
5A		5B
4A		4B
3A		3B
2A		2B
1A		**1B**
0A		0B

1B. FREQUENCY THERAPY

Eliminates all species of Parasites (1A) from all locations. Clean, quick, comprehensive and free of side effects, it is **the future of human healthcare.**

7

Muscle Testing
Healing Compounds

I t might be stated without exaggeration that the whole history of human health has been building up to the questions posed in this chapter.

We understand from The Health Ladder that 1A Parasites are the likely root cause of medical conditions and that 1B Frequency Therapy is the only way past The Dosage Toxicity Problem. However, it is apparent from MT the existing FQs in use that nobody has cracked the chaos code to identify a single, finite solution.

But what if somebody had? What if they had gone so far down this rabbit hole that they had emerged in some Wonderland where the answer to the infinitely dynamical FQ question was clear? They would encounter a problem that nobody has yet confronted: that even if we had the perfect FQ, it wouldn't work on its own.

The ultimate question is as simple as it is unprecedented: What factor is needed to facilitate the delivery of the FQ to the location?

Quantifying the Question

As outlined previously, a solution is defined as one that results in a particular outcome, not merely a MT correspondence.

Are we defining the outcome correctly? The original question was: How can we use a FQ to bring about a state where we can no longer find praz 11 in a location? If this were the ultimate outcome then we wouldn't have been brought to this stage in the consideration process, since that question has a simpler answer.

Instead, praz 11 is just the starting point. When we eliminate praz 11 (with a chemical FQ or an electrical FQ), a MT analysis indicates the presence of praz 18. When we eliminate praz 18 we find praz 33. How high does praz go? That's the first question. 44, 51, 70, 100, 350, 1000, 10,000, 20,000, 50,000, 100,000? It goes that high.

But we could only begin to isolate the higher praz values (44 to 100,000), presumed to represent distinct parasites, if we could conclusively eliminate praz 44, and 44 is already a near-lethal dose of praz. It also represents the finite limit of what an electrical FQ can achieve due to the body's own limitation in how much voltage it can handle.

At 10 volts an electrical FQ isn't strong enough to work and at 11 volts the body starts to get an electricity burn. The nerves aren't built to handle more than 10 volts. That is why even though the FQ in your home electrical wiring is safe at 60 Hz, it is lethal at 120 volts.

So now we have numerically quantified the question: How can we deliver an electrical FQ to the body to eliminate praz 44 (and all praz values above 44) when a chemical FQ is too high-dosage to work and an electrical FQ would need to be too high-voltage to work?

We can only arrive at a consideration process where we are clear that the final question depends upon eliminating praz 100,000 if we can get through all the praz values between 44 and 100,000.

To achieve this requires a shift in perspective from simply MT the presence of the parasite, and from simply finding the perfect FQ, to the rather challenging issue of how to facilitate the delivery of the perfect FQ to the location without using more voltage.

This is the question that has never been asked, or answered.

Muscle Testing Magnetism

In general, the health claims about magnets are based on a misconception. Magnets can and do support the human bioelectric field, this is why a muscle that tests weak will MT strong if a magnet is held near to it, a fact that has accomplished little more than contributing to the sale of magnetic bracelets at health trade shows.

The problem is that a magnetic field is universally supportive of all life, parasite and bacterial life included. The desired outcome might be that the magnet supports us but not the parasite. Magnetism doesn't work that way, it non-selectively supports all life. A rising tide lifts all boats, as the expression goes, and we're no closer to healing.

However, if we move on from the misconception that a magnet could have a healing (i.e., parasite killing) effect, we can ask a more specific, functional question about magnetism: can a **passive magnetic field** facilitate the delivery of a FQ to a location in the body?

The standard unit of magnetism is 1 Tesla (T) and that is also the average strength of a coin-sized N52 neodymium disc magnet. Could the act of holding a 1T magnet near the body during a FQ treatment enhance the delivery of the FQ?

This results in the familiar MT correspondence but not an outcome. Even 500 x 1T magnets all stacked together fail to produce an outcome.

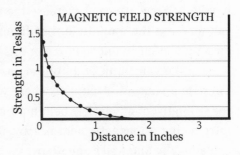

This is because the magnetic field exponentially decreases proportionate with the distance from its surface. At the surface it can be up to 1.4T but even 3 inches away it can be 0T.

Since our bodies are only about 12 inches thick, we might wonder whether an industrial strength natural magnet could provide the needed depth, but the risks aren't worth the reward: there is the real danger that the magnet could attract a metal object to itself, and if your body was in the way it would impale, crush or kill you.

Muscle Testing Electromagnetism

Could pulsed electromagnetism (PEMF) hold the answer? This would bypass the safety concerns and an **active magnetic field** can be much stronger and is much safer than a passive (natural) magnetic field.

In pulsed magnetic technology an electrical signal (the 60 Hz sine wave in a North American power grid) is pulsed through a copper coil. The number of pulses per second is the FQ it is pulsing at. Most of these devices are programmable by pulses per second and range from 1 to 60 Hz. By increasing the voltage or the number of coils (or both) we can increase the strength in T of the magnet.

The purpose of the pulsing is to dissipate heat. If it pulses too fast it is no longer a pulsed magnet, it becomes a continuous electromagnet and very quickly generates too much heat.

The strength of a pulsed magnet varies based on its size and cost. A home unit might produce 0.8T and cost $5,000 while an MRI, essentially a giant pulsed magnet, might be 3T to 9T and cost $2 million.

We understand now that we cannot facilitate the delivery of the FQ to the location using voltage because our nerves can't handle it. Since we can't increase the voltage of the FQ, perhaps we can increase the amplitude. But function generators don't have an amplitude adjustment so how can this be accomplished?

We can think of amplitude as the volume dial on a stereo. There is a concept in physics where we can increase the amplitude (or strength) of an electric field not by increasing the voltage but by introducing a magnetic field nearby. This is explained by Maxwell's equations.

James Clerk Maxwell (1831-1879) was a Scottish physicist who may have been smarter than Einstein. In a famous set of equations he demonstrated that we can increase an electric charge by introducing a magnetic field, or vice versa. In other words, magnetism is proportionate with electricity. This is the

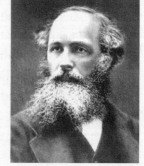

basis for what you will know of as an electromagnet.

Since we can't get the electric charge of a FQ stronger by increasing the voltage, is it possible to get it stronger by introducing a pulsed electromagnetic field? Yes.

Unlike a 1T natural magnet that exponentially diminishes in strength proportionate with the distance from it, a pulsed electromagnet can maintain its field strength for 10 feet or more.

We find that if we turn on a 0.8T pulse magnet nearby while a FQ is wired into a location we are able to eliminate praz 44 and 51. In theory this is significant but in practice the progress is too small to be substantial. We still have praz 70 and beyond. On the rationale that if some magnetism helps some, more might help more, we can try a stronger magnet. They are sold commercially as strong as 1.2T and cost between $7,500 and $20,000. Unfortunately, what we find is that the results are not significantly greater than the 0.8T model.

By this calculation we would need something above 5T to reach the higher praz values. The only pulsed electromagnet that produces this strength is an MRI. MRIs are not made for this purpose: they have the same safety concerns as high-tesla natural magnets and are not comfortable to lie in at the best of times, let alone for the years of 14-hour days needed to run antiparasitic FQ clinical trials.

An additional factor with a pulsed magnet concerns the pulse rate itself. This has to do with the problems of chaos and nonlinearity explored further in Pt3-Ch34. By pulsing at a linear rate, the magnet de-syncs in the same way a linear FQ does, and needs to be re-synced every 3-5 minutes for the duration of the treatment. This is not practical.

The end conclusion is that 1.2T pulse magnets can amplify the strength of an electrical FQ up to a point (praz 51), but that the level of magnetism needed to address higher praz dosages (up to 100,000) would probably exceed 5T and would require a product that is neither commercially available, practical, comfortable nor safe.

So, delivery is still an issue and now it is confirmed that natural magnets won't work as a carrier and pulse magnets aren't practical. If there is a solution to this issue, it is not to be found in magnetism.

Muscle Testing Light

We might consider whether a **carrier wave** in the spectrum of visible light can improve upon magnetism to conduct the 1B Frequency deeper into the body's bioelectric field. This can be explored with MT.

Light is part of the spectrum of radiation but visible light is only a small slice of that spectrum. Light is referred to as being a **wavelength**. The unit used to measure a wavelength is the nanometer (nm).

Some common examples of nm are blue light (450 nm), green light (520 nm) and red light (700 nm). When we reach 800 nm we pass into the infrared spectrum which isn't visible to the human eye.

WAVELENGTH in NM OF VISIBLE LIGHT

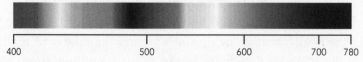

| 400 | 500 | 600 | 700 | 780 |

Visible light can be MT against organ locations. Specific wavelengths will MT positive or negative. The questions are then:
1. Will any specific wavelengths of light MT against an organ location with a known parasite?
2. Will introducing that wavelength in a FQ treatment result in a more effective outcome than the FQ alone?

We can quantify which nm wavelength MT the best against a target location with a variable digital wavelength generator.

We find that the optimal range is around 580 nm, which is quite close to the color of the sun. However, when we introduce this wavelength in an experimental clinical setting, it becomes clear that like magnetism, light isn't strong enough to be sufficiently effective.

MT Protocol For Light Against A Location

1. Start with a baseline.
2. MT the location, find the weak MT response.
3. Then introduce different wavelengths of light to see which nm value cancels out the weak location.

A: If the nm cancels out the weak MT, you have found a correspondence.
B: If it doesn't, you haven't.

Muscle Testing LEDs

The problem with using visible light therapeutically is that it exists on a **wavelength curvature**. When we see yellow light (580 nm), it appears yellow because there is more yellow in it than anything else but it also contains blue, green, orange, red and infrared. This **wavelength density** means that there is a lot of information, so to speak, in visible light. These extra wavelengths make it hot.

This is a problem because in a clinical setting where the goal is to use light as a carrier for a FQ, the heat of the light prevents us from making it bright enough for it to be strong enough to work.

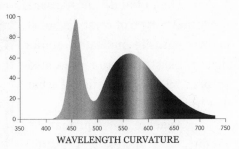

WAVELENGTH CURVATURE

If we switch gears from visible light to infrared, the wavelength density still makes it too hot only now we can't see it happening.

One thought process was to use custom-made LEDs in the near infrared spectrum that are tailored to produce a single **wavelength spike**. This was explored with a specialty company in Japan that manufactured custom LEDs in the 800 to 1650 nanometer range.

This theory seemed the most promising. The wavelength spike was narrow enough that there was no extraneous heat, but the problem now became a technological issue: any input intensity higher than 1 amp (A) burnt them out. Since the minimum power requirement for an LED above the 1000nm range to act as a carrier is between 5A and 10A, it wasn't technologically possible to run enough power through an 800+nm LED to translate into a clinical outcome.

So, it was lights out on that idea.

This is a reinforcement of the MT problem of correspondence. Correspondences are easy enough to find but it is important to remember that they identify a relationship only, not an outcome.

The objective, then, was to find a technology that could both handle the high amps and produce a tailored wavelength spike.

Muscle Testing Crystals

Crystals were the likeliest candidates to be structurally strong enough to overcome the intensity limitations of custom LEDs while still possessing unique wavelength spike properties.

This isn't a stretch of the imagination. There is a thriving industry of crystals in the world. They are used for many industrial purposes, so why not this?

The initial diagnostic screen involved MT sizable samples of every major type of crystal against known parasite indicator points that at this stage were represented by praz 70. Here is a list of what was tested:

Angelite, aquamarine, bornite, calcite, celestite, chrysoprase, danburite, diamond, emerald, iron ferrite, jade, jasper, jet, kunzite, kyanite, labradorite, lapis lazuli, lepidolite, petrified wood, quartz (clear, pink and brown), rhodonite, ruby, sapphire, septarian, seraphinite, serpentine, shattuckite, stromatolite, topaz, tourmaline and petrified wood.

> **MT Protocol For Crystals Against A Location**
>
> 1. Start with a baseline.
> 2. Find a location that MT weak.
> 3. Confirm a type and quantity of antiparasitic medication that cancels out the location.
> 4. Go back to step 2. Hold various crystal samples near your abdomen and see which ones cancel out the weak location.
>
> **A:** If the crystal cancels out the weak location, there is a correspondence.
> **B:** If it doesn't, there isn't.
> Note: Crystal size is a factor.

Of this whole group only the quartzes MT strong. This narrowed things down nicely because quartz is silicon dioxide (SiO_2) which gives us something to work with that has clear scientific implications.

After experimenting with quartzes and various forms of electric currents it became apparent that this had already been perfected in the industry of quartz infrared heaters.

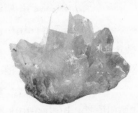

This leads us back to infrared wavelengths.

Muscle Testing Infrared Light Sources

Quartz infrared heaters produce an orangey-red glow that is in the visible spectrum, but the associated heat comes from the near and short wave infrared spectrums. This wavelength MT as a correspondence.

To our delight, we find that this wavelength is an effective enough delivery system to allow the FQ to eliminate praz 70 and praz 100 but to our disappointment, this is when it becomes apparent that praz 350 is in the background.

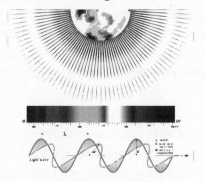

Trying to increase the wattage (W) doesn't work. A 1500W unit is not sufficient against praz 350 and produces so much heat it risks burning the skin. The problem with upgrading to a 4000W model is that the exact same limitation arises but from farther away.

The wavelength curvature analysis of a quartz IR heater looks so close to sunlight that it even makes sense to try using the sun as the heat generator. Perhaps the sun projecting off sand (a naturally occurring form of quartz) might be the solution and might explain why beaches are so therapeutic.

To explore this, I went somewhere that the sun was nice and hot (Goa, India) and lay out on the beach for a couple of hours at noon wired up with a function generator to see what would happen. It didn't work, but I got quite the sunburn, and also a reminder from my wife that when normal people go to Goa, they don't get sunburns because they wired themselves up with a function generator on a beach at noon to see if the wavelength produced by the sun would act as a carrier wave for a parasite killing FQ targeting praz 350. I didn't have any defense to this: it was true, I wasn't a normal person.

But the bigger problem was that running electricity through quartz to replicate a sun-like wavelength curvature as a carrier wave produced an intensity that was too hot for the skin to handle.

What the Solution is Not

Here is a summary of what the solution is not, and why:

Electricity The required voltage is too high for the body to handle.

Natural Magnetism Tapers down to 0T, stronger is too dangerous.

Electromagnetism Too large, expensive, uncomfortable, impractical.

Light Not strong enough or too hot for the skin.

Custom Infrared LEDs Can't handle the necessary amps.

Crystals Only quartz MT, not workable in naturally occurring form.

Quartz Infrared Burns the skin before it gets in deep enough to work.

This rules out every so-called healing device on the market today. These devices were doomed from the outset since they are all based on the misconception that healing is even possible at the level of the carrier wave alone. Electricity, magnetism, lights, infrared, even radio waves are only carriers. They need to be carrying something. We don't sit back and listen to radio waves, we listen to sound waves that are embedded in the radio. The sound wave is the FQ.

How can a carrier heal unless it has a parasite killing FQ to carry? How can it work unless it delivers the FQ to the right location? It can't. Then, when we consider that none of these technologies is able to bridge the voltage and temperature limitations of the human body it is clear why they are ineffective even as carriers.

We have to understand that parasites have evolved (or were created, if you prefer) to be in us. There is perfect biological compatibility. As far as parasites are concerned, if we don't like it, that's our problem. The existence of parasites throughout time has been predicated on the assumption that anything that is strong enough to kill them would have to kill us too, so they are safe.

What we want to do from a healing standpoint has never been possible: kill the worst parasites the body hosts. And we can now see that this is defined as the outcome of eliminating parasites we can't even find by using a carrier wave that doesn't exist to deliver a FQ nobody has discovered into a location nobody is MT at a dosage of medication nobody understands they should be looking for.

And we wonder why we're lost in a desert.

Further Reading on Healing Compounds

The Complete Muscle Testing Series: *Book 7 Muscle Testing Healing Compounds* contains an expanded presentation of this material. It also includes an outline of the methodology needed to quantify solutions to the problems posed in this chapter.

Part 1 surveys the physics of the electromagnetic spectrum but from the perspective of wavelength, not of frequencies. These are two sides of the same coin but different sides with different interpretations.

Part 2 analyzes the biology of wavelengths with a focus on how various electromagnetic emanations are able to penetrate human tissue and more important, parasite tissue. The core of this science is unexplored, so the bulk of this information is new and unprecedented.

This is a summary of the latest science of bioelectrochemical engineering, without which no solution to treating parasites with frequencies will be possible.

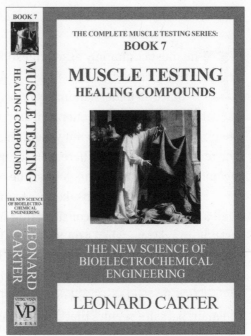

0A. THE VECTOR

All animals in nature are the primary or intermediate hosts to various species of Parasites (1A), many of which can infect humans.

0B. AWARENESS

Educate yourself. Start by reading *Experiments in Muscle Testing* by Leonard Carter. Then, apply what you learn.

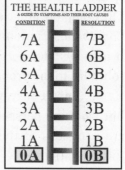

THE HEALTH LADDER
A GUIDE TO SYMPTOMS AND THEIR ROOT CAUSES

CONDITION		RESOLUTION
7A		7B
6A		6B
5A		5B
4A		4B
3A		3B
2A		2B
1A		1B
0A		0B

8

Muscle Testing
Parasite Vectors

The most commonly asked question about parasites is: Where do they come from?

Since an understanding of parasites is intrinsic to The Health Ladder and to health in general, it is vital to explore where we get them from. Otherwise, even if we eliminate them we'll pick up more. The term that describes where we acquire a parasite from is **vector**, meaning the direction or angle that the organism attacks us from.

It is common to mistakenly assume that we have no parasites at all and only to begin to consider that we may have picked up one—just one, mind you—when a 6A Symptom becomes chronic or invasive. Once we reach this awareness, it is natural to assume that we could only have picked it up on a trip to somewhere tropical, never at home.

In this chapter we will examine why this is a myth and explore the main parasite vectors that affect human populations.

Parasite Life Cycles

The central principle to understanding parasites is the life cycle.

Each species of parasite has its own **life cycle**, which is a set of stages that it goes through from egg to maturity. Parasite life cycle charts are readily available on the internet though not always accurate. Exposure to the vector is often deemphasized or placed in a limited geographical context.

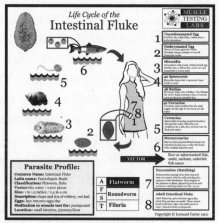

At Muscle Testing Labs, we have developed our own life cycle charts that set the record straight on a number of points.

Examining such charts is revealing. They tell a story that is happening all around us—and inside us—in the microcosmos.

The life cycle chart seen here is of the fish intestinal fluke.

Flukes can lay up to 100,000 eggs at once but none of them hatches in us because 100,000 flukes hatching at once would overwhelm our immune systems, killing us and the parasite. To prevent this from happening, the eggs can only hatch in—of all things—a snail. Once inside the snail they go through three distinct growth stages before they are ready to move on. They emerge as free-swimming cercariae whose job is to find a fish. The cercaria swims into the fish as it filters water through its gills. Once in the fish, it changes into a metacercaria (*meta* means changed) which is an encysted stage, a sort of parasite hibernation that can last for years. It is waiting for the fish to be eaten.

When we eat sushi, the metacercarial cyst, thought of by us as a parasite egg, hatches on contact with stomach acid and migrates to the small intestine. When it can finally lay its first batch of 100,000 eggs, it has completed its life cycle. All parasites must complete their life cycle to survive. This is what we might be finding when we MT for praz 33, whereas the bovine intestinal fluke tends to MT for praz 11.

The Language of Parasites

There is a funny way of naming flukes and roundworms. Flukes (identified by MT a location for praz) are named after the organ we find them in, while roundworms (MT for meb) are named after the animal we think we got them from.

So, there are lung flukes, intestinal flukes and liver flukes, and then pork roundworms, fish roundworms and cow roundworms.

This overlooks the fact that there is almost unlimited parasite variation. Every single mammal species hosts both flukes and roundworms. The Jersey cow intestinal fluke could be different from the Holstein cow intestinal fluke. One Holstein cow intestinal fluke could cause celiac, another could cause fibromyalgia. There is simply no biomedical language to summarize this with because it would require information we don't have: the subspecies (or serotype) of the organism, which bacteria it excretes into us, how those bacteria interact with our other parasites and how they interact with our own bacteria, our own immune system and our own genetics.

There simply isn't a **language of parasites**, and while hiding this by referring to them in Latin might sound impressive (e.g., one lung fluke is *paragonimus westermani*, another is *paragonimus kellicotti*), there is no way of understanding which medical conditions they may or may not give rise to, which is the only thing a non-biologist cares about.

More often than not, your doctor will simply tell you that your stool test (that screened for bacteria only) found no parasites and that therefore, you don't have any; that absence of proof is proof of absence.

In the 22nd century, 3D microwave computer imaging diagnostics might make it possible to see the parasite in the human body on some *Star Trek* type video screen.

The only 21st century solution is to quantify parasites by the various doses of medication that they MT for. If you are MT for praz 11, you must have some kind of fluke. If praz 50,000, you've found some other fluke. At least this gives us a numeric frame of reference: a common language of parasites to move forward with.

The Vector Blind Spot

The problem with vector analysis has to do with a **vector blind spot**. Upon examination it becomes clear that we are living according to a particular interpretation of vectors that is contradictory.

The official story of parasites is that they are only acquired by accident, from eating unwashed food or if someone somewhere didn't wash their hands. From insects, certainly, but only certain insects. We don't get them from our mothers, from crop oils or syrups, sushi, deli meats, spices or milk products. These things are certified safe. It's okay to eat raw fish, rare beef and pasteurization doesn't need to reach the boiling point because milk doesn't have parasite eggs.

This set of misconceptions is too comprehensive to be anything but one of the biggest and oldest blind spots in the human psyche, one that stretches all the way back to a time when we didn't know parasites existed. According to this blind spot, they still don't.

Quite another interpretation arises when we perform a MT analysis of milk, sushi, vegetable oils, corn syrup, raw fish, deli meats, spices, insects and, for that matter, breast milk. Here, we find what, to a biologist at least, should make a lot more sense: that there are parasite eggs in absolutely everything.

We find standard values of praz 1-33, meb 1-30, alb 1-10, iver 1-10 and metro 1-4 in every food source listed above. Some foods appear to have been brought to a safe temperature by cooking but in cases where it hasn't, the parasite egg is apparent with a simple MT.

If they're all so safe, why do they MT for antiparasitic medications?

We see here with vector analysis the same sort of clash of world views that arises in other areas when we compare the process of orbiting the data around our opinions (the confirmation bias) to the process of orbiting our opinions around the data we find in a MT.

What follows is a vector analysis based not on historical precedent, opinion or studies, but on MT. Something is understood to be a vector when it produces a weak MT response that is cancelled out by a dose of antiparasitic medication, indicating the presence of a biologically viable parasite egg that is capable of hatching in us.

Parasite Vectors

We can divide human parasite vectors into 6 main categories: 1) Our mother's milk 2) Cow's (and other) milk 3) Manure based dietary sources 4) Raw meat 5) Insect bites 6) Natural exposure.

1. Our Mother's Milk The first species of parasites we acquire are filaria, which are picked up in utero. This can be confirmed by MT newborn infants at various indicator points along the spine for ivermectin. If they don't have filaria, why do they MT for ivermectin mere days after birth?

Male semen also MT for ivermectin so we can infer that there is a component of transmission from the father at conception. It may be of interest to know that this factor explains why some women are allergic to some semen. They are reacting to the microfilaria in it.

An analysis of breast milk samples from different mothers has indicated the presence of flatworm (MT for praz) and roundworm (MT for meb) eggs but not filaria (MT for iver). Presumably then, these larger organisms (e.g., flatworm and roundworm) are acquired from our mothers' milk while filaria are acquired in utero.

The implications of this data are clear. In the womb we pick up filaria. Upon emerging and taking our first drink of milk we pick up various species of flatworm and roundworm. The acquisition of these organisms gives us some immunity to our environment which is also saturated by parasite eggs. Acting as placeholders (via The Motel Room Concept) they appear to play a role in preventing us from getting certain post-natal parasites when we are at an age where we might not have the immunity to handle them.

2. Cow's (and other) milk It is an interesting fact that raw milk is agreed to contain almost every bacterial species from here to Mars, but isn't thought to have a single parasite egg, or if a parasite is found, it is only single-celled like an amoeba, never the multi-celled organisms like roundworm, fluke or tapeworm.

The contradictory fact is that all unboiled milk MT for various doses of antiparasitic medicines (at least praz 11, meb 8 and alb 2).

The principle that this seeming contradiction rests on is the idea that parasite eggs can only come to maturity when they pass through multiple **intermediate hosts**, such as those outlined in the parasite life cycle above (e.g., a snail and fish). This is certainly the case in most instances, but if it is exclusively the case then the parasite eggs in milk that MT for praz 11 cannot hatch in us even though they are in the milk. But then why do they MT for praz 11?

There are a few possibilities. The MT may only be finding some electromagnetic echo of the parasite eggs, they may not be there. But then why does the milk no longer MT for praz 11 when it is brought to a boil? Alternatively, they may be there but not be biologically viable. But then why does someone who is praz 11 free (e.g., someone who has been treated for praz 11) exhibit symptoms and MT evidence of praz 11 shortly after they consume this milk?

You may well ask why everyone doesn't get sick when they consume dairy. This question has the easiest answer: The Motel Room Concept. Once everyone has praz 11 already, they are immune to praz 11 and can live under the illusion that there are no parasite eggs in their milk.

This is problematic because the dairy pasteurization process used around the world fails to bring dairy to a boil. If the historical precedent is valid, we don't need to boil dairy. If the MT of praz 11 is valid, we do. This is a simple matter for some biologist to confirm: Can they find biologically viable fluke eggs in a milk sample using a microscope? I hope I am not the only one who has done this test.

The microbiological question is that of whether there is some unknown or poorly understood stage in the life cycle of some flukes and roundworms where they can propagate directly through milk during lactation, and at that time can bypass the intermediate hosts.

The evidence that various doses of antiparasitic medication MT against unboiled milk samples seems to confirm that this is the case, but the reader should understand that this needs to be, can be, and should be confirmed in a laboratory setting.

Since there is enough empirical evidence to support the idea we will proceed on the assumption that it is the case.

3. Manure based dietary sources It is an accepted fact in biology that once some parasite eggs wash out into nature through urine or feces, they are able to mature into an infective form.

This happens by exposure to soil minerals or sunlight in the case of whipworm, hookworm and ascaris (i.e., soil-transmitted helminths) or by moving through an intermediate host like a garden snail. In either case, soil is a major vector for parasite eggs.

Because we have a manure based agricultural system, these infectious eggs are transported directly to primary food sources: oil crops, syrup crops, spices and grains. Vegetables are the least of the problem because they at least can be washed. Can you wash your flour? The argument might be made that we bake flour, and we do. But do we bake vegetable oil or corn syrup? Do we bake black pepper before sprinkling it on our food? Pepper is often dried on soil.

A close look at the agricultural process reveals that everybody thinks it's somebody's job, anybody could do it but nobody does.

Crop oils and syrups are subject to the same misconception as dairy pasteurization: that they can be rendered safe at temperatures below the boiling point. This simply doesn't line up with the basics of parasite biology. Unboiled oils and syrups represent an unbroken chain from the cow's feces to the field (as manure) to the crop to the harvest to the refining process to the food production plant to the grocery store to your table. Some parasite eggs are alive, well and biologically viable (infectious) by the time they arrive.

This is confirmed in a MT analysis of various syrups, oils, spices and condiments. The vector in this case is the manure and our lack of understanding of how to safely handle manure is a blind spot.

4. Raw meat It would be unusual not to have been taught as a child never to eat raw pork but somehow deli meats have slipped under the radar as have rare beef and sushi.

These MT for various doses of antiparasitic medications and it goes without saying that we are finding biologically viable eggs because muscle tissue is the final stage of most parasite eggs before reinfection. Deli meats, raw beef and raw fish are all vectors.

5. Insect bites All insects MT for ivermectin and therefore host a particular type of parasite called filaria. This applies literally to all insects but in the case of non-biting creatures like moths and butterflies, we wouldn't need to know this because they don't bite us.

With biting insects, the parasite is transmitted during their bite, whether from venom in the case of bees, wasps, hornets, ants, scorpions and spiders or in the anesthetic fluid we are injected with when being feasted on by a tick, mosquito, sandfly, flea, bed bug or kissing bug. In addition to insects, the venom from snakes, jelly fish and probably Komodo dragons infects us with filaria.

Filaria are among the most vicious and serious parasites we can get. Of all the parasite species in the biosphere these are the only ones that can (and often do) autopopulate inside of us, meaning if we pick up a subspecies of them from an insect (or other) bite, they can multiply over time, causing progressively worse symptoms.

In addition to the problems they create on their own, many subspecies of filaria host their own single-celled parasites and bacteria that can cause other pathologies. For the filaria that live in a tick, we have Lyme disease. For those in the flea, bubonic plague. For the sandfly, leishmaniasis. For the kissing bug, chagas. For the tsetse fly, trypanosoma (sleeping sickness). For the mosquito, malaria and separately, elephantiasis.

The missing root cause of many of these well-known conditions and the protozoans that we know produce the symptoms is the filarial parasite that hosts and poops out the protozoan.

The only reason we don't develop some major pathology every time we are bitten by an insect is that we already have our own species of filaria that we picked up from our parents, or from the mosquitoes in our childhood towns. These act as placeholders via The Motel Room Concept, protecting us to a certain extent from getting a full-blown medical condition on a random Tuesday from some innocuous insect bite.

All insect bites and all types of venom are parasite vectors and some of these can have more serious consequences than others.

6. Natural exposure By the time we have picked up parasites from all the vectors listed above there isn't generally space, microbiologically speaking, in our internal ecosystems to get parasites from accidental exposure.

It can happen. Some forms of tapeworm can be inhaled from the dust made by mouse feces, so if you're an exterminator or doing repair work in walls, attics, basements or barns it's probably a good idea to wear a mask.

Exposure to the feces of deer, wild pig and raccoon in a child's sandbox can present challenges for infants, particularly when they have a tendency to put their hands in their mouths.

Household pets can be a source of parasites, though less frequently than suspected. Puppies can spread a type of roundworm in their saliva and we can get toxoplasmosis from a cat's litter box.

There is always that once in a lifetime exposure to some unusual species that causes a clear symptom of a parasite, and we know when this has happened. More often than not it is while on vacation, precisely because other parts of the world contain parasites that we have no prior exposure to and therefore no protection from. There is always a motel room open for a guest we've never seen before.

At such a time it is important not to misinterpret what we have picked up as a 2A Bad Bacteria alone, such as salmonella, E.coli or listeria. It is wise to remember that all 2A Bad Bacteria come from a 1A Parasite in the same way that when you have found mouse feces in your basement, somewhere there must be a mouse as well.

Summary Vectors are impossible to avoid and most species of parasites are already in us. The size of the blind spot created by the parasite Motel Room Concept should not be underestimated. The challenge in coming to an understanding of this information lies in overcoming the psychological barrier of not having any reason to believe the data until a medical condition has developed, and then getting so caught up in the 7A Name of the 6A Symptom that there isn't time or mental clarity to look for a more proactive solution.

Muscle Testing Parasite Vectors

To a biologist or amateur scientist, this is a fascinating field. All that's needed is a Parasite MT Kit. Any sample from any vector can be MT. Food forms are easy enough to acquire and analyze. In the case of an insect, it can be MT alive or dead.

All vectors will MT weak. The diagnostic process involves identifying which antiparasitic medication cancels out the weak response to the vector. In this way we can logically infer which species of parasite the sample is a vector of (e.g., praz=fluke).

Quantifying parasites in their vectors using pharmacology is relevant for the purpose of generalization. For example, all insects MT for ivermectin, and since ivermectin treats filaria we can infer that all insects host a filarial parasite.

> **MT Protocol For Finding A Parasite In A Vector**
>
> 1. Start with a baseline.
> 2. MT the vector, it should MT weak. If it doesn't, try again.
> 3. MT one of the antiparasitic medications against the weak response to the vector.
>
> **A:** If weak test plus medication still tests weak, no correlation.
> **B:** If weak test plus medication now tests strong, you can infer the vector hosts whatever parasite that medication treats.

The complexity arises when it becomes apparent that every sample will MT for the same few doses of antiparasitic medications. Here pharmacology has its limits. A mosquito carrying a harmless strain of microfilaria will MT for ivermectin 12mg x 6 pills. Then another mosquito carrying a deadly strain of filaria that excretes dengue fever into us will also MT for ivermectin 12mg x 6 pills.

Clearly then, multiple species of parasites are blanketed by the same numbers of pills. This means that we can use the pills to confirm the presence of the parasite, but not to quantify other factors such as how harmful the organism would be should we be infected by it.

If you've been bitten, this technique can be quite useful to analyze what species of parasite your vector has given you. The dosage of medication can be used against the bite for diagnostic purposes and can also act as a feedback loop to see if the treatment has worked.

Further Reading on Parasite Vectors

An expanded form of this chapter, The Complete Muscle Testing Series: *Book 8 Muscle Testing Parasite Vectors* provides an analysis of vectors that combines accepted biology with MT evidence that hasn't previously been available.

The information is presented in a format that is accessible to biologists and researchers as well as amateurs.

Part 1 covers a years-long pet project of extrapolating the paleobiology of parasite evolution from the available evidence in the fossil record to determine which parasites really came first.

Part 2 analyzes the parasites passed on at birth in much greater detail as well as the bacterial process by which they confer immunity.

Part 3 explores some well-known and lesser-known modes of transmission from our food chain with an emphasis on the parasite egg and how it survives the manufacturing process.

Part 4 follows in the great tradition of the 18th century amateur biologists. I have spent some time traveling around the world analyzing filarial species in insect populations. I present my findings in detail.

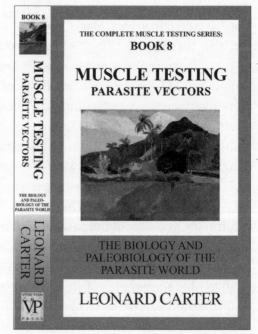

Part 5 assesses the vector of human contact in greater detail, allowing for an analysis of fertility issues and sexually transmitted diseases with implications in virology.

Part 6 is an encyclopedic list of the Muscle Testing Labs parasite vector charts.

4A. FUNGUS / VIRUS

Fungus: your best friend, helps you break down Bad Bacteria (2A).

Virus: your worst enemy, thrives in an environment of Metal Toxicity (3A).

2A. BAD BACTERIA

At some stage all Bad Bacteria (2A) come from a Parasite (1A). Once excreted into your body they circulate everywhere, causing inflammation and tissue damage.

THE HEALTH LADDER	
A GUIDE TO SYMPTOMS AND THEIR ROOT CAUSES	
CONDITION	RESOLUTION
7A	7B
6A	6B
5A	5B
4A	4B
3A	3B
2A	2B
1A	1B
0A	0B

9

Muscle Testing

Bacteria, Fungi and Viruses

The challenge in MT for bacteria, fungi and viruses is that, like a dog chasing his tail, we might actually find one, think we've found the root problem and bite down on it.

Every educated adult knows what bacteria are but few can explain the chemical difference between good and bad bacteria and even fewer understand that 2A Bad Bacteria originate almost exclusively from the feces of a 1A Parasite already living in the body.

Likewise with fungi, everyone knows the term fungus but few if any understand the beneficial role that fungi play in helping us break down 3A Metal Toxicities and 2A Bad Bacteria.

Viruses present their own unique challenges and as we saw in the 2020 lockdowns, the main ones lie in not knowing whether we have picked one up or what it will do to us if we get it.

In the chapter below we will explore these questions.

Understanding Bacteria

The best way to understand bacteria is to take everything you think you know about them and assume that it's only half the story.

The other half is explained by the fact that all Bad Bacteria found in humans comes from a parasite at some stage. This concept is summarized as: **Bad Bacteria comes from a parasite.**

We have inherited the idea from the 18th to 20th centuries that certain bacteria are out there and they're bad for us—that the bacteria themselves are the problem. This is a definite upgrade from the 17th century when the human race didn't yet understand that bacteria or the microscopic world existed. Now, we do.

The dreaded bubonic plague is caused by the bacterium *Yersinia pestis*, cholera by the bacterium *Vibrio cholerae*, leprosy by *Mycobacterium leprae*. The list goes on and includes more common 2A Bad Bacteria like H.pylori, E.coli, C.difficile, Salmonella and Listeria.

They are what they are, but they don't cause themselves. Once afloat in our systems, they are engulfed by our white blood cells and evacuated. To persist in our bodies then, something needs to regenerate their numbers. That's where the 1A Parasite comes in.

2A Bad Bacteria live inside a parasite. They're probably good for it in the same way our naturally occurring acidophilus bacteria are good for us. But when the parasite excretes bacteria in its waste, its good bacteria becomes our 2A Bad Bacteria.

The more common 2A Bad Bacteria like H.pylori, E.coli, C.difficile, Salmonella and Listeria come from the more common parasites: tapeworm, roundworm, fluke and whipworm. The less common bacteria like Yersinia (the plague) and M.leprae (leprosy) come from the filarial family. Interestingly enough this makes sense. The known 0A Vector for the plague is a flea bite. A flea is an insect, all insects are vectors for filaria, some filaria carry Yersinia.

It appears that biologists have been finding bacteria because they could, and missing the parasite host because they weren't looking for it. This is why focus needs to shift from finding the 2A Bad Bacteria to treating the 1A Parasite that is propagating it.

Q: Don't you get bacteria from not washing your hands?

A: Not the ones we're talking about. With your clean, washed hands you take some milk or a piece of cheese out of the fridge and drink or eat it. There are thousands of parasite eggs suspended in milk products because dairies around the world don't understand the need to boil milk above 100°C/212°F. Bad bacteria leaches out of the parasite egg, souring the milk. That's why it needs to be refrigerated and has an expiry date. When we drink the milk, the eggs hatch on contact with our stomach acids, the parasite larva emerges, begins to feed and excretes more bacteria. If several thousand larvae do this at once the bacterial surge is overwhelming and we call it food poisoning (as if this were still Renaissance Italy and people poisoned food). In cases where it is identified that there is a 2A Bad Bacteria involved in this process (E.coli, Salmonella, C.difficile) we assume that someone, somewhere has not washed their hands.

This principle equally applies to any crop (condiment, oil, syrup, grain, bean) grown in manure. Where milk is one 0A Vector, manure is another and of course all insect bites are a third.

Q: But I got a bacterium from drinking water so I know it's bacterial.

A: It's not a case of either/or, bacteria or parasite, it is always a case of both. It's difficult to keep water away from feces. We have runoff from farmers' fields, municipal sewage seepage, animal feces washing into water sources upstream, bird and fish poop collecting in reservoirs. Every single ounce of feces in the world contains multiple species of parasite eggs. Some countries add chlorine to their water which helps, but it's not a perfect system and developing countries barely do that much. When you have picked up a 2A Bad Bacteria from drinking water you have also acquired a 1A Parasite egg.

Q: Can I only have a bacterium and not the parasite it came from?

A: There are rare occasions where this is possible but that probably wouldn't cause enough of a symptom to get your attention. If your white blood cells have not cleared the bacterial infection in a day or two, there is most likely a parasite generating more 2A Bad Bacteria.

Q: So why do people feel better after taking antibiotics?

A: Sometimes wiping out enough of the bacteria enables your immune system to find a better balance with what's left. Other times, as you probably know, antibiotics don't help at all. The fact is that 2B Antibiotics kill some 2A Bad Bacteria but never the 1A Parasite.

Q: My doctor told me I have a chronic stomach bacterial problem (H.pylori), so how can that be a parasite?

A: How can there not be a parasite? If it were a self-contained colony of H.pylori, your white blood cells or vitamin D stores would have eliminated it long ago. This elimination process is continuous and effective. A bacterial colony can only survive if it is being replenished by a parasite living in you. A continuous H.pylori infection indicates continuous parasite defecation.

Q: I was told I had a bacterial infection in my lungs, how could that be a parasite?

A: Some parasites live in the lung tissue, others pass through the lungs on their way somewhere else and still others live elsewhere but their bacteria washes into the lungs where the body tries to evacuate it. If you have a bacterial lung infection, you have a parasite somewhere.

2A Bad Bacteria are alive for a while once they are excreted into us. To stay alive as long as possible they will uptake metals they are specifically adapted to as a cofactor in their energy metabolism. In the same way that humans use phosphorus (P#15) to metabolize energy in our ATP cycle, bacteria will uptake elements like arsenic (As#33), lead (Pb#82) and mercury (Hg#80). These metals make some bacteria highly toxic for us. The more preexisting 3A Metal Toxicity we have in our systems from environmental sources, smoking, pollution, etc., the more and the longer these bacteria will thrive.

Their waste has a suppressing effect on our natural (good) bacteria and is highly inflammatory. As they and their waste move throughout our circulatory and lymphatic systems, cerebrospinal fluid and bone marrow, we can experience swelling, burning, pain, tissue damage, ulceration, localized nutrient deficiencies and many other 6A Symptoms. Modern medicine really is correct that 2A Bad Bacteria are found at the root of all medical conditions, but we can see from The Health Ladder that there is a deeper root cause as well.

A useful medical application for doctors and surgeons is to tailor a 2B Antibiotic to a 5A Location using MT. Symptomatic locations (lungs, stomach, intestines, etc.) will MT for specific antibiotics. In time-sensitive cases like a surgery, this is better than a guess and can save a life.

Understanding Fungi

The best way to understand fungi is to take most of what you think you know about them and assume that the exact opposite is true.

The role of a 4A Fungus is to help us break down the waste material from 2A Bad Bacteria. But isn't that the job of our white blood cells? It is, so the first question we should be asking is that of why our white blood cells aren't doing their jobs.

When we have ruled out low white blood cell count or blood disorders as obvious suspects, we can think through the remaining possibilities logically: white blood cells should be clearing out the waste material from 2A Bad Bacteria but they're not. Why not? The most likely scenario is that they are doing their jobs but are overwhelmed.

Think about a forest. Every day millions of leaves fall, and let's imagine that there are 10 leaf rakers whose job it is to rake up the leaves. The forest floor stays clean. But what happens in the autumn? Now tens of millions of leaves fall, hundreds of millions. And let's imagine there are still only 10 leaf rakers. They can only rake so much each day, so what happens to all the extra leaves? They pile up, and the ones on the bottom get damp and start to rot. The agent that causes a leaf to rot is a fungus. It assists the leaf rakers.

Fungi exist throughout nature and in every case their role is to rot dead material. If this didn't happen in a forest, the leaves would soon pile up in a soggy mess, the trees would get buried and the forest would die. If this didn't happen in us, we would get blood poisoning and die. The trees are our parasites, the leaves are our 2A Bad Bacteria and the leaf rakers are our white blood cells, which we only have a finite quantity of. If too much waste built up in our bodies, particularly in moist areas like the mouth and genitals but also the skin, it would soon poison us and those areas would rot.

Fungi help us break down excess 2A Bad Bacteria. **Fungi are friends not foes**. When we need them, they appear. When we don't, they're gone. And we already know where the bacteria are coming from.

We need to come to a new understanding of the fact that a fungal infection is indicative of a dangerously high 1A Parasite load.

Fungi Q & A

Q: What product can we use to MT for the presence of fungi?
A: There are 3 main products: fluconazole (which is over-the-counter), ketoconazole and itraconazole. They each indicate different types of fungi. Whereas with 3A Metal Toxicity, we test for the metal by using the metal itself (e.g., we test for mercury using pure mercury), when we are MT for fungi, we can only logically infer their presence. See the adjacent MT Protocol for specifics.

Q: If a fungal infection is not the root problem, why is fluconazole so effective on candida and yeast infections?
A: The fungus itself can cause its own symptoms. Sometimes those are so extreme that the body needs a full reset. However, the pitfall lies in thinking that by resetting the fungus you have solved the root problem.

Q: Are there good and bad fungi, and isn't candida bad?
A: Not exactly. Biologically they're good for you because they prevent you from getting blood poisoning. Medically they're bad for you because they represent a deeper problem. The two main fungi are candida (white mold) and aspergillus (black mold). Of the two, aspergillus can hurt you, particularly from inhalant exposure. It seems to thrive in bodies that are high in 2-valence metal toxicity (mercury, Hg#80 and cadmium, Cd#48). So if you're exposed, and have the right toxicity profile it can make things worse, but believing that years later aspergillus is still causing your lung problem misses the point: roundworms excrete the bacteria aspergillus feeds on. Roundworms are your lung problem.

MT Protocol For Fungi

1. Start with a baseline.
2. MT the symptomatic area to find a weak response.
3. Put the anti-fungal into the bioelectric field, redo the MT and see if the anti-fungal cancels the weak response out.

A: If it doesn't, there is no evidence of a fungus, or the product you're using is the wrong anti-fungal.

B: If it does, you have found two things: 1) a fungus and 2) the appropriate antifungal medication.

Understanding Viruses

Anyone reading this section after the 2020 coronavirus pandemic and shutdown will have a unique perspective on the incapacitating fear that a virus can cause when it gets out in to a population.

Had there been a simple button to press to eliminate the Wuhan virus, or even a MT to identify an infected person, trillions of dollars and a hundred thousand lives could have been saved, not to mention lost livelihoods, businesses, homes and a way of life.

One of the factors that makes a virus so complex is that it isn't actually alive. All of the evidence points to them being spontaneously assembling protein structures that self-read off the DNA strand. How can we kill something that isn't alive to begin with? We can't.

This is where we should begin when trying to understand viruses. We need to change our mentality from killing a virus to altering the climate in which it can spontaneously assemble.

There is MT evidence that **viruses thrive in an environment of metal toxicity**. There is a way to use a MT analysis to determine which virus feeds on which metal. It is quite specific.

There are 2 steps to this:
1. Confirm the presence of the virus MT an antiviral medication like valacyclovir against a viral indicator (this can be anything from a body location to a stool or blood sample, sputum, an oral swab or a parasite sample). If the antiviral cancels out the weak MT response produced by the indicator location or by the sample, you have found a correspondence.

This simple technique in itself could have made it unnecessary for the world to go through the 2020 shutdown.

> **MT Protocol For Viruses**
>
> 1. Start with a baseline.
> 2. MT the symptomatic area, or indicator (like a parasite sample), find a weak response.
> 3. MT a general antiviral medication like valacyclovir against the negative indicator, see if it cancels out the weak response.
>
> **A:** If it does, you've found a virus.
> **B:** If it doesn't, you have failed to find a virus.

2. Isolate the metal toxicity

Using the positive viral indicator as a reference, introduce various element samples from the 76 possibilities to see which one cancels out the indicator. In this way we can identify a correspondence at Rung 3A.

It should be noted that if the viral indicator is general, the correspondence will not be guaranteed to have a specific causal relationship.

Examples of positive causal relationships are shingles which MT against tungsten (W#74) and oral herpes (cold sores) which MT against mercury (#80). Although a MT only indicates a correspondence, there has been some evidence in a clinical setting that active, symptomatic cases of shingles have spontaneously resolved during a 1B Frequency Therapy treatment.

> **MT Protocol For A Virus Against A Metal**
>
> 1. Start with a baseline.
> 2. Confirm the viral indicator.
> 3. MT various pure element samples against the viral indicator, see which one cancels it out.
>
> **A:** If one does, you have found a correspondence with the virus.
> **B:** If one doesn't, you haven't, but more likely you're doing it wrong. There is always a heavy metal correspondence.

This allows for a multi-leveled understanding of The Health Ladder. Since 3A tungsten (W#74) would only stick to someone who had a high count of 2A tungsten-loving bacteria, and since it is the case that tungsten-loving bacteria only live in certain species of 1A filarial parasite, we can draw a tentative conclusion about a causal relationship between 1A filaria and 4A shingles. This might explain why the symptoms of shingles are so intrinsically neurological (many microfilarial species live in the cerebrospinal fluid in the vertebral foramen of the spinal column).

The outcome necessary to confirm this causal association is that cases of shingles, ideally currently symptomatic, should resolve in the presence of an effective 1B Frequency Therapy treatment of the filarial species, and this is what we observe. Upon the death of the parasite, the location no longer MT for the antiviral indicator.

Muscle Testing Face Masks

The iconic and horrific symbol of World War 1 was the gas mask. A little over a century later, the face mask is the symbol of the 2020 pandemic. This was the World War 1 of the 21st century. It was a war not of territory or attrition but for health, awareness and information.

There are two layers of consideration with face masks: 1) Are they effective? and 2) Are they healthy for us?

We don't need a MT to evaluate this, we can look at the numbers: The mesh size of a standard face mask is 2 to 5 microns. A coronavirus, at 1 micron, would get through. Then, these masks don't seal tightly to the face and so, are not even mechanically effective.

It is notable that when the health regulatory authorities in Canada were conducting telephone interviews to screen for contact tracing, if the respondent stated that they had been wearing a standard face mask (i.e., not an N95 mask), they were marked down as having worn no mask at all. If regular masks didn't even count as masks, then why did we all have to wear them? There is no simple answer to that.

Whether a face mask is healthy however, can be MT. It will be found that after breathing through a mask for as few as four breaths, the nervous system will express a weak MT response.

> **MT Protocol For Your Face Mask**
>
> 1. Start with a baseline.
> 2. Put on a face mask, breathe through it for 60 seconds.
> 3. Then redo the baseline.
>
> **A:** If step 3 is a strong test, the mask is probably fine for you.
>
> **B:** If step 3 provokes a weak MT, you have identified that breathing through the mask is a nervous system stressor.

This is due to one of the primary functions of breathing, which is to rid the body of toxic bacteria and other waste. By collecting all of that waste in a layer of fabric over the mouth, we are forcing our lungs to re-inhale what was just evacuated. It is extraordinarily unhealthy to do this for more than a few minutes. When we consider that wearing face masks was the norm for hours at a time, we can imagine what problems this would have led to.

The End of Pandemics

"What if the pandemic doesn't end?" That was the title of a *Financial Post* article from Feb 9, 2021. An old virus mutates into a new variant, a new lockdown, it goes on forever and in the process, society ends.

In 2020, we lost our way of life to fear. Then, when we allowed certain virologists to become public spokespersons, they didn't help with this—they stoked the fear. They started by contradicting their own proclamations and ended by contradicting the evidence. "Two weeks to flatten the curve" became a neverending process. A life-saving vaccine became a political play for totalitarianism.

I've got some bad news for you: We are all absolutely going to die. The question is, do we live a full, happy life first? A social life? A free life? Or do we die after having been locked down in our houses for years, afraid to step outside without a mask or a vaccine passport?

Isn't the reward of living free worth the risk of living free? Every generation needs to ask, and answer, this question, as we do.

I'm not a specialist in virology and maybe that's a good thing: if all you have is a hammer, you'll see everything as a nail. In my limited experience with viruses, I have seen shingles resolve during a 1B Frequency treatment. Could the factor that renders it inactive be a common denominator to other viruses? That question leads to these ones:
1. To what extent does a 4A Virus depend upon a 3A Metal Toxicity?
2. Is the parasite-bacteria-element-virus relationship the reason that some people suffer and die from viruses while others are immune?
3. If we eliminate some 1A Parasites can we be free from some viruses?
4. Is mass-immunity to viruses possible by mass-treating parasites?
5. Is this why antimalarial hydroxychloroquine helped with the Wuhan virus?

The unknown has always been a source of fear. The only way out of this is to quantify it. Make the unknown known—with a MT. What are the 3A Metal Toxicities behind the worst viruses in the world: SARS, H1N1, dengue, West Nile, typhoid fever, yellow fever, smallpox, HIV, Marburg and Ebola? Herein might lie a cure to all viruses.

Using MT to understand viruses is the most effective way for our society to remember that freedom is a right, and move forward.

Further Reading on Bacteria, Fungi and Viruses

The three fields outlined in this chapter are expanded in The Complete Muscle Testing Series: *Book 9 Muscle Testing for Bacteria, Fungi and Viruses.*

Part 1 Bacteriology examines the fields of antibiotics and probiotics in more detail, with an emphasis on MT these products against various 5A Locations.

This section also addresses the extent to which 2A Bad Bacteria are good for the parasite, as well as how they metabolize specific 3A Metal Toxicities as cofactors in their metabolism. The data is addressed to the general reader but summarized in a form that bacteriologists and researchers can work with and reproduce.

Part 2 Fungal Biology delves into the biological functioning and helpful role that fungi play in the human health ecosystem.

Part 3 Virology explores in greater detail the relationship between viruses and the elements. The core question of whether it is possible to render a virus inert by altering the biochemical climate in which it functions is intrinsic to virology and is addressed using MT correspondences and clinical research. This section also goes into a detailed analysis of the Wuhan virus and evaluates various responses to it from around the world.

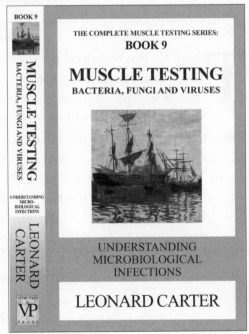

BOOK 9

THE COMPLETE MUSCLE TESTING SERIES:
BOOK 9

MUSCLE TESTING
BACTERIA, FUNGI AND VIRUSES

UNDERSTANDING
MICROBIOLOGICAL
INFECTIONS

LEONARD CARTER

MUSCLE TESTING BACTERIA, FUNGI AND VIRUSES

UNDERSTANDING MICRO-BIOLOGICAL INFECTIONS

LEONARD CARTER

VITRUVIAN
VP
PRESS

0A. THE VECTOR

All animals in nature are the primary or intermediate hosts to various species of Parasites (1A), many of which can infect humans.

0B. AWARENESS

Educate yourself. Start by reading *Experiments in Muscle Testing* by Leonard Carter. Then, apply what you learn.

THE HEALTH LADDER
A GUIDE TO SYMPTOMS AND THEIR ROOT CAUSES

CONDITION		RESOLUTION
7A		7B
6A		6B
5A		5B
4A		4B
3A		3B
2A		2B
1A		1B
0A		0B

10

Muscle Testing

Your Food

There are two reasons that food will MT weak on us:

1. There are parasite eggs in it.

2. It is feeding a parasite that is in us.

In this chapter we will touch on point 1: The foods that have parasite eggs in them. We need to dispel the absurd myth that a lack of hand washing causes contamination. How many news articles about parasites in food start (or end) with the admonition that hands not being properly washed was the cause of contamination? For goodness' sake! Do you have any idea how many trillions of parasite eggs would need to be on someone's hands for their lack of adequate washing to contaminate whole batches of food in industrial production facilities? An actual handful of feces would barely be sufficient for this purpose.

No, the parasite eggs are already in the food.

Top Sources of Parasites in Your Life

It will help to understand the magnitude of the following list if we can agree that every species of animal on the planet hosts parasites. The shock of where all these parasites are coming from is replaced with the Rung 0B Awareness that parasites are the norm, which paves the way to view the following list as a matter of fact, versus a sensationalized account of biology.

1. Milk products Milk MT for all the parasites a cow has: praz 11, 18, 20, meb 8, alb 4, 8. This can easily be verified with a Parasite MT Kit.

The reason for this is that dairies rarely cook their milk at 100°C/212°F. The most common form of pasteurization, called vat pasteurization, takes place as low as 63°C/145°F. The method we all assume is happening, where the milk is brought to 100°C/212°F, only leaves it there for 0.01 seconds. That's simply not enough time to kill parasite eggs and frankly, such a duration doesn't seem plausible.

Dairies fail to boil their milk because they don't know any better. The benefit of low temp. pasteurization is that it allows for different milk consistencies, particularly with creams and cheeses.

Parasite eggs are the reason why milk goes sour and needs to be refrigerated in the first place. This applies to all milk products: cream, butter, yogurt, ice cream, whipped cream, cheese, uncooked cheese products, powdered cheese on chips and many whey and milk-based protein powders (though not milk chocolate, which is usually cooked). Yogurt generally can't be boiled as the high temperature would kill the bacterial culture.

In parasite biology there isn't an acceptance of the fact that parasite eggs are transmitted during lactation, probably because it is assumed that these parasites have a life cycle that requires an intermediate host. Since the MT evidence strongly supports the assertions made here, it must be the case that some parasite eggs can bypass the intermediate host requirement.

That is a prediction for a biologist to confirm.

2. Manure-based vegetable oils Parasite eggs come in with the harvest and after lying in the soil are fully infectious. Oil seeds aren't washed upon harvest, they are at most blow-dried in the processing plant and the particulate filters in the expeller presses are too large to catch 10-40 nanometer parasite eggs.

Oil extraction from the seed generally takes place at 88°C/190°F which is not a sufficient temperature to render the oil safe. Production facilities don't bring oil to a boil as this takes time, money and makes the oil taste bitter.

Consumer goods that contain crop oils (canola/ sunflower/soybean/safflower/ corn) that are not brought to a boil include all condiments (ketchup, mustard, relish, barbecue sauce, mayonnaise, salad dressing), margarine, fake sliced cheeses and the many hundreds of sauces sold around the world including hot sauce.

> **MT Protocol For Your Food**
>
> 1. Start with a baseline.
> 2. Place the product in your bioelectric field and MT it, ideally at the stomach. Remember that you can MT through plastic and glass but you can't MT through metal.
>
> **A:** If product = strong then it's fine.
> **B:** If product = weak then either there are parasite eggs in it or it is feeding parasites in you. To rule this out, cook it and retest.

We associate the word processed with unhealthy but clearly these oils aren't processed enough. Olive oil is not exempt from this problem. Most mass-market companies dilute their olive with canola to save money.

3. Manure-based vegetable syrups For the same reason as vegetable oils above, corn syrup is a condensed source of parasite eggs. On the one hand, bringing syrups to a boil presents the risk of spoiling the batch or reducing it too much. On the other, food manufacturers assume it is safe and often add it to their own products without further boiling. This includes sauces, condiments, many soft candies, table syrup, cough syrup and those little square plastic containers you get at hotels that say maple syrup.

4. Sushi While the existence of parasite eggs in dairy calls into question the orthodoxy that all species always require an intermediate host, no such limitation applies to fish. We know from even a basic understanding of parasite life cycles that by the time the cercaria has reached the fish and encysted, it is at a stage that is unquestionably infectious to humans.

There is no justification for national health guidelines in Canada and around the world to state that it is safe to eat raw fish. The guideline is that if fish is frozen below -20°C/-4°F for 7 days or -35°C/-31°F for 24 hours, the parasite eggs in the fish's flesh have been killed. This just doesn't line up with the MT evidence. A MT of sushi frozen to these parameters indicates that the eggs are alive and well. To cross-check this, experiments in MT have been done where raw fish was left outside for 24 hours at -45°C/-49°F in central Alberta in winter. The next-day MT of the frozen fish indicated biologically viable parasite eggs. The lethal temperature is probably around -100°C/ -148°F which isn't happening. All fish MT for praz, meb and ivermectin.

5. Deli meats Various forms of deli meats are assumed to be safe because they have been smoked. However, the smoke temperature, even when it is above the boiling point, does not always penetrate to the center of the meat pan, so for dietary purposes deli meats can be considered completely raw. This is confirmed in a MT analysis.

6. Other Additional food sources of parasites are presented without any explanation: soy sauce, hot sauce, so-called smoked fish and meats, soft drinks from a fast food soda fountain, flavoring on chips, jams, nuts, pasta and pizza sauces, raw chicken eggs, children's gummy bear vitamins, cough medicine, spices like pepper, vegan protein powders, raw grain flours, bottled water and for infants, a mother's breast milk.

In short, dairy, manure-based oils and syrups, sushi, deli meats and a number of lesser contributors that are consequences of the above factors are the leading sources of parasites in the Western diet.

If we think fruits and vegetables are the problem, we're looking in the wrong place: washing works nicely for most of them.

Dietary Philosophies

Raw Due to parasites, eating raw food is the most dangerous thing we can do. This applies to feeding raw food to pets as well.

Organic and vegan diets These are just as high in parasites as a processed-food diet. Parasites are themselves organic, and vegan food is grown in parasite-egg-rich soil (most soil will MT weak).

Dirt If you endorse the idea that a little bit of soil in your diet is good for you, particularly for vegetarians who feel they need more vitamin B12, at least make sure you cook your soil...

Junk We can now we can see the problem with junk food in perspective: it is not so much the salt, saturated fat, refined carbohydrates, processed meats or preservatives that make people sick as the roundworm, whipworm, fluke and tapeworm eggs in the condiments, sauces, cheeses and milk products. Vegan kale chips can be worse for you than a hamburger if the burger is at least cooked and if the kale chips have a raw corn syrup-based powdered flavoring.

GMO There is no MT evidence that GMO presents a dietary problem.

Rendering Food Safe

There are four simple ways to kill the parasite eggs in your food.

1. Temperature Parasite eggs are ruptured above 100°C/212°F which is why we cook our food. Microwaving also works just fine. Microwaves may denature some of the nutrients in that one meal but some parasites can live in you for 80 years, so pick your priority.

2. Alcohol Something soaked in alcohol for long enough (this depends on size) will probably have no live parasite eggs in it. This is why it is much safer to drink beer on vacation than water.

3. Carbonation Carbonic acid kills parasite eggs in an hour, so a corn syrup drink from a soda fountain would need to sit for a while.

4. Vinegar Pickling kills parasite eggs in about an hour but the vinegar concentration will be a factor. The vinegar in condiments is not concentrated enough to render them safe.

5. Hot Peppers This is a huge myth. Hot peppers don't kill parasites.

Food Poisoning

Food poisoning is a misnomer. This isn't the Italian Renaissance, nobody has poisoned your food. If we get sick from eating something, there were parasites eggs in it. The egg hatches on contact with saliva or our stomach acid. The larva emerges from the egg and starts to eat and poop. The poop is full of 2A Bad Bacteria, which causes instant nausea and a biological flushing response. If the larvae hatch in our stomach we will have the urge to vomit; if they end up in the intestines, there will be diarrhea.

Either way, these responses rarely flush out the organism. Once it hatches in us, it can stay alive for between 2 and 80 years.

Every food poisoning incident is a unique parasite infection event. If you want to understand how many times you have picked up a parasite this way, count the number of times in your life you have had food poisoning. Rung 2B Antibiotics wouldn't have helped because antibiotics don't kill parasites.

No Vacancy

As per The Motel Room Concept, better a 4-foot human tapeworm in our small intestine that steals 5% of our lunch than a 60-foot fish tapeworm that steals 90% of our calories and starves us to death.

The role parasites play in our internal ecosystems is to excrete a bacterium in their waste that contains a chemical message that prevents same-species eggs from hatching. This serves the dual purpose of preventing us from picking up so many parasites from our diet that we die, and also allowing us to consume that diet moving forward without further ill effects (after the initial infection event).

This is what enables carnivores to eat raw meat and what allows herbivores to chew grass full of feces without getting sick. It is how fish are able to breathe water full of cercaria and why you can eat fast food—or any food, without constantly throwing up.

There is no point in trying to avoid these foods unless there has been an effective parasite treatment. If you're not actually sick, having no vacancy is biologically better than some vacancy.

Further Reading on Muscle Testing Food

The Complete Muscle Testing Series: *Book 10 Muscle Testing Your Food* contains the following ingredients:

Part 1 starts with an examination of the leading diet philosophies from the parasite perspective. It demonstrates the limitations of any dietary agenda that fails to take parasites into account in its formulation.

Part 2 provides a complete breakdown of all the common foods we find parasite eggs in and an explanation of how they got there.

Part 3 covers MT for chefs, cooks, mothers and the rest of us. There is also a detailed explanation of how to prepare meals in a culture that doesn't understand parasite vectors.

Part 4 offers a set of proposals for the food manufacturing industry and national health regulatory agencies on simple steps that can be taken to render foods parasite free once and for all.

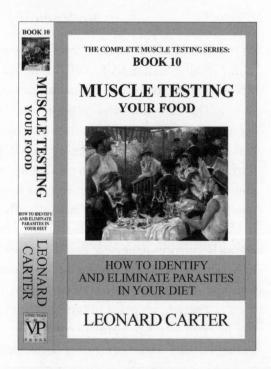

7A. THE NAME

The word agreed upon to summarize the Symptom (6A), that historically was also presumed to cause it.

6A. SYMPTOM

The expression of RUNGS 1A–5A at a level that can be perceived or measured.

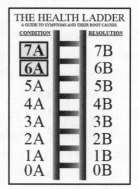

THE HEALTH LADDER		
A GUIDE TO SYMPTOMS AND THEIR ROOT CAUSES		
CONDITION		RESOLUTION
7A		7B
6A		6B
5A		5B
4A		4B
3A		3B
2A		2B
1A		1B
0A		0B

11

Muscle Testing
For Food Allergies

As already stated, there are two reasons that a food will MT weak: 1) There are parasite eggs in it 2) It is feeding a parasite that is in us. We can rule out parasite eggs in the food by cooking and retesting it. Point 2 is the remaining possibility.

We call this second phenomenon a food allergy but this is a misleading term because it places emphasis on the food or on our immune system, while overlooking the parasite that causes the reactivity. In fact, every food allergy is caused by a parasite: sometimes a unique parasite for each food, sometimes the same parasite for multiple foods.

In this chapter we will examine the methodology of using MT to equate the food someone is reacting to with the parasite causing the reactivity. We will also touch on permanent allergy elimination.

Parasites and Food Allergies

The relationship between a parasite and a food allergy is obvious: someone eats a food and then gets the symptom of a parasite—bloating, vomiting, diarrhea, swelling, itching and a headache. If this happens every time with the same food we call it a food allergy. But why don't we call it a parasite?

It wasn't obvious to me for years. I started suffering from a gluten allergy in my mid-20s and dealt with it for about 10 years. At one stage my reactivity got so severe that I couldn't breathe when I had the slightest bit of flour in a sauce. I didn't understand that parasites were doing this. The allergy had built up so slowly, and it so encompassed my five senses that something as simple as a parasite just didn't seem to explain the severity.

This was reinforced by society. Every doctor (traditional and alternative) confirmed that my 6A Symptom was a 7A Name: a gluten allergy. After all, there are gluten free expos, celiac societies, companies dedicated to gluten free food products. The momentum of the whole world seemed caught up in food allergies, who was I to think otherwise? So, I thought what I was taught.

But I never stopped trying to resolve it and one day I did. I had been MT various antiparasitic medications against my small intestine for a couple of months, and every time I found a dose that I MT for, I would take it. I MT for alb 4 so I took alb 4. Then one day I MT for praz 11 so I took the whole 11 pills...and nothing happened. The next day when I retested, I needed another praz 11. This made sense because praziquantel (fluke medicine) is usually consumed for two days in a row. I took the praz again. This was at 9 a.m.. At 2 p.m., I needed an urgent visit to the washroom and out came about 20 large flukes. They were flat and all different shapes but generally the size of a bunch of wet leaves.

Right then, at 2:05 p.m. I went and MT for gluten. It MT just fine. I ate some and felt fantastic. I have been eating it (and breathing) every day since.

The Confirmation Triangle

We already understand that there is a way to MT which parasites we have (Pt3-Ch5). This is how I knew that I had praz 11 in the preceding example. Now we will examine a way of using MT to equate the parasite with the food allergy. This is called **The Confirmation Triangle.**

The way MT works is that an indicator muscle will exhibit positive or negative neurological responses to a stimulus. Positive is not morally good, negative is not morally bad, it just means that whatever stimulus we have introduced has provoked a corresponding muscular response. Since the response is very conveniently binary (always either positive or negative) we can now make a logical value judgement about the MT. The reasoning goes like this:

- If gluten MT negative
- and if stomach (ST) MT negative
- AND if gluten plus ST at the same time MT positive
- then we can infer a correspondence between gluten and ST.

This is called a **double negative** (a positive MT that is only arrived at by combining two negatives).

We aren't yet sure of the meaning of the correspondence, but if both charges cancel each other out, there is a definite relationship. This can be represented graphically as follows:

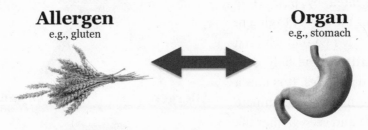

Allergen
e.g., gluten

Organ
e.g., stomach

We can now expand on this and MT various antiparasitic medications against the stomach until we find a correspondence. Say we find praz 11:

Antiparasitic Medicine
e.g., praz 11

Organ
e.g., stomach

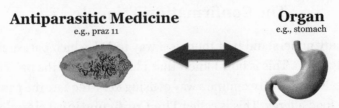

Since we know that praziquantel is fluke medicine and that flukes are often found in the stomach, what we are identifying in the MT is reasonable (it's not like we're finding a Volkswagen in there).

Now we can forget about the stomach for the moment and using the body's own bioelectric field as the connector, place gluten somewhere on the body and see which antiparasitic medication cancels out gluten. It is common to find different values but for the sake of this explanation, let's say we find a correspondence between gluten and praz 11.

Antiparasitic Medicine
e.g., praz 11

Allergen
e.g., gluten

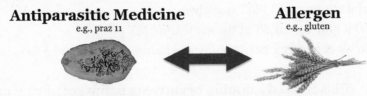

There is a way to logically connect these MT. If gluten=ST, ST=praz 11 and praz 11=gluten then we have a Confirmation Triangle. From this we can now infer an extremely important fact:

It appears that a fluke in the stomach represented by praz 11 is causing the allergy to gluten.

Establishing **causality** is the holy grail of food allergies. It is now a simple matter to eliminate praz 11 and see whether the 6A Symptom resolves itself.

If it does, there it is.

Antiparasitic Medicine
e.g., praz 11

Allergen
e.g., gluten

Organ
e.g., stomach

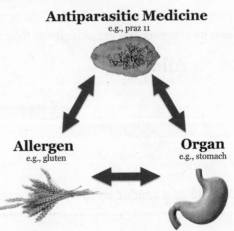

Applying the Confirmation Triangle

Eliminating a food allergy using antiparasitic medication is rarely simple. When I eliminated praz 11 I could eat gluten, but this is not always so simply reproducible. The process is often much more complicated. Here are some technicalities that we might encounter:

Multiple praz values for flukes: Every celiac MT for at least praz 11, but it is also common for the same person to MT for additional values of praz such as praz 20, praz 33 and even praz 100, praz 350 and praz 600. Since 33 is the maximum amount of praz someone can take (probably about 50 praz would be lethal), what can they do about the other parasites? This is where and why 1B Frequency Therapy is the only solution.

Multiple values for other medicines: It is quite common for someone with gluten reactivity to have a Confirmation Triangle that shows, in addition to the praz, correspondences with alb 2-20 and meb 4-6000. Less commonly (we see this more often in cases of ulcerative colitis), it will require as many as meb 7000 to cancel out gluten.

Keep in mind that a highly symptomatic person could have 5 praz values, 3 alb values and 15 meb values. Thus it becomes apparent why nobody has ever found a repeatable cure to a food allergy - how could they eliminate the medication values above the safe doses? How could we even know if that was going to work?

Last, there is a technicality that has to do with **waking parasites up**. It is common to notice during a 1B Frequency Therapy against celiac and other forms of gluten reactivity that the person will appear to MT clear around the 2-hour mark, but as soon as we introduce gluten, within minutes they are MT negative for it again. Upon MT the antiparasitic medications to quantify what is happening, a new value will show up higher than we previously found. If praz 33 was eliminated, some other value would show up in the Confirmation Triangle. By prolonging the treatment, these also die but lead to yet another wakeup round. We can observe as many as six wakeup rounds. This process is only feasible when using a FQ because of the medication toxicity issue. These are clinical distinctions but important ones.

Other Food Allergies

First, we start by MT the food and confirm we're getting a negative MT response to it. When filling in the Confirmation Triangle for a food allergy, the patterns are relatively simple and repeat themselves. Here are the most common patterns at the low doses of medications:

Gluten: praz 11, 20, 33; alb 4, 8; meb 4, 6, 8, 10; iver 2-30

Dairy: praz 18, 33; alb 4, 8; meb 8

Beef: praz 18, 20; meb 8

Eggs: meb 2, 10

Shellfish, Peanuts, Eggs: doses of praz and meb above 1000

The point isn't to try to spell out every allergy there is. The intention is to teach the principle of the Confirmation Triangle and then it can be applied in each new case. Just remember two things:

> **MT Protocol For A Food Allergy**
>
> 1. Start with a baseline.
> 2. MT the food.
>
> **A:** If it MT strong, great.
> **B:** If it MT weak, cook the food and retest.
> **C:** If still weak after cooking, you have found something that indicates a parasite in you, call it an allergy if you like.

1. If we're not finding a correspondence with an antiparasitic medication we're either not MT the right medication or not enough pills.
2. We can't eliminate the organisms at the toxic doses without a 1B Frequency Therapy alternative to the medications.

Food Allergies and The Health Ladder

Rung 7A: The Name	Celiac
Rung 6A: Symptom	Bloating reaction to gluten
Rung 5A: Location	Stomach, Small intestines
Rung 4A: Fungus/Virus	Candida-like symptoms could be fungus
Rung 3A: Metal Toxicity	Confirmation Triangle = arsenic
Rung 2A: Bad Bacteria	Confirmation Triangle = penicillin
Rung 1A: Parasites	Various values of praz, meb, alb, iver
Rung 0A: The Vector	Various food sources over time

Further Reading on Food Allergies

More detail on food allergies can be found in The Complete Muscle Testing Series: *Book 11 Muscle Testing for Food Allergies.*

The following topics are addressed:

Part 1 explores the physiology of food allergies and how they express themselves in us. It answers questions such as what is happening bacteriologically? What activates the immune system response to the food? Why do different parasites cause different allergies? If everyone has parasites why do only some people get allergies? How can an allergy disappear on its own over time?

Part 2 examines inhalant (seasonal) allergies and their difference from food allergies.

Part 3 presents a number of important case studies in allergy elimination including gluten, dairy, peanut, shellfish and bee sting, along with others.

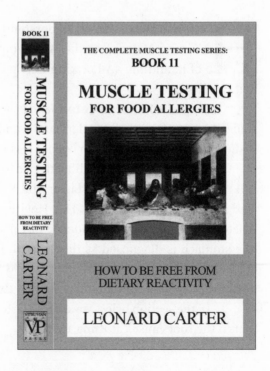

6A. SYMPTOM

The expression of RUNGS 1A–5A at a level that can be perceived or measured.

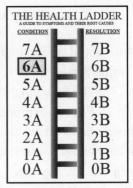

THE HEALTH LADDER
A GUIDE TO SYMPTOMS AND THEIR ROOT CAUSES

CONDITION		RESOLUTION
7A		7B
6A		6B
5A		5B
4A		4B
3A		3B
2A		2B
1A		1B
0A		0B

12

Muscle Testing
Your Physical Symptoms

How much do we really understand about our 6A Symptoms? The 7A Name describes the symptom but is not the cause of it, and the 5A Location may tell us where the problem is, but rarely what.

Only when we are able to analyze the 6A Symptom at Rungs 4A and below can we actually understand it and knowing this, sometimes a shortcut to 1A Parasites can bypass less relevant information.

It was the historic difficulty in quantifying parasites that led medical researchers like Lister and Pasteur to assume that they had reached the bottom of The Health Ladder at Rung 2A Bad Bacteria. We can still see evidence of this today when a problem in the stomach is diagnosed as the bacteria H.pylori or E.coli, or with major infectious diseases like leprosy and the bubonic plague which are both still talked about and named at Rung 2A only.

In the section below we are interested not only in the symptom but in the root causes at Rung 1A.

Understanding Your Symptoms

The important thing to remember with 6A Symptoms is not to mistake your experience of the symptom for your understanding of the cause of the symptom.

For example, you will know very well that you have a sore throat. You will be quite confident that 7A The Name sore throat is the best description of the 6A Symptom of throat pain. It is obvious then that the 5A Location is the throat itself but this is where things stop being obvious. Can you fill in any rungs below 5A? The 4A Fungus/Virus? The 3A Metal Toxicity? The 2A Bad Bacteria? The 1A Parasite? Do you know which 0A Vector you got the parasite eggs from? Suddenly a sore throat isn't making nearly as much sense.

The question with understanding symptoms is not that of how we know what we know. That's obvious: we know it, and we don't need a MT to tell us otherwise. The real question is how can we know what we don't know? Were you aware that you needed to know what 1A Parasite was causing your sore throat?

We have been conditioned to use what we might call **Horizontal Thinking** about health issues. The Health Ladder takes this into account in that Rung 6A has a Rung 6B that is horizontal to it and represents that best action we can take at that level of thinking. The 5A Location needs a 5B Therapy, which is horizontal thinking but it doesn't presuppose understanding. To understand, we need to use **Vertical Thinking** and move from 6A downward to Rung 0A.

For this reason, it helps to be in the habit of using the positions on The Health Ladder (2A, 1A, 0A) as empty placeholders. We can fill in the blanks we do know for each symptom, and when we can't fill in a blank, we have identified that we don't know something.

The most essential rung to be understood is Rung 1A: What Parasite do you have that is vertical to the 6A Symptom? This can be challenging to quantify but deserves primary focus nonetheless.

Rung 1A: Parasites: **fill in the blank**

Let us keep this consideration in mind as we review the following examples.

Health Ladder Profiles of Common Symptoms

Health Ladder Profile for: **A Sore Throat**

Rung 7A: The Name	Sore Throat
Rung 6A: Symptom	Throat pain
Rung 5A: Location	Trachea or esophagus
Rung 4A: Fungus/Virus	Could be a virus
Rung 3A: Metal Toxicity	Can be MT if you have element samples
Rung 2A: Bad Bacteria	Probably. Could MT for which antibiotic
Rung 1A: Parasites	Will test for: alb 4 / praz 18 / meb 4
Rung 0A: The Vector	Got it from...the mayo you just bought

Explanation: It is very common for a sore throat to MT for praz 18. This is an esophagus fluke. Thousands of fluke eggs are in your mayonnaise which is 0A The Vector. Our 0B Awareness is that they got there from unboiled canola oil via cow manure.

Then at 1A Parasites, the larva emerges from the egg on contact with the saliva in your throat and instantly starts to burrow into the 5A Location, the tissue wall of your esophagus. This hurts and registers as 6A The Symptom. You will call it a 7A Sore Throat and may think that you have a 2A Bad Bacteria or a 4A Virus.

A throat exam by a doctor may show little white staphylococcus spots, reinforcing their understanding that you have picked up a 2A Bad Bacteria. With a serious tone and 14 years of medical school behind them, they tell you that you've got a staph infection and need to go on 2B Antibiotics. You take this new 7A Name, Staph, back to your friends and family and they give you 7B Social Support: sympathy and maybe a mug of hot lemon and honey.

Within a week, the esophagus flukes have burrowed to their desired depth and have manufactured proteins on their outer skin to mimic your immune system tags, so now to your immune system they look like...you! The attack is over, your 6A Symptom subsides, the flukes are safe, and now they have years to grow to full size and start causing a real medical condition like anaphylactic shock to nuts.

It's a good thing you took those 2B Antibiotics...

Health Ladder Profile for: **Traveler's Diarrhea**

Rung 7A: The Name	Traveler's Diarrhea
Rung 6A: Symptom	Loose stools, bloating
Rung 5A: Location	Large intestine
Rung 4A: Fungus/Virus	Sure, there could be a virus
Rung 3A: Metal Toxicity	MT will show multiple values...
Rung 2A: Bad Bacteria	Certainly. Could MT for which antibiotic
Rung 1A: Parasites	Will test for: alb / praz / meb
Rung 0A: The Vector	Deli meat

Explanation: During an episode of diarrhea, your descending colon can MT for various antiparasitic medication values: meb 4, praz 11, praz 20, alb 4, 8. Many different parasites can cause the same symptom.

You've eaten some 0A Vector, goodness knows what, maybe a deli meat sandwich. The parasite eggs were adapted to wait to hatch until they reached the alkaline environment of your large intestine.

Tens to hundreds of 1A Parasite larvae emerge from their eggs like tadpoles in a pond and immediately start fighting their way into your microbiome. Their waste as they feed and excrete has its own battle with your good bacteria and you lose, your bacteria die off in droves and stop solidifying your feces. The liquid waste sits there, not being solidified or broken down. When peristalsis pushes it to the sigmoid colon and rectum, it is flushed out in a watery mess and is full of 2A Bad Bacteria. There is no point in doing a stool test for this 6A Symptom because the 1A Parasite larvae are safe inside of you, burrowing to their 5A Location: the mucosal lining of the colon.

You will call this a 7A Name, let's say traveler's diarrhea because it happened while you were traveling. You see your doctor who recommends some 2B Probiotic like *Saccharomyces Boulardii*. This helps to repopulate some of your good bacteria which the 2A Bad Bacteria from the parasite have wiped out during their invasion.

Eventually they burrow to their desired depth and manufacture proteins on their outer skin to mimic your immune system tags, so now your immune system leaves them alone. Your stools may or may not return to their former solidity.

Health Ladder Profile for: **A Chest Cold**

Rung 7A: The Name	Chest Cold
Rung 6A: Symptom	Coughing
Rung 5A: Location	Lungs, Trachea
Rung 4A: Fungus/Virus	Sure, there could be a virus
Rung 3A: Metal Toxicity	MT will show multiple values...
Rung 2A: Bad Bacteria	Certainly. Could MT for which antibiotic
Rung 1A: Parasites	Will test for: alb / praz / meb
Rung 0A: The Vector	You were out for dinner so no idea

Explanation: One of the most common parasites found at the root of a cold is praz 17 the lung fluke, but don't rule out meb 8 or alb 4. You can MT this at the lungs or where it hurts when you cough.

You've eaten something again. Maybe the 0A Vector was the cream sauce on your fettuccine, which isn't boiled, maybe it was the parmesan cheese, maybe the butter on the bread or the dairy in the dessert. There would have been parasite eggs in all four but whatever hatched in you was something your existing parasite load wasn't excreting a bacterium to protect you from. Perhaps some 10 million year old strain of lung fluke that was in a cow from Sardinia where they got the milk to make that parmesan cheese. And now it's in you.

It circulates through the body and ends up in the oxygen-rich mucosal lining of the lungs, a 5A Location that would be toxic for most other parasites but they are specialized for it. The 1A Parasite larvae emerge and start pooping 2A Bad Bacteria. Maybe the bacteria sticks around a little longer than usual because your lungs have a 3A Metal Toxicity like lead (Pb#82) from your perfume. Now there's a bacterial party going on and who joins the party? A 4A Virus that thrives in an environment of lead. Now it's a full-blown body wide fever.

You see your doctor and they put you on a 4B Antiviral which doesn't help much. After a week off work it's back to just a 7A Name, a cough. The 5A Location burns and hurts and the 6A Symptom lasts an entire month. You get lots of 7B Social Support, everyone is worried about you. Eventually it goes away and 10-20 surviving lung flukes have found a new home. Watch out for asthma down the road.

Application

Try to get in the habit of thinking of the positions on The Health Ladder as blank placeholders, and then fill in the blanks that you know. Particularly when it's something you're eating at home, it is important to identify the 0A Vector as often as possible.

Health Ladder for: **Enter what you know for your symptom**

Rung 7A: The Name   fill in the blank
Rung 6A: Symptom   fill in the blank
Rung 5A: Location   fill in the blank
Rung 4A: Fungus/Virus   fill in the blank if you can
Rung 3A: Metal Toxicity   fill in the blank if you can
Rung 2A: Bad Bacteria   fill in the blank if you can
Rung 1A: Parasites   MT for alb / praz / meb / iver
Rung 0A: The Vector   MT what's in your fridge if you can

Here is a short list of common symptoms that a parasite will cause when it is newly acquired: cold/flu, headache, constipation, shortness of breath, pain everywhere, insomnia, sweating at night, new skin rash, new unusual moodiness, itching, heartburn, bloating/gassiness.

These things may be caused by a parasite you have just picked up or they could be the 6A Symptom of a 1A Parasite you have been hosting for some time. Either way, you will need 1B Frequency Therapy to resolve it. This can take place as a chemical FQ or if it is available, as an electrical FQ.

It is worthy of note that newly acquired parasites usually respond well to low (safe) dose chemical FQs, whereas longstanding infections sometimes won't respond as well to a chemical FQ.

Further Reading on Physical Symptoms

Symptoms are relevant because eventually, we will all live with them and suffer from them. So much of being free from a symptom has to do with psychological freedom—with simply understanding it.

The Complete Muscle Testing Series: *Book 12 Muscle Testing Your Physical Symptoms* is written with this in mind.

Part 1 evaluates the physiology of symptomatology from the lymphatic and inflammatory to the circulatory and anatomical perspectives.

Part 2 studies The Health Ladder profiles for top 200 symptoms. This facilitates an understanding of the contributions of Rungs 1-5A to the 6A Symptom and allows the reader to become free from the misconception of 20th century medical science that the symptom is somehow caused by the 7A Name or the 2A Bad Bacteria.

The top 200 symptoms are chosen from a longer list, since many of the more serious symptoms represent full-blown medical conditions that we will address separately in the next chapter.

Part 3 explores the pathways whereby a symptom can resolve once the associated 1A Parasite is eliminated.

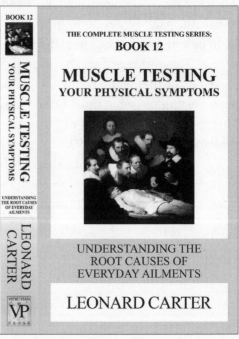

BOOK 12

MUSCLE TESTING YOUR PHYSICAL SYMPTOMS

UNDERSTANDING THE ROOT CAUSES OF EVERYDAY AILMENTS

LEONARD CARTER

THE COMPLETE MUSCLE TESTING SERIES:
BOOK 12

MUSCLE TESTING
YOUR PHYSICAL SYMPTOMS

UNDERSTANDING THE
ROOT CAUSES OF
EVERYDAY AILMENTS

LEONARD CARTER

VP
PRESS

7A. THE NAME

The word agreed upon to summarize the Symptom (6A), that historically was also presumed to cause it.

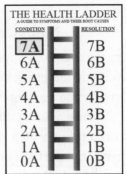

THE HEALTH LADDER
A GUIDE TO SYMPTOMS AND THEIR ROOT CAUSES

CONDITION	RESOLUTION
7A	7B
6A	6B
5A	5B
4A	4B
3A	3B
2A	2B
1A	1B
0A	0B

13

Muscle Testing
Medical Conditions

When a 6A Symptom becomes prolonged, invasive or life threatening, it is necessary to name it. This determines which 6B Treatment will be implemented and paves the way for much-needed 7B Social Support. Everyone can support you better when they know the 7A Name that summarizes your symptoms, if only just to give you a hug.

But does this classify as understanding? Why did the 6A Symptom arise? What is wrong with the 5A Location? Did a 4A Virus have anything to do with it? How about a 3A Metal Toxicity, a 2A Bad Bacteria or a 1A Parasite? If so, what 0A Vector did you get it from?

The standard answer is: we don't know.

The Health Ladder provides us with a way out of this impasse, not only by clarifying actions that we can take at the lower rungs, such as 3B Metal Detox, 2B Probiotics or 1B Frequency Therapy, but by creating a context in which real understanding can take place.

We will only be truly free from medical conditions when we learn to interpret them using The Health Ladder as a conceptual framework.

Measuring Medical Conditions

There are countless ways to measure a 6A Symptom. The challenge lies in correctly assigning causality to what we find, since only when we understand how a symptom originated can we begin to try to collapse it.

If we assume that there is a 1A Parasite in every case, we will be correct, but which one? You could have hundreds of species of parasites but perhaps only one is causing a particular 6A Symptom.

The best strategy is to start at 3A Metal Toxicity. Every symptomatic location will be cancelled out by a predominant element. Since there are only 76 elements to keep track of, this is a short search and it underscores the benefit of having access to a Periodic Table MT Kit. Refer to Pt3-Ch4 for how to MT a location for a metal.

The chart below contains some common patterns to look for.

Metals in Medical Conditions		
Rheumatoid Arthritis	Tin, Arsenic	MT for: Alb, Praz
Arthritis	Iron	MT for: Meb
Gout	Silver	MT for: Iver
Anxiety	Mercury	MT for: Meb
Migraines	Manganese	MT for: Praz
Alzheimer's	Aluminum	MT for: Praz
Parkinson's	Thallium	MT for: Praz
Multiple sclerosis	Selenium	MT for: Iver
Asthma	Arsenic	MT for: Praz
Diabetes	Chromium	MT for: Iver
Tooth Decay	Fluorine	MT for: Iver

Once we have identified a metal associated with a condition we can move to the next consideration and try to use the metal to quantify which parasite appears to be causing the condition.

The MT is simple: it involves determining which antiparasitic medication cancels out the metal toxicity we have found. This information is included in the above chart and it tells us which parasite is likely to be at the root of a particular symptom.

This works because parasites host specially adapted bacteria and we can use the metals to find them. This allows us to target individual parasites to see if the medical condition resolves.

The Health Ladder Profile for Diabetes

Rung 7A: The Name Diabetes

Rung 6A: Symptom Lack of insulin metabolism, neuropathy

Rung 5A: Location Pancreas, sensory nerves, circulatory system

Rung 4A: Fungus/Virus Hard to quantify which one if any

Rung 3A: Metal Toxicity Lead, arsenic, mercury, aluminum, chromium

Rung 2A: Bad Bacteria Certainly, but antibiotics won't help

Rung 1A: Parasites Alb 4, meb 2, praz 33, praz 500, iver 4

Rung 0A: The Vector No way to know this so long after the fact

The core question with diabetes is causality. Which parasite is causing the 6A Symptom? This can be a frustrating question because with diabetics, the 5A Location will MT for multiple 3A-1B-1A combinations. Lead-albendazole-whipworm; mercury-mebendazole-roundworm; arsenic-praziquantel-flatworm; chromium-ivermectin-filaria. Which one is it? Or are all of them putting the person over some tipping point?

We can rule out whipworm, roundworm and flatworm because when they are eliminated, the 6A Symptom fails to resolve. This places emphasis on filaria and explains a lot of things about diabetes, such as how it can be passed on from parents (some species of filaria are acquired in the womb) and also how it can manifest in someone without a prior health history (the wrong mosquito bite could do it).

However, we are led back to The Dosage Toxicity Problem explored previously, where the number of pills of ivermectin required to cancel out 3A elemental chromium when MT against the 5A pancreas of a 7A diabetic will far exceed the safe dose.

Resolving this becomes not a medical issue per se but a technological issue. Can we introduce a 1B Frequency Therapy that replicates the action of hundreds of pills of ivermectin so that we can explore whether diabetes resolves upon the elimination of the filaria we find in the pancreas of diabetics? Subordinate questions to this are do we have the right math to mesh with the body, do we have the right delivery system, do we have the right electrical engineering? These are physics questions; a doctor would be out of their depth here.

The Health Ladder Profile for Lyme Disease

Rung 7A: The Name Lyme Disease
Rung 6A: Symptom Progressively worse neurological issues
Rung 5A: Location MT brain? Probably the cerebrospinal fluid (CSF)
Rung 4A: Fungus/Virus Periodic viruses are an issue
Rung 3A: Metal Toxicity 6-valence metals like sulphur, selenium
Rung 2A: Bad Bacteria Borrelia and others. MT for doxycycline
Rung 1A: Parasites Babesia but also MT for ivermectin (filaria)
Rung 0A: The Vector A tick bite

In Lyme disease, the vector is easy to identify: a tick bite. What we are missing with this condition is the knowledge that the tick vector has not only injected us with the single-celled parasite babesia, and the bacterium borrelia, but also with a microfilarial parasite. Remember from Pt3-Ch8, all insect bites are vectors of filarial parasites.

Superimposing an awareness of filaria on what we already know about Lyme, a number of answers fall into place. Lyme symptoms are predominantly neurological, filaria can migrate to the CSF. Filaria can autopopulate: might this explain why Lyme symptoms never seem to go away? Most filaria require a stronger dose of medication than it is safe to take. Could this explain why Lyme doesn't respond to iver 1 (1x12mg) even though ivermectin treats filaria?

Understanding this, we can see a causal relationship between filaria and babesia, something that is not currently even suspected. Then, whether the filaria are the true host of borrelia or whether the babesia is responsible for it, we can see why medicating the babesia directly (with atovaquone) or the borrelia (with doxycycline) would not work. Treating a single-celled parasite, even though it is classified at 1A on The Health Ladder, is only one step removed from treating a 2A Bad Bacteria like borrelia. We must treat the multi-celled 1A Parasite.

This holds the promise of a permanent cure to Lyme but as always, we are brought back to the need for a 1B Frequency Therapy that can solve The Dosage Toxicity Problem with ivermectin, where 1x12mg is a safe dose, but where tick bites will MT for 6 to 50 pills, or higher.

The Health Ladder Profile for Multiple Sclerosis

Rung 7A: The Name   Multiple sclerosis
Rung 6A: Symptom   Deterioration of the myelin sheath
Rung 5A: Location   Nerve axons in the brain, body and spine
Rung 4A: Fungus/Virus No evidence of this
Rung 3A: Metal Toxicity Tellurium or selenium
Rung 2A: Bad Bacteria MT the patient for clindamycin/lincomycin
Rung 1A: Parasites   Filaria, MT for ivermectin
Rung 0A: The Vector   Possibly black flies

The vector in MS is not understood. In fairness, we cannot be sure that it is the black fly, a mosquito, a spider or even filaria as the 1A Parasite. MT analyses indicate a relationship with filaria so this is most likely, but more research is needed on this condition. What a MT makes clear is that some species of parasite is rampant in each case, that it has something to do with tellurium or selenium and that the arginine-rich myelin sheath seems to be consumed as a food source.

A characteristic of MS is a system-wide degeneration of the myelin sheath. Filaria travel throughout the body, so this lines up. Myelin is composed partly of arginine. Could this particular species of filaria be chewing away at the myelin sheath to get an arginine-rich lunch? In cases of MS, we find a MT correspondence between 3A tellurium, 1B ivermectin and 5B arginine. Is this worth closer examination?

If there were a set of cures for MS in place then I, admittedly not a credentialed neuroimmunologist, would hesitate to offer my opinion on the disease. However, when the best that the philosophy of diagnosis can come up with is that one 7A Name (MS) is caused by another (autoimmune), I think that at the very least, MS patients deserve to know whether anyone is exploring the filarial angle.

As always, we are brought back to the need for a 1B Frequency Therapy that can bypass The Dosage Toxicity Problem with ivermectin.

An additional concern with MS is that once the myelin sheath has been chewed away, it may not spontaneously regenerate. This is where a 5B Therapy like amino acid supplementation might be appropriate, and would be a great subject for an experiment in MT.

The Health Ladder Profile for Alzheimer's

Rung 7A: The Name   Alzheimer's disease
Rung 6A: Symptom   Loss of memory and identity, dementia
Rung 5A: Location   Hippocampus, amygdala, prefrontal cortex
Rung 4A: Fungus/Virus Autopsies reveal a fungal mat on the brain
Rung 3A: Metal Toxicity Aluminum. This is well-documented.
Rung 2A: Bad Bacteria MT for penicillin, amoxicillin
Rung 1A: Parasites   Tapeworms or large flukes in the digestive tract
Rung 0A: The Vector   Milk products, crop oils, syrups, deli meats

Establishing causality with Alzheimer's is complex and thankless. A MT analysis of the hippocampus will indicate aluminum; a MT of human parasite samples, cross referenced with Periodic Table MT Kit confirms that aluminum is the 3A Metal Toxicity with flukes. But are flukes the causal 1A Parasite for Alzheimer's? This is by no means certain and if so, the relationship is probably indirect.

For example, a fluke in the digestive tract could excrete an amoeba from the tissue-destroying category (E.Histolytica, for example) that could circulate through the body, end up in the brain and over a period of years, chew it into Swiss cheese, metaphorically speaking. When we contrast this with the action of another known brain eating amoeba, Naegleria fowleri, we can see that it is not unprecedented in nature for an amoeba to have a histolytic effect on brain tissue, with the distinction that some are slower than others.

However, it is just as possible that aluminum shows up in the hippocampus by coincidence, or via some shared metabolic pathway, but that it has no causal relationship with Alzheimer's. This reinforces a primary concern with MT, as with traditional biomedicine, namely that of differentiating correspondence from outcome.

Since most quantities of praziquantel, the medication that MT against aluminum, indicate values far above the safe dose, it would only be possible to explore whether the aluminum/fluke theory in Alzheimer's was correct by implementing a 1B Frequency Therapy that bypassed The Dosage Toxicity Problem with praziquantel.

Muscle Testing Cancer

We encounter a number of problems when trying to MT cancer.

First, since no MT will tell us that we have cancer, no MT can tell us that it's gone. Without this necessary feedback loop, we can't know whether anything we're MT is quantifying or working on cancer.

We can MT a location if we know where an already-cancerous tumor is but again, a random lump on the body that MT weak cannot be assumed to be cancerous just because it provoked a weak neurological response. A tissue biopsy would need to confirm that the lump was cancerous to begin with. We could then try to build on this.

Second, even if we are MT a medically proven cancerous indicator, (i.e., a lump that has been biopsied and diagnosed as cancerous) then we are back to the problem of correspondence versus outcome where we cannot be sure of causality. Several 3A Metal Toxicities will MT against a tumor (aluminum, arsenic, mercury, lead and selenium) and these will each indicate a different species of parasite (e.g., mercury is roundworm, aluminum is fluke, lead is whipworm) but can we blame one of these parasites over the others as the cause of the cancerous indicator? We cannot. There is no way to establish causality. Even if we eliminated every parasite in the host, extrapolating which parasite was the actual causal agent after the fact would be impossible.

The fact is, the body circulates 2A Bad Bacteria everywhere, but we cannot confidently blame the bacteria we find in a particular location for the 6A Symptom in that location.

It is most likely that cancer represents some sort of tipping point that the body has reached. If this is the case, it might be possible through eliminating enough 1A Parasites to bring the immune system back on the good side of the tipping point, and in such a case it may transpire that the cancer no longer expresses itself.

If a 1B Frequency Therapy were completely effective and if it were performed on someone with cancer, would it be possible for them to still have cancer when their parasite count was at zero? This is the question, but being technology dependent, it remains to be proven.

Further Reading on Medical Conditions

MT medical conditions is an advanced application. A number of details and exceptions will inevitably arise.

An expanded form of this information might be valuable not only to the patient suffering from the condition but also to physicians, pathologists, biologists and researchers who desire a MT perspective on their field. Several thousands of hours of data on The Health Ladder profiles for various medical conditions has been assembled for this purpose. These notes are presented in The Complete Muscle Testing Series: *Book 13 Muscle Testing Medical Conditions*.

Part 1 scrutinizes the physiology of medical conditions from tissue nutrient deficiency to a breakdown of lymphatic drainage, cellular repair and tumor formation.

Part 2 investigates The Health Ladder Profiles for the top 200 medical conditions with an emphasis on the role of the 1A Parasite and the 2A Bad Bacteria in the development of the pathology.

Part 3 outlines the process of a medical condition resolving itself once the underlying causes are eliminated and is a summary of the pathway to physical healing.

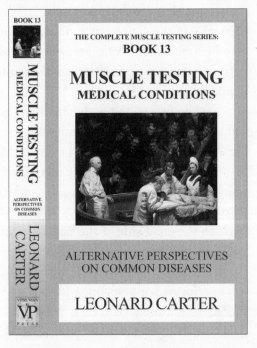

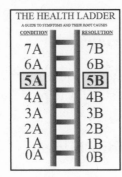

THE HEALTH LADDER	
A GUIDE TO SYMPTOMS AND THEIR ROOT CAUSES	
CONDITION	RESOLUTION
7A	7B
6A	6B
5A	5B
4A	4B
3A	3B
2A	2B
1A	1B
0A	0B

5A. LOCATION

The regions of the body that manifest the stress from RUNGS 1A–4A, often below the awareness threshold.

5B. THERAPY

RUNG 5B Therapy is support-focused: vitamins, supplements, herbs and some manual treatments attempt to heal the Location (5A).

14

Muscle Testing
Your Children

A s soon as a parent learns that MT can be used to quantify important health factors, their first impulse is to want to know how to apply it to the ones they love the most: their children.

This isn't only loving behavior, it is very intelligent behavior. Many of the parents I have taught MT to over the years have been among the smartest people I have met.

They are not dissuaded by MT's shady history, where it was misused to sell magnetic bracelets in trade shows or where major medical misdiagnoses were arrived at using Truth Testing. Parents understand one need: to fulfill their responsibility for the life and wellbeing of their child and it is obvious that MT, when correctly done, can provide a level of certainty not easily found elsewhere.

What parent hasn't spent hours in a waiting room with a sick child and weeks waiting for test results only to be told there is nothing wrong when the 6A Symptom is as clear as day? Or worse, that the cause of the 6A Symptom is the 7A Name. How frustrating is that? MT and The Health Ladder provide a way out of this desert.

Surrogate Testing Review

Children under 10 years of age are generally going to require Surrogate Testing. They rarely have the strength or joint stability to produce an accurate neurological response. (See pages 78, 89.)

Health Ladder Applications for Children

The multilayered perspective of The Health Ladder makes it clear that we aren't obligated to interpret a 6A Symptom at one rung only but can appreciate that all 8 rungs are factors simultaneously.

Focus naturally moves to the rung that we are able to have the most control over but this doesn't detract from an awareness of the other aspects of the condition.

Prioritization is given to the most effective action available. 1B Frequency Therapy as an electromagnetic technology, if it is effective, is the most ideal. A pharmaceutical form of a 1B Frequency such as an antiparasitic drug may also help. After that, a 2B Antibiotic is the next best thing. Then, 3B Metal Detox will have limited effect but might help. A 4B Antiviral medication can be indispensable in a state of crisis and a 5B Therapy is a good fallback plan. A 6B Treatment is not ideal but as a last resort can be the difference between life and death. At 7B, Social Support is a fair consolation prize but it often means the worst has already happened or is in the process of happening.

This describes the biomedical terrain a parent must navigate in the process of managing the health of their child. None of these options except the electromagnetic form of 1B Frequency Therapy is ideal, but needing to contend with the imperfect alternatives has been the human condition throughout time. It may take some time yet for the human race to arrive at a point where we even have a context in which to define and recognize perfection in healthcare (e.g., a child passes a MT organ exam with no parasites). This is partly technology dependent, and also subject to approval at various organizational and administrative levels of society, including political, regulatory, institutional, legal, socioeconomic and logistical.

Top 20 Childhood Medical Symptoms

What follows is a list of the most common 6A Symptoms that will affect a child. Divided into five main categories based on symptom groupings, the descriptions below place emphasis on understanding the critical point in each case. Taking an effective course of action will necessarily be dependent upon the resources available to the parents at the time.

Various Health Ladder applications from Rungs 1B to 6B can be MT for efficacy with each of these conditions. Some will be more effective than others, and unfortunately a MT will not indicate priority. As a reminder, a MT correspondence does not guarantee an outcome.

Eyes, Ears, Nose and Throat Symptoms:

1. Eye and vision issues The eye itself can play host to various parasite species, such as filaria or the dog roundworm, which children have exposure to. At 1B MT meb 200mg, various doses of ivermectin.

For a deterioration in vision (Pt3-Ch20), understand that the retinol that fuels the eyes can run low when there is a large worm in the digestive tract siphoning off the body's beta carotene. At 1B MT stomach and small intestine for various doses of antiparasitic medications. At 5B MT beta carotene or lutein. At 6B get eye glasses.

2. Ear aches This happens when 2A Bad Bacteria has clogged the lymphatic drainage passages below the ears. At 1B MT the small intestine or cerebrospinal fluid for parasites. At 2B MT antibiotics against the sore spot below the ear. At 3B find a metal detox binder. At 5B try vitamin D for its antibacterial properties.

3. Stuffy nose The lymphatic system is overwhelmed with 2A Bad Bacteria, the excess is flowing out through the sinuses. At 1B MT for any parasite in the throat, lungs or intestines. At 2B MT antibiotics. At 5B try vitamin D for antibacterial or vitamin C for tissue support.

4. Sore throat This is almost universally caused by a parasite in the throat tissue itself. If caught early with a 1B screen for parasite meds, they tend to be easier to eliminate when newly acquired.

Breathing Symptoms:

5. Breathing problems Shortness of breath and pulmonary inflammation are always the direct result of 2A Bad Bacteria. 2B Antibiotics are generally ineffective because they fail to address the chronic root cause but at 6B a corticosteroid inhaler (puffer) will suppress the immune response to the bacteria. At 1B MT the lungs and small intestines for roundworms and flukes or the circulatory system for albendazole. At 5B MT the lungs for beta carotene or lutein for mucosal support, or vitamin C for tissue support.

6. Cough More acute inflammation causing coughing can be a 4A virus or an invasive form of 2A Bad Bacteria. At 1B MT the lungs and small intestines for parasites or a 4B Antiviral. Sometimes a 2B Antibiotic will kill the bacteria that is causing the 3A Metal Toxicity. Since it is this that the 4A Virus is feeding on, this may address a general susceptibility to viruses.

Digestive Tract Symptoms:

7. Food allergies These are always caused by a parasite, usually in the intestines or stomach (Pt3-Ch11). However, these particular organisms are generally only identified by MT ultra-high doses of antiparasitic medications (in the thousands of pills) creating the limitation that only a 1B Frequency Therapy capable of replicating such a dosage of medication can eliminate them. The only other alternative is avoidance or a 6B treatment like an Epi-pen.

8. Stomach ache Either parasites have chewed away the mucosal layer in the stomach so that digestive acids are burning into the organ tissue or there are organisms physically burrowing into the tissue, excreting bacteria as they feed, all of which burns and hurts. Try MT for 1B antiparasitic medication doses, or at 5B MT the stomach for beta carotene or lutein to replenish the mucosal layer.

9. Vomiting In this case, toxic 2A Bad Bacteria from parasites is being excreted in or close enough to the stomach that the nervous system periodically engages in the vomiting response to get it out.

Try MT for 1B antiparasitic medications to quantify the organism. A 2B Probiotic might help if it is taken regularly or 5B beta carotene or vitamin C might support the mucosal lining.

10. Constipation Look for a severe mucosal lining deficiency in the large intestine. Parasites, generally inside the colon organ tissue, will siphon off the mucosal layer as a food source. The result is that the body lacks the lubrication to pass the feces out in a comfortable manner. At 1B MT the large intestine indicator areas for the organisms. At 2B a probiotic might help. At 5B ongoing beta carotene supplementation will top up the nutrients. Since beta carotene is an up-regulator of mucous production in the intestinal tract, it is possible to supplement with enough of it, in the short-term at least, to **pay the parasite mafia**, so to speak, and live relatively free from symptoms. However, beware of supplementing with beta carotene over the long term due to fat-soluble vitamin toxicity.

11. Diarrhea The evacuation of large amounts of 2A Bad Bacteria will alter the pH balance inside the small and large intestines. The altered pH causes the short-term suppression of your good bacteria. These can then no longer solidify the feces, which comes out in liquid form. At 1B MT the intestines for parasites. At 2B MT for a probiotic. At 5B MT the intestines for a digestive enzyme or vitamin C, which is toxic to parasites, or try drinking carbonated water for the same reason.

12. Acne Excessive 2A Bad Bacteria in the lymphatic system comes out in the form of pimples on the face and torso. During puberty, growth hormones speed up this process causing cosmetic concerns. At 1B MT the intestines, throat and sinuses for parasites. At 3B Metal Detox try some chelators or MT soap, toothpaste and other products to avoid certain metals. At 5B, try MT for vitamin C (tissue support) or vitamin D (antibacterial support).

13. Urinary Tract Infections Most UTIs have to do with 2A Bad Bacteria from parasites in the intestines washing through the bladder. At 1B MT the intestines for parasites but also the bladder itself. At 5B, try powdered cranberry, it seems to MT well against this.

Neurological Symptoms:

14. Headaches A common cause is an increase in intracranial pressure from 2A Bad Bacteria that has filled the cerebrospinal fluid (CSF). These bacteria can originate from a parasite in the digestive tract or from microfilaria living in the CSF which everyone hosts. A 3B Metal Detox binder can greatly help. At 5B MT for minerals like manganese and selenium but watch for over-supplementation (as a reminder of why, see p.117-118).

15. Dandruff Excess 2A Bad Bacteria in the CSF (see point 14 above) is often evacuated through the scalp as dandruff. 3B Metal Detox binders are a significant help but won't address the source of the bacteria. Focus should be on identifying the causal parasite.

16. Nightmares and insomnia Elevated levels of 2A Bad Bacteria in the CSF can directly impact the pineal gland, undermining normal functionality. To MT the pineal gland, see Pt3-Ch25, p.315)

17. Irritability and anxiety issues Elevated levels of 2A Bad Bacteria in the CSF can undermine functioning of the brain structures responsible for normal emotional behavior: the thalamus, hypothalamus, amygdala, hippocampus and prefrontal cortex. Narrowing down which 1A Parasite this is, using 1B antiparasitic medications, can be a challenge due to the child MT for overlapping dosages. There isn't a simple solution beyond eliminating everything with a blanket 1B Frequency Therapy treatment. Try MT for 3B Metal Detox, but it will only be a band-aid. Be cautious when MT for 5B brain-specific amino acids or omega oils to not create toxicity.

18. Learning difficulties Whether diagnosed with 7A Names like autism, ADD, ADHD or some other combination of letters, if the core symptom is that a behavior is out of control, look for the influence of a 2A Bad Bacteria. Narrowing down which 1A Parasite is excreting this can be a challenge as it may result from a combination of organisms. Try MT for 1B antiparasitic medications or a 3B Metal Detox binder. Remember that learning and behavior are also subject to non-parasite factors.

Metabolic Symptoms:

19. Overweight A tendency to carry a higher body fat level does not have to do with caloric intake, though exercise can be a factor. It is rooted in hosting a particular parasite that causes a deficiency in carnitine, the amino acid that allows us to metabolize fat. These could be the largest parasites in the body or the smallest. At 1B MT for roundworm, tapeworm or microfilaria but don't expect antiparasitic medications to be strong enough to eliminate them.

20. Underweight Difficulty in putting on weight tends to be the result of a higher than average parasite load siphoning off the nutrients before they can be converted into muscle and tissue. At 1B MT for any parasite you can find and do your best to eliminate it. When the body is past a tipping point, every improvement helps.

Other pediatric concerns: **Vaccines**

A MT analysis of a small number of vaccines has failed to indicate that any of them were an obvious nervous system stressor. If something about a particular vaccine were detrimental, this would show up as a weak MT.

In such a case it would be appropriate to refuse it and either find an alternative vaccine or make alternative plans.

It is a simple enough matter to MT a vaccine as the body's bioelectric field easily passes through the glass or plastic container.

> ### MT Protocol For Vaccines
>
> 1. Start with a baseline.
> 2. Hold the vaccine into your bioelectric field or that of the person being vaccinated and retest. Ensure that it is not in a metal casing.
>
> **A:** If the vaccine MT weak, avoid it.
> **B:** If the vaccine MT strong, there is no evidence of a problem with it.

The concern that a vaccine could cause autism doesn't line up with a Health Ladder interpretation of autism (i.e., Rung 4A is not 1A). However, it is theoretically possible that an engineered virus could negatively effect how a 2A Bad Bacteria expresses itself. A MT should pick up this potentiality in advance of the reaction happening.

Childcare Products to MT and Why

There are two reasons for any product MT weak: 1) It has 1A Parasite eggs in it, 2) It contains 3A Metals that are feeding 2A Bad Bacteria from parasites the child already hosts. You may not know whether you've found a metal or a parasite so follow The Golden Rule of MT: If it MT weak, don't use it.

Here is a short list of things you should MT, with notes on what I've periodically identified in these items.

Infants:

1. **Diapers** Often MT for copper or silver for its antimicrobial properties. These can cause diaper rash in some babies.
2. **Baby wipes** Same as the diapers above.
3. **Baby formula** Generally MT okay but you should be checking this.
4. **Laundry detergent** May contain metals that provoke a reaction.
5. **Dryer sheets** Same concern as laundry detergent.
6. **Soap** Can use MT to find one that agrees with the child.

Children:

7. **Child's gummy vitamins** MT for parasites eggs, these are in the unboiled corn syrup they're made with.
8. **Cough syrup** Also MT for various parasites from the corn syrup.
9. **Shampoo** Can use MT to find one that agrees with the child.
10. **Toothpaste** Can use MT to find one that agrees with the child.
11. **Sheets and blankets** Can use MT to screen for metal toxicity.
12. **Room paint and air fresheners** Can contain aerosol metals.

Adolescents:

13. **Deodorant** Screen for metal toxicity.
14. **Perfumes** Screen for metal toxicity, often cause headaches.
15. **Makeup** Screen for metal toxicity, can cause acne, headaches.

Hopefully this can get you thinking about other things to check. Remember, the point isn't to avoid these things per se, it is to be empowered to identify any potential negative health influences.

Further Reading on Muscle Testing Children

Because parents naturally love their children so much, and since the energy field of lovingness (Hawkins cal. 500) has more power than reason (Hawkins cal. 400-499), we see a greater open mindedness toward Health Ladder applications in pediatric conditions than we do when the matter concerns ourselves. The spirit rebels at the idea that a child should develop an adult medical condition. There is an intuitive recognition of the fundamental falsity of the interpretation that the 7A Name has caused the 6A Symptom in a child.

To strengthen this growing awareness in our society and to support parents in taking a more proactive role in managing the health of their children, The Complete Muscle Testing Series: *Book 14 Muscle Testing Your Children* is focused on elucidating the root causes of childhood medical conditions.

Part 1 is a summary of the basics of in utero, infant and childhood physiology.

Part 2 is a detailed outline of how parasites affect children in the early stages of their lives with an emphasis on pediatric immunology and endocrinology.

Part 3 covers The Health Ladder profiles for 100 of the most common pediatric medical conditions. This includes food allergies, digestive conditions, skeletal imbalances, breathing and inflammatory pathologies, vision issues, neurological and endocrine disorders, behavioral problems and learning disabilities.

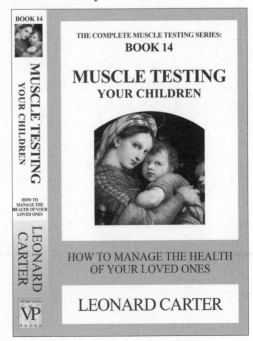

BOOK 14

THE COMPLETE MUSCLE TESTING SERIES:
BOOK 14

MUSCLE TESTING
YOUR CHILDREN

HOW TO MANAGE THE HEALTH
OF YOUR LOVED ONES

LEONARD CARTER

MUSCLE TESTING
YOUR CHILDREN

HOW TO
MANAGE THE
HEALTH OF YOUR
LOVED ONES

LEONARD CARTER

VITRUVIAN
VP
PRESS

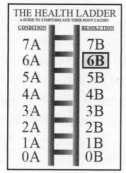

THE HEALTH LADDER	
A GUIDE TO SYMPTOMS AND THEIR ROOT CAUSES	
CONDITION	RESOLUTION
7A	7B
6A	6B
5A	5B
4A	4B
3A	3B
2A	2B
1A	1B
0A	0B

6B. TREATMENT

RUNG 6B Treatment is symptom-focused: surgery, drugs and some manual modalities are all designed to suppress the Symptom (6A).

15

Muscle Testing

The Elderly

Someone is elderly when they have reached both an age and a time when they require more care. They are typically incapacitated or at least have limited mobility. Degenerative medical conditions and pain management become a primary focus for themselves and those caring for them which is a pity, because with all those years of experience, a lifetime of knowledge and hearts filled with a love of existence, they should be running the world, not stuck in a bed somewhere.

The question, in cases like these, is that if we did know what we didn't know about their symptoms, could that information potentially help us to help them reduce their pain or degeneration?

The answer is yes, but of course this depends on what we need to know. There are a number of ways that a MT analysis can help to quantify degenerative issues.

We will explore these variables below.

What is Degeneration?

It is a misconception that we have a whole new body every 7 to 10 years. Our cells die at different rates. Cells in the colon die in 4 days. White blood cells last 2 weeks, red blood cells live for 4 months. A liver cell can survive for 18 months, some bone cells last 50 years.

However long they live, eventually all cells die and to ensure that you don't die with them, they copy themselves. But like an artist copying a masterpiece, the replica never looks the same. Whether this is caused by chemicals in the mitochondria, shortening telomeres, loss of stem cells or more obvious factors like deficiencies in proteins, fats, vitamins and minerals, emotional stress, air pollution, food quality, chemical exposure or lack of sleep, sunlight or fluoride, the fact is that cell copies don't quite match the original.

That is degeneration. A common estimate is that the human body can degenerate for a maximum of 130 years before it dies.

The problem is that nobody is getting there to prove whether this is accurate or not. We are degenerating faster than that. You can't see your liver aging but you can see it happening on your face. If you compare pictures of yourself 10 years apart, that's probably a good visual representation of your internal degeneration.

Researchers in senescence, the field of aging physiology, take a very intelligent approach to this. A lot of importance is placed on 5A Locations like the mitochondria, methyl accumulation in the DNA itself, protein degeneration in the telomeres or loss of stem cells. This is medical science at its best.

What you will not find, however, are studies on how 1A Parasites and their 2A Bad Bacteria facilitate degeneration at the 5A Location. This comes back to the problem that scientists haven't had an effective methodology of finding parasites in the human host and even if they did, there has been no 1B Frequency Therapy solution to The Dosage Toxicity Problem, so nobody can get them out. This is why so many cases of parasitosis have to end in surgery.

Ironically, some senescence researchers are studying the effect of aging on worms but not the effect of worms on aging.

Muscle Testing the Elderly

By the time someone is classified as elderly their nervous system will generally be functioning at a very low level. This means they will usually only be able to perform three to five MT before experiencing neurological fatigue. We see the same thing with younger people who are sick or have been diagnosed with autoimmune conditions, where they are only strong enough for a few MT and then everything stays weak.

A further issue with the elderly is that they rarely have the joint stability to be tested without hurting themselves. This is a different factor, though related, to neurological fatigue.

The solution is Surrogate Testing. As with infants and the very sick, elderly people should be surrogate tested at all times. This means that their care giver will always need a MT helper.

In the sections below, it will be assumed that the recommended MT for the elderly are being done via Surrogate Testing.

Health Ladder Applications

6B Treatment Do they need all those medications? With an elderly patient whose health is already fragile, a doctor can cause harm by guessing about medications and their dosages. This can be avoided by MT the medication against the target location and doing quantity testing to clarify the correct dosage. Ideally this would be done by the doctor but a concerned caregiver can also use this technique to check the doctor's advice, particularly when it is many months old.

Interestingly, a MT also identifies negative drug interactions. In a crisis, such as during an operation, it can be used to determine in seconds which drugs are needed. Anesthesiologists and oncologists in particular will find this information relevant and should be using it.

5B Therapy In an elderly person, all the 5A Locations will typically MT weak. A supplement regimen can be tailored to their needs using Surrogate Testing. This will both limit deficiency-related problems and minimize toxicity from incorrect or over-supplementing. See Pt3-Ch2 for more detailed information.

231

4A Fungus/Virus Although heartbreaking to see, it was not surprising that during the 2020 coronavirus pandemic, elderly populations were the most at risk and the hardest hit. A virus flourishes in a body high in 3A Metal Toxicity and someone with a lifetime of untreated 1A Parasites excreting 2A Bad Bacteria is going to be much more susceptible.

If there had been a MT protocol available to screen for the virus (a simple, general MT for valacyclovir would have been a good place to start) we might have avoided a lot of infections at retirement homes, for example, from visitors and in-house care givers.

Or what if society understood the need for 1B Frequency Therapy and this technology had become part of the culture? It is interesting to estimate how many lives might have been saved if we could have had a wireless antiparasitic frequency generator in the common room of every retirement home. Might this be something we could coordinate before the next pandemic comes along?

3B Metal Detox While 3A Metal Toxicity itself can be measured, the most effective action at Rung 3 would be taking a 3B binder to attempt to prevent the metal from allowing a 4A Virus to flourish.

It is not uncommon when performing a heavy metal analysis of an elderly person to see off-the-charts levels of particular elements. It is common to observe levels of chromium, arsenic, mercury, thallium and lead that would make your hair curl. Interestingly enough, personal care products such as hair dye are frequently the sources of such elevated quantities of these metals. While it is true that the metal sticks to the host because of their 2A Bad bacteria, we can still use a metal analysis to help minimize further exposure, and then a MT to select products that are less stressful for each person.

2B Pro/Antibiotics MT which antibiotic is needed is a great way of tailoring the medication to the patient, particularly in surgery when there isn't time to grow a culture in a petri dish.

Another application at Rung 2B is with probiotics. MT the right probiotic at the right quantity to the right elderly person can help them to better maintain their own inner bacterial balance.

1A Parasites A MT analysis of parasites in the elderly isn't different in concept from the rest of the population. In practice, however, we encounter a different consideration: the **parasite tipping point**.

While it is rare for a younger person to reach a tipping point of parasites, by definition someone in the 60+ year old category will be closest to that point. This is a function of 4 factors:

1. Size Most parasites grow in size over the years and the larger they become, the more 2A Bad Bacteria they can excrete.

2. Number of species We continually pick up new species as we age. The older we get, the more species we have had time to be exposed to.

3. Adaptation Parasites excrete bacteria and chemicals that modify our bodies to be more favorable to them. A higher level of arsenic is an example of this. The longer we host them, the more time these changes have to take place and affect us.

4. Auto-population Everyone hosts parasites from the microfilarial family. They autopopulate, and the more years they live in us, the longer they have to fill every available niche in our health ecosystems.

One of the reasons an elderly person's health is so fragile is that when they are already at the 4-factor parasite tipping point, they can't afford to pick up a single new species. Yet they do, anyway.

We have all seen someone in this age range go from healthy and balanced to very sick, very fast, and then they die. It is the sudden slippery slope many elderly people fear. When I have had the opportunity to MT someone in this position, I have always found what looked like a new parasite in the person, usually in the digestive tract. A concerned caregiver should be looking out for this.

0A The Vector The source of the new parasite that puts an elderly person over the tipping point will depend on the species. The worst group, filaria, almost universally come from mosquito or insect bites, though black pepper and other spices grown in tropical manures are a source as well. Picking up parasites like roundworm, fluke or tapeworm after a certain age can result in hospitalization due to their growth rate and these come from the same simple sources you would expect. It's just bad luck which subspecies (serotype) someone gets.

Diagnosis Versus Treatment

When we are able to move past the conceptual limitation of placing undue importance on the 7A Name of medical issues in the elderly, or for that matter on the 6A Symptom, focus moves to addressing the root cause. Since this is understood to be 1A Parasites, the question of how to treat the parasite becomes of paramount importance.

A stark look at the numbers tells us that as a form of 1B Frequency Therapy, chemical FQs (pharmaceutical antiparasitic medications) are effective on fewer than 10% of the parasites a host is likely to have. It was the personal experience of the author that medications worked on fewer than 1% of his own collection.

This brings up 2 treatment concerns for the elderly.

1. Medication toxicity Even the 1-10% of parasites an elderly person hosts that a medication might eliminate can't be treated if they cannot take the pills. There are numerous concerns: drug interactions, cost, lack of diagnosis or medical supervision, risk of secondary complications or just not being physically strong enough to handle the nausea, vomiting and neurological side effects of the medications. And remember, we are still only talking about the parasites a medication could eliminate.

2. Medication insufficiency The larger concern is that 90% of the parasites in an elderly person can't be eliminated even if they take pills. What can they do in a case like this? For that matter, what can any of us do? Nothing. It has been the human condition throughout the ages to suffer from parasites and not be able to do anything.

The development of a 1B Frequency Therapy technology that uses clean electricity with no pharmaceutical side effects is obviously of great interest to the entire human race, and the elderly are no exception. The difference is that the elderly need it more because getting the right parasite out can actually save their lives.

It is a prediction that the urgent nature of geriatric medical conditions will be one of the factors that creates pressure for approval of 1B Frequency Therapy in medical systems around the world.

Top 10 Degenerative Conditions

Here is a list in random order of the conditions that tend to express themselves as the aging process advances. Included is a short physiological explanation of how parasites contribute to each condition.

1. Arthritis Look for the following combination of indicators: a species of filaria that has got into the arthritic bones (MT the bone for high doses of ivermectin) and a larger flatworm or roundworm in the digestive tract contributing its portion of the bacterial equation.

2. Bladder control This tends to be the result of a tipping point of bacteria from various parasite species inflaming the bladder tissue.

3. Insomnia Any 2A Bad Bacteria in the cerebrospinal fluid can potentially inflame the pineal gland. See Pt3-Ch25 for more specifics.

4. Hair loss This is the result of widespread protein deficiency, usually from a parasite tipping point. See Pt3-Ch19 for more specifics.

5. Loss of mucosal linings This is the parasite tipping point causing widespread deficiency in vitamin A and beta carotene. It can be supported with high dose supplementation over the short term.

6. Poor eyesight A combination of vitamin A deficiency and bacterial inflammation inside the eye itself, both caused by a parasite tipping point. See Pt3-Ch20 for more specifics.

7. Loss of hearing Look for high levels of 2A Bad Bacteria in the lymphatic system, especially in the cerebrospinal fluid (Pt3-Ch20).

8. Loss of taste, smell These have the same root cause as hearing loss (above). It is common for these to return if the parasite is eliminated.

9. Loss of sexual arousal A combination of loss of circulation, reduced sex hormones, an increase in 2A Bad Bacteria and the tryptophan-serotonin pathway (outlined on p.325).

10. Cognitive degeneration This is caused by high levels of 2A Bad Bacteria in the ventricular system (p.317), usually from microfilaria.

Some common denominators in each of these conditions are:
1) Microfilaria 2) Time to cause damage 3) The parasite tipping point
    This doesn't have to be the human condition. An understanding of the variables clarifies the need for a 1B solution.

Further Reading on Muscle Testing the Elderly

Caring for the elderly presents the unique challenge of not wanting to do anything to hurt them and not wanting to do nothing. The Complete Muscle Testing Series: *Book 15 Muscle Testing the Elderly* creates a context for these decisions.

To support their direct caregivers as well as geriatric medical practitioners and retirement home staff, this book is a condensed outline of the MT someone would need to understand to manage the health of an elderly person.

Part 1 is a review of the physiology of the aging process and which MT to use to quantify age-related medical conditions, along with an examination of the benefits of high-dose supplementation to offset specific deficiencies.

Part 2 outlines how parasites can affect seniors with special emphasis on immunological interactions between different parasite species in the host.

Part 3 explores The Health Ladder profiles for 200 of the top geriatric medical conditions.

One of the aims of this book is that it can get the right information to people in their 50s-80s who are merely aging, and help them to make decisions that can hold off the time when they become elderly and need other people to care for them.

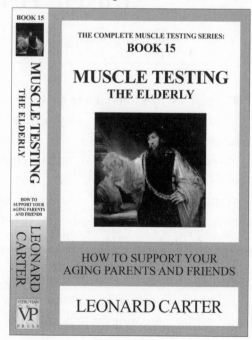

THE HEALTH LADDER

A GUIDE TO SYMPTOMS AND THEIR ROOT CAUSES

CONDITION	RESOLUTION
7A	7B
6A	6B
5A	5B
4A	4B
3A	3B
2A	2B
1A	1B
0A	0B

5A. LOCATION

The regions of the body that manifest the stress from RUNGS 1A–4A, often below the awareness threshold.

5B. THERAPY

RUNG 5B Therapy is support-focused: vitamins, supplements, herbs and some manual treatments attempt to heal the Location (5A).

16

Muscle Testing

Dogs, Cats and Other Pets

I f you are lucky enough to have earned the love of a pet then you know what other people probably do not: that the bond with an animal is the purest way to experience unconditional love (Hawkins cal. 540). It is natural to reciprocate this, and to want your pet to be as happy and healthy as possible. But health deteriorates over time, and eventually every pet owner will come to understand the feeling of helplessness when their pet gets sick.

Is there a way to use MT to help? Absolutely.

In this section we will examine various applications of MT for pets. My primary experience is with dogs, having had a Collie and an English Springer Spaniel, but the concepts transfer easily to cats and with a little more thought to horses, birds and other animals.

Surrogate Testing Your Pets

It is the case that all pets host multiple species of parasites. The 0A Vectors are impossible for animals to avoid: They acquire the first few species from their mother's milk and the rest from chewing dirty sticks, picking up balls from the mud, all rawhide bones, many contaminated treats and, of course, all insect bites.

However, to understand what is going on biologically with your pet, whether your focus is at the 6A Symptom or the 1A Parasite, you will need to gather information from the 5A Location. For this process to be effective, your pet needs to be MT and as with children and the elderly, the only way to do this is through Surrogate Testing.

Any location can be MT: the eyes, the snout, the tongue, the paws, the fur or the organs. If you are familiar with human organ MT, you will find that the locations are similar. Refer to the chart below for the most common MT points on dogs and cats.

Organ Locations for a Pet

1. STOMACH **Where** Soft tissue just below the ribs. **Function** Begins digestion, timed release of food into the small intestine. **Dysfunctions** Vomiting, itching, stomach ache, cramps, hiccoughs, ulcers, initial allergic responses to foods.	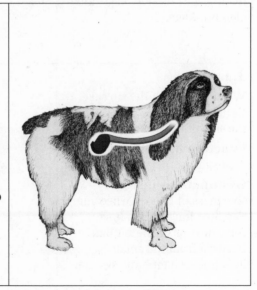

2. SMALL INTESTINE

Where Soft tissue from the stomach to between the back legs.

Function Digestion and nutrient absorption.

Dysfunctions Diarrhea, skin rashes, food allergies, bloating, gas, 2A Bad Bacteria that circulates elsewhere in the body, such as the lungs or ears.

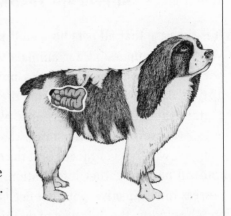

3. LARGE INTESTINE /RECTUM

Where Easiest to access by MT the soft tissue around the anus, or above the back haunches underneath the spine.

Function Solidifies and evacuates feces.

Dysfunctions Diarrhea, itching, gas, fecal leakage, anal gland leakage.

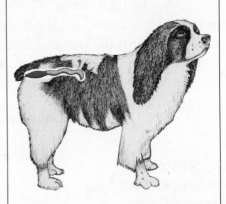

4. LUNGS

Where Beneath the rib cage. Easiest to MT each lung from the side of the torso.

Function Breathing, expelling waste gases.

Dysfunctions Cough, shortness of breath, wheezing. Can host lung flukes, lung roundworms or the 2A Bad Bacteria from the small intestine or lymphatic system.

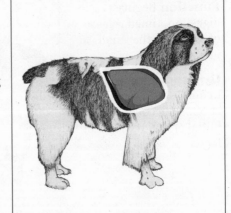

Top 10 Parasites That Pets Have

	Name	0A Vector	What is it? (Pathology)	Medication to MT for
1	**Toxoplasma Gondii** (Toxoplasmosis)	Cats, Raw meat	Single-celled parasite that can get into our CSF and cause neurological issues	**Pyri-methamine** (Sulfadoxine)
2	**Tapeworm 1** (Cystic/Alveolar Echinococcosis)	Dogs	The smallest tapeworms you can get: 1mm-7mm, but their eggs encyst and can kill humans	MT for **Praziquantel** dosage varies
3	**Tapeworm 2** (Dipylidium caninum)	Fleas and Lice	When dogs, cats or humans accidentally ingest a flea or louse, a 2-foot tapeworm can grow in the intestines	MT pets and humans for **Praziquantel** dosage varies
4	**Toxocara Canis, Toxocara Cati** (Toxocariasis)	Dog and Cat feces	Roundworms that burrow through tissues. They like the eyes. Eggs become infectious after 2 weeks in nature	MT Pets for **Fenbendazole** MT humans: **Mebendazole**
5	**Whipworm** (Trichuriasis)	Any feces (dog, cat, human, cow, pig)	Eggs in soil become infectious after 1 month, grow into 2-inch worm, lives in the intestines for 1 year	MT Pets for **Fenbendazole** MT humans: **Mebendazole**
6	**Hookworm**	Feces	Soil-transmitted worms that live in the intestines and drink blood through the venous tissue wall	MT Pets for **Fenbendazole** MT humans: **Mebendazole**
7	**Fluke** (Various species)	Snails, Soil	Flatworms that are adapted to live in every organ causing local dysfunction	MT for **Praziquantel** dosage varies
8	**Rat Lungworm** (Angiostrongyliasis)	Snails, Water	Roundworm can cause a cough or bacterial meningitis	No known treatment
9	**Heartworm** (Dirofilariasis, esp. Dirofilaria Immitis)	Mos-quitoes	Roundworm in dogs that fills the veins leading to the heart. In cats it doesn't come to full maturity but still causes lung issues. In humans it can hatch in the blood vessels, face or eyes	**Ivermectin** (MT for ultra-high dose, antigens may show up in blood test)
10	**Giardia Lamblia** (Giardiasis)	Water, Feces	A single-celled parasite found in all water. Cannot be avoided, only minimized	MT Pets and humans for **Metronidazole** 250mg

The Logic of Antiparasitic Medications

Your instinct will be to assume that your pet is free from all of the above parasites. After all, you love them and you have a clean house and parasites are dirty and only infect unloved pets, right?

This is precisely why your pet has at least half of the parasites on the above list, if not all of them. Pet owners are so certain parasites are not there that they're not even looking for them.

The way to make sure that your pet is actually parasite free is to be scientific and methodical with a MT analysis of the organ locations, cross referenced with the antiparasitic medications. Then, use simple logic: If a negative lung MT is turned back to a positive with fenbendazole, it is reasonable to conclude that the lungs must (or at the very least, may) be hosting something that fenbendazole treats. This applies to all organs.

> **MT Protocol**
> **For Parasites In Pets**
> 1. Surrogate test a baseline.
> 2. Find an organ location indicator that MT weak.
> 3. Place an antiparasite medication on the pet and redo the step 2 above.
>
> **A:** If the meds plus indicator still MT weak, no correlation.
> **B:** If the meds plus indicator now MT strong, your pet must have whatever parasite the meds are designed to treat.

Pet Antiparasitic Medications

There are only 4 main antiparasitic medications you need to understand to be able to use basic logic in a MT analysis of your pet:

1	Fenbendazole	Treats and therefore indicates roundworm (in pets)
2	Praziquantel	Treats and therefore indicates fluke and tapeworm
3	Ivermectin	Treats and therefore indicates filaria and dirofilaria
4	Metronidazole	Treats and therefore indicates amoeba and giardia

At this stage of understanding, the medicine will not tell you which species you have found, just what category the parasite falls in. This allows you to decide which course of treatment to follow.

1B Frequency for Pets: Medication

The problem with treating a pet for worms is that every bite of nature is chock-full of parasite eggs. As with human physiology, the parasites they already have protect them from simply getting more. At this level of thinking, deworming is futile unless there is a crisis.

In a crisis, a parasite has progressed from neutral to harmful. Full deworming would be counter-productive, taking away all of your pet's protection from their environment but is partial deworming possible? Can you target the single organism causing the problem?

You can try. The paradox is that by the time it has become a problem, a parasite will probably need a dosage of medication too toxic for your pet to handle. You can quantity test antiparasitic medications against the symptomatic location but there is no guarantee that the parasite you find in your MT is the one causing the symptom. If you think this sounds random and frustrating, that's pharmacology for you.

1B Frequency for Pets: Bioelectromagnetism

This paves the way for an understanding of the need for a clean, comprehensive 1B Frequency Therapy. Just imagine if you could turn on a frequency generator and eliminate all parasites in your pet and the medical symptoms they cause. This is a higher level of thinking but it comes with a cost: your pet will have lost all of their protection.

Now, every time they have a contaminated treat, eat a wild animal, chew on a bone or some rawhide, or so much as pick up a ball out of the mud, they will vomit or have diarrhea as the new organism hatches. And then you have the filarial and dirofilarial classes of parasites to think about from every insect bite. The Parasite Motel Rooms are all vacant.

If it were possible to have an effective, wireless 1B Frequency Therapy running continuously in the room where your pet slept, reinfection wouldn't matter, as they would get a physiological reset every night. This would be ideal but isn't technologically feasible at this stage and will probably only begin to be available when we as a society become aware that such a technology is needed.

The Health Ladder for Pets

If the root cause of the 6A Symptom can be eliminated at Rung 1B, then your pet is off The Health Ladder and out of the desert.

If it can't, you will need to manage the 2A Bad Bacteria that is constantly being reproduced, which is at the source of inflammation, bad breath, limping, lameness, fur and skin conditions, mucous, dental problems, deteriorating eyesight, snoring, constipation, diarrhea, loose stools and every other symptom they have.

For pets, it is second-most effective to treat this at Rung 3B: Metal Detox. While humans usually MT for needing mineral chelators like magnesium, pets need MSM and the greens chelators: barley grass, chlorella, spirulina, wheat grass. These are essential components to every Pet MT Kit. Don't worry about compliance: offered a binder that they need, your pet will consider it a treat. They know exactly what they need.

Misconceptions About Parasites and Pets

1. You get parasites from petting them This is not likely. It is possible to inhale parasite eggs from dust, or to accidentally swallow them but based on experience with this issue it is extremely uncommon. Hookworm can infect you through your skin but you would feel it happening. It would start as an itch and then burn for hours. Rubbing alcohol would kill it if caught before it burrowed too deep.

Remember that most parasite eggs need to go through an intermediate host like a snail, flea, black fly, louse or mosquito before becoming an infection risk to you. Insect vectors present a very grave health risk and should be taken extremely seriously but this can be a problem even if you're not a pet owner. If you redirected all your concern about getting parasites from pets to the insect world, your fears would be justified and your attention better spent.

2. Raw diets are healthy for animals The misguided idea is that since wild animals eat raw food, domesticated breeds can (and should) as well. This is probably the best way to kill your pet as early as possible. All raw meat (100%) carries multiple species of parasite eggs. In nature, this exposure leads to natural selection: The animals that can handle all these parasites survive while the ones that can't, die early. However, even the survivors have a much shorter life span than domestic animals. As with humans, a raw diet ensures a maximum parasite burden which increases the likelihood of an early death.

3. One yearly deworming pill kills all parasites As with humans, the 3 main categories of parasites a pet will host are flatworm (tapeworm, fluke), roundworm and filaria. No single medication works on all categories, some species can't be killed by pills at all and when they can the dosage is usually too low to work. Then, many dog and cat medicines treat fleas only. Do the math. At the very least you need to MT this.

4. Medication spacing It is a mistake to believe that a medication is only effective if it is re-administered a second time 1 to 4 weeks after the first dosage. This doesn't match the MT evidence, which indicates that the medication is needed for 2 to 5 consecutive days. This myth is probably perpetuated because of the belief that newly laid parasite eggs hatch in the body at a later date, but any first-year biology student knows that these organisms can't autopopulate because they require an intermediate host outside your pet to complete their life cycle.

MT Applications for Your Pets

1. MT (on them, not yourself) their brand of pet food. Can vary by bag.
2. MT their brand of daily treats. Can vary by bag.
3. MT rawhide bones and food-based chew toys to avoid parasite eggs.
4. MT garden fertilizer if you use it, to avoid covering your back yard in parasite eggs your pet will consume or track into the house.
5. MT any vaccine before they're injected.
6. MT which antiparasitic medicine to give them.
7. MT their vomit or stools (if runny) against the pet antiparasitic medications to see what they have just picked up.
8. MT which 3B binder to give them to support an ongoing condition.
9. MT a household food you want to give them and aren't sure about.
10. Teach your pet how to MT you. It won't work, but it's cute.

Further Reading on Muscle Testing Pets

Pets can pick up many of the same parasites that we can but also quite a number that we can't. This requires different avoidance and treatment strategies.

The Complete Muscle Testing Series: *Book 16 Muscle Testing Dogs, Cats and Other Pets* compresses all of these details into a single volume.

Part 1 provides a complete outline of canine and feline anatomy with the appropriate MT points to make location-specific distinctions. We touch briefly on supplementation for pets but it isn't generally recommended.

Part 2 lists the top species of parasites that dogs and cats fall prey to. This is relevant for understanding specific medical pathologies in pets and may help to resolve the symptom or at least support them better. Emphasis is placed on environmental and insect vectors as these are the primary modes of infection.

Part 3 includes a series of Health Ladder profiles for various pet medical conditions, both for my own dogs and for the other pets I have worked with over the years.

They're cute little things, let's keep them as healthy as possible.

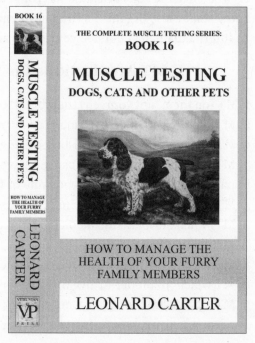

BOOK 16

THE COMPLETE MUSCLE TESTING SERIES:
BOOK 16

MUSCLE TESTING
DOGS, CATS AND OTHER PETS

MUSCLE TESTING DOGS, CATS AND OTHER PETS

HOW TO MANAGE
THE HEALTH OF
YOUR FURRY
FAMILY MEMBERS

HOW TO MANAGE THE
HEALTH OF YOUR FURRY
FAMILY MEMBERS

LEONARD CARTER

LEONARD CARTER

VITRUVIAN
VP
PRESS

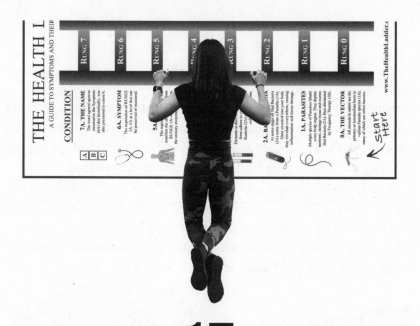

17

Muscle Testing

Your Workout Program

Working out isn't a rung on The Health Ladder, it's what we do when we're finally healthy enough to get off the ladder.

This is the major misconception of the fitness industry-more of a deception, really: that if one is out of shape, exercise will get them back into shape and all that's needed is a little motivation.

In fact, fat gain is more often the result of carnitine deficiency, muscle loss is general amino acid deficiency and an inability to move quickly or lift heavy weights is the result of weakness, pain and inflammation, all of which are caused by parasites, not laziness.

If we try to push through the above factors we run into the real problems: 1) Loose tendons and ligaments 2) Bad form in our exercises. Between the two, we have a recipe for injury.

We will explore these issues in the sections below.

Tendons and Ligaments: Connective Tissues

For those not fluent in muscle anatomy, **tendons** connect muscle to bone, **ligaments** connect bone to bone. If these connective tissues are loose (lax) our muscles will be weak and our joints will get injured when we put them under load. Body weight counts as load.

There is a simple test you can do to evaluate the tightness or laxity of your connective tissues: try to gently bend one of your fingers backwards at the middle joint. Under pressure, it should remain at a flat 180° angle. If it moves into the 190° range or greater, that is happening because of tendon and ligament laxity.

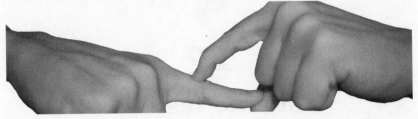

Laxity can be analyzed at different levels. There will be a mineral deficiency, often manganese, and also an amino acid deficiency, often collagen. This can be MT. But why are you deficient? Only parasites could have such a system-wide impact. This means that without addressing your parasites, the underlying laxity will persist.

Where does that leave you? Whether you have eliminated your parasites and need a year for your connective tissues to tighten up, or whether you still have the parasites and therefore the deficiencies and the consequent laxity, you need to be careful with your exercise form or you'll get microtears in your tendons.

> **MT Protocol For Tendons and Ligaments**
>
> 1. Start with a MT baseline.
> 2. Firmly bend a finger ligament backwards, then quickly have someone perform a MT on an indicator muscle.
>
> **A:** If strong, good.
> **B:** If weak, hold collagen or manganese against your bioelectric field and redo the MT. If one of them cancels out the weak MT, quantity test for dosage.

Microtears in the Tendons

Correct exercise form ensures that all the weight you're lifting goes on your muscles, not your connective tissues. This tonifies the muscles, strengthens you and is a great stress reliever. It also ensures that your joints stay safe.

With incorrect form, you're lifting the same amount of weight but the portion that the muscles aren't absorbing goes onto the tendons and ligaments. This strains them.

When you're young they can handle this strain but as you age, the cumulative impact of nutrient deficiency and years of bad form takes its toll on your tendons and ligaments. They become lax and develop what are called **microtears**. Imagine little strands of a rope fraying and then finally, over the years, the rope breaks. Same idea.

This is probably the leading cause of all exercise-related injury. It is also the main reason that young people are more effective athletes and soldiers, and why free weight rooms in gyms tend to be devoid of seniors.

Therefore, whether you are exercising to get healthy or stay healthy, correct exercise form is absolutely essential.

My Exercise History

I have a personal interest in the matter of exercise form.

In my teens I was preparing to study philosophy at university. When I was diagnosed with ulcerative colitis at 16, it caused a shift in how I thought about health. At the time I didn't know that my condition was caused by a parasite but I found that I could keep the symptoms under control if I lifted weights. Weight lifting became my first priority because it was made clear by my gastroenterologist that if the ulceration got any worse, they'd have to cut my colon out.

I went to university but for a number of reasons, my health being one of them, I dropped out and got a job in a gym. Looking back, I probably made better money than I would have in philosophy and since that was where I learned about MT, it was for the best.

248

Over time, I got the colitis under control but an older, more debilitating problem started to become more severe: nerve pinching. From 13 years old I had suffered from sudden unexpected impingement. With weight lifting as an adult, the degree of impingement worsened. No longer a little pinch or a sore muscle, my neck or back experienced such a severe spasm from an impingement that I would be paralyzed for a week. Each breath was excruciating, movement was impossible. It is difficult to communicate in writing a level of pain that requires absolute immobility for a week.

And all of this came from doing a simple bench press, a shoulder press or a squat. I would exercise for 2 months, pinch a nerve and spend a week paralyzed, then take 3 weeks to recover and do it all over again. I tried to be careful, that's why it only happened every third month. I would have stopped lifting weights entirely but then it happened from other things like opening a door or looking over my shoulder while walking.

This made no sense because X-rays showed nothing wrong with my spine and by this time my exercise form was textbook perfect. And of course there was no MT analysis available yet to tell me that the impingement was the result of increased pressure from 2A Bad Bacteria in the cerebrospinal fluid along my vertebral foramen. I always suspected my exercise form was making an underlying problem worse, but I could never isolate exactly how.

When I was finally introduced to MT, it became clear that one application was to evaluate the effect of exercise form on my nervous system. I did a thorough analysis and the results were troubling. I wasn't just doing a couple of exercises wrong: my form was wrong on all of them. For someone who had been working in the health club industry as a personal trainer and manager for the preceding 10 years by this time, this was mind boggling. I and my colleagues were the arbiters of correct form. For my form to be wrong, that meant the textbooks had the wrong form as did the entire fitness industry and by extension, the world. No wonder I was hurting myself.

The question became how to fix the problem.

Where Does Correct Form Come From?

To start, where does bad form come from? The original way of exercising was introduced by the first fitness gurus in the early to mid 20th century, people like Frank Zane, Jack Lalanne and Joe Weider. They were icons, certainly, but not specialists in biomechanics. In fairness, there was no such thing back then. Their misconceptions were perpetuated by the next generation of fitness competitors and from there, the wrong form became dogma and moved into academia.

We can see the effect of this when the body building greats of yesterday are interviewed. Schwarzenegger has lost all of his muscle mass. Dorian Yates only does yoga. Ronnie Coleman is in a wheel chair.

If correct form were a simple matter of consulting with a personal trainer, I would suggest it, but trainers don't understand this any better than you do. Having hired hundreds of them in my health clubs over the years and eventually having run a national seminar company specializing in biomechanics, Vitruvian Training, I can verify that personal trainers are subject to the same misconceptions as everybody else and in fact seem to be quite receptive to embracing new misconceptions that the rest of us haven't heard of yet.

And who can blame them when every exercise science textbook and certification manual reinforces poor form? Not only do instructional pictures on the exercise machines demonstrate the wrong form, the machines themselves are designed around mistaken ideas about what constitutes correct form. To be clear, most exercises aren't off by much. An inch too low here, an internal rotation there, the feet six inches closer than they should be and the effect is that everything looks fine until a tendon pops off and you're on crutches for three months. In your teens and 20s this won't matter because your ligaments are tight. After 30 it is a concern and since exercise should take place into your 100s, it is a real issue.

There is a universal correct form but it doesn't come from a textbook, the picture on the machine, your personal trainer or the way it has been done for 100 years. It is confirmed in only one way: MT the effect of the exercise on your own nervous system.

Muscle Testing Exercise Form

Exercise form is not relative, it is absolute because we all have the same basic biomechanical makeup. The most effective way of confirming this is to base your understanding of correct form on a MT.

If the MT is strong, that set of variables (form, weight, range of motion, speed) is safe. If instead the MT is weak, you have identified something about the exercise that is placing excessive load on your tendons, ligaments and nerves. Either it's the wrong form or it's too heavy or you did it too fast. By using a slower speed and a lighter weight, we can isolate for exercise form only and with some experimentation, we can use MT as a feedback loop to tell us the correct form.

> ### MT Protocol For Exercise Form
>
> 1. Start with a baseline.
> 2. Perform 1 repetition of the exercise in question.
> 3. Then within 3-5 seconds, have someone MT you and compare to the baseline.
>
> **A:** If the MT is strong, your form is probably fine.
> **B:** If there is an exercise shut-off, your form is wrong.
> **C:** Keep retesting until you get it right.

The conscious mind will not notice this minute level of stress but a MT will pick it up. We can call this the **Exercise Shut-off Concept** and it would be wise to interpret it to indicate that micro-tears are happening.

A full MT analysis of all exercises indicates that traditional form will almost universally provoke a weak response. This includes the core exercises in any gym: squat, dead lift, bench press, pull ups. It applies equally to free weights and machines.

While the purpose of exercise is to strengthen, poor form only weakens. The desire is to feel good but this process leads to pain and injury. The goal is longevity but this hastens the aging process.

In the sections that follow we will examine a few examples of exercises that are being done incorrectly with an explanation of how to improve your form to ensure safety. You are encouraged to apply MT to these exercises to confirm the information.

The Squat: Leg Spacing

Works: quads, glutes, hamstrings, calves

Incorrect Spacing *(too wide)*

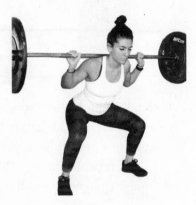

Most squat spacing is either too wide or too narrow. This forces the femur to rotate in the pelvic socket at an angle that doesn't allow the quads or glutes to fire fully, stressing the spine.

With body weight this won't cause injury, but when squatting a heavy load or landing from a jump it is a recipe for a back or knee injury.

It will also prevent you from ever reaching your full squat potential.

Correct Spacing

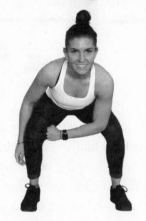

If you place your fist and forearm between your knees, as shown in the attached image, this provides the natural, anatomically correct spacing for your legs when doing a squat.

If you try this you should find that it MT strong. Then, move your foot even an inch out of alignment and retest it. It should MT weak. Check your spacing with this method every time you squat until your foot placement is intuitive.

Comments: This method of leg spacing is not only the best way to avoid injury, it has the potential to increase the amount of load you can squat by up to 50%. If you know anything about weight lifting you'll know that's unheard of. The problem is that most seated squat machines don't have a foot placement pad that is wide enough for correct spacing. Don't trust the machine design. MT it for yourself.

| The Bench Press: Depth | Works: pecs, shoulders, triceps |

Incorrect Form

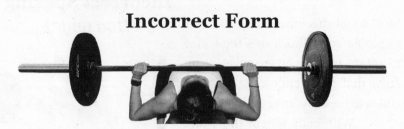

Bringing the bar down to your chest hyperextends the shoulder joint. The pec muscles are no longer bearing all the load. This increases the likelihood of a pectoralis major tear and a shoulder capsule injury.

The misconception is that this form gives you a deeper workout and builds stronger pecs. All it really does is cause microtears.

Correct Form

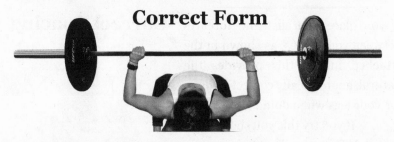

While it is counterintuitive that only moving your pecs through (what seems like) half the range of motion gives you a better workout, the fact is that keeping your arm (the humerus) parallel with the floor is the only way to ensure that the pecs bear the load. Move the elbow another inch lower and the exercise MT weak. The load needs to stay on your pecs and off your tendons, rotator cuff and shoulder capsule.

Comments: From body builders to personal trainers to exercise science textbooks, bringing the bar down to your chest is unquestioned common sense. It must be right because it has always been done that way. Then, when there is a pec tear, which is inevitable, the bizarre rationalization is that you must have gone too heavy.

The Lat Pulldown: Arm Spacing

Works: lats, rhomboids, mid-trapezius, biceps, forearms

When your arms are angled out too wide it puts strain on the shoulder capsule and destabilizes the joint.

The misconception is that a wider grip gives you wider lats. This is not true. All it does is predispose you to dislocating your shoulder.

Don't trust the instructional picture that is pasted on the machine, its design is based on this misconception. MT it for yourself and see.

Incorrect Form

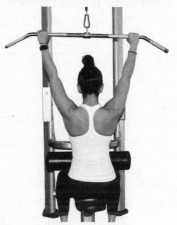

If you place your arms straight over your head and then angle them out six inches each, this lines them up with the muscle fibers in your lats. By placing the load in a lat pulldown on the lat itself, and not on the shoulder capsule, this is both the safest form and will give you the best lat workout.

Make sure to only pull the bar in front of your head, not behind the neck, which will also MT weak.

Correct Form

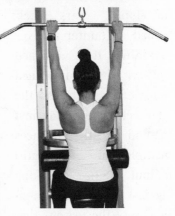

Comments: One day in the gym I was waiting to use the lat pulldown machine. A trainer was instructing a gentleman in his mid-40s that the best way to get nice, wide lats was to grip the bar as widely as possible. Part way through the set, out popped the poor guy's arm from its shoulder capsule. Just brutal. He was taken away on a stretcher. What we need to understand isn't that bad form is bad, it's that what we assume is good form is bad form.

Further Reading on Muscle Testing Workouts

With correct form, you should be able to lift weights well into your 100s and never injure yourself, assuming that you are off The Health Ladder and able to exercise.

There are quite a number of applications of MT to exercise form. It used to take an 8-hr day to teach all of it to personal trainers. This was day-1 from the 3-day VTS Level 1 course that I taught through my old seminar company.

A complete outline of all the exercise techniques in that course is presented in The Complete Muscle Testing Series: *Book 17 Muscle Testing Your Workout Program*.

Part 1 clarifies the physiology of exercise form including the motor neuronal system, joint stability, cartilage support and ligament and tendon activation.

Part 2 specifies the correct form for 100 of the most common exercises.

Part 3 incorporates a neurological training system that I developed years back, called Counter Lever Training. It is designed to work with the ingrained muscle firing patterns of the gait cycle instead of against it and greatly enhances neurological (strength) output. Since working against the nervous system is one of the reasons that people need to stop weight lifting as they age, this is a vital component to every exercise program that has longevity as its goal.

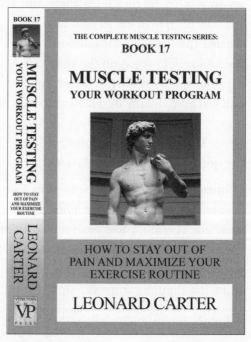

BOOK 17

MUSCLE TESTING YOUR WORKOUT PROGRAM

HOW TO STAY OUT OF PAIN AND MAXIMIZE YOUR EXERCISE ROUTINE

LEONARD CARTER

THE COMPLETE MUSCLE TESTING SERIES:
BOOK 17

MUSCLE TESTING
YOUR WORKOUT PROGRAM

HOW TO STAY OUT OF
PAIN AND MAXIMIZE YOUR
EXERCISE ROUTINE

LEONARD CARTER

VITRUVIAN
VP
PRESS

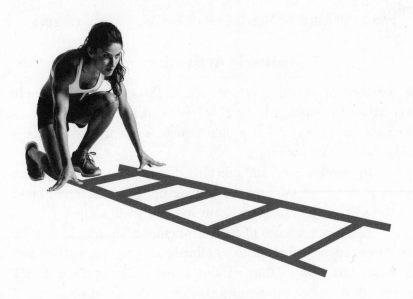

18

Muscle Testing

For Athletic Performance

A thletic performance isn't what we do to get fit and healthy, it's what we do once we've already been working out and are in good shape.

While the main concerns for a workout program are having good flexibility, healthy tendons and ligaments and maintaining correct form, with athletic performance the requirements are more specific:

1. Muscle activation If our muscles are not activated they can't perform the way we need them to. This needs to be MT.

2. An understanding of biomechanics If we place more load on our activated muscles than they can handle, such as jumping, swinging or other plyometric activities, injury will follow.

In this chapter we will explore how to use MT to measure, modify and manage these variables.

Muscle Activation

At the core of athletic performance is the concept of **muscle activation.** A muscle can be activated or deactivated because its electrical functioning is like a light switch. A deactivated muscle is said to be "off" or "not firing."

If a muscle is off and it is placed under load anyway, it isn't simply a matter of the tendons picking up the slack. First, other muscles will compensate. Then, pain and injury will ensue.

There is a science of testing whether each muscle is firing and if this is done before the day's athletic activities begin, there will be virtually no injury. Athletic trainers who understand how to MT whether muscles are firing move quickly to the top of their field. I noticed this time and again with students in my VTS Level 2 courses.

But the underlying reason that a muscle will cease to fire is that its corresponding organ has an imbalance. There are **organ-muscle relationships**. This principle is not widely understood: If an organ is off, a muscle that has a relationship with it won't fire properly even if there is nothing wrong with the muscle itself.

We already understand that an organ can be MT (Pt3-Ch2), that it can be temporarily reactivated by supplementation (Pt3-Ch3) and that a 1A Parasite is the root cause of the inhibition (Pt3-Ch5). To answer the question of why particular muscles are deactivated, we simply need to understand which organs shut off which muscles. I designed a course called VTS Level 3 to cover this information. It was unique in the athletic and fitness industries.

Below are some common organ-muscle relationships:

Area	Muscle	Organ
Chest	Pectoralis major	Lungs or Stomach
Upper back	Mid trapezius, Rhomboids	Lungs
Mid back	Iliocostalis, Longissimus	Stomach, Small intestines
Low back	Quadratus lumborum	Large, Small intestines
Neck	Upper trapezius, Levator scapulae	Small intestine
Elbow, Wrists	Extensor carpi ulnaris, Flexor carpi radialis longus	Lungs or Stomach
Knees	Quadriceps, Hamstrings	Large, Small intestines

Specific Muscle Tests

Here are the two most fundamental MT for athletic performance,
reprinted from the VTS Level 2 training manual.

Pectoralis Major (pec, pecs, chest)

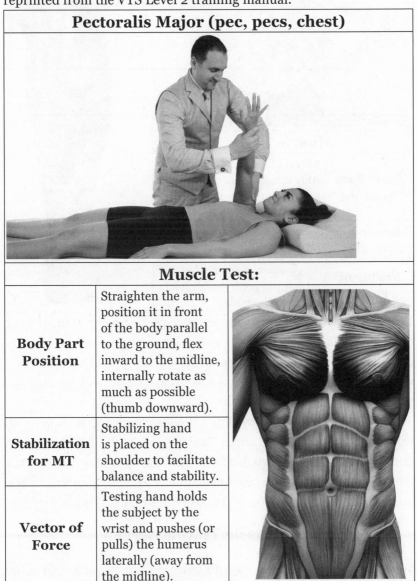

Muscle Test:

Body Part Position	Straighten the arm, position it in front of the body parallel to the ground, flex inward to the midline, internally rotate as much as possible (thumb downward).	
Stabilization for MT	Stabilizing hand is placed on the shoulder to facilitate balance and stability.	
Vector of Force	Testing hand holds the subject by the wrist and pushes (or pulls) the humerus laterally (away from the midline).	

If the pec isn't firing, your upper body won't be able to bear load.
There go your bench press, push-ups and running cycle.

Rectus Femoris (quadriceps, quads, legs)

Muscle Test:

Body Part Position	Lie on your back with knee fully extended, foot and knee pointing straight up. Lift leg to a 40° angle.
Stabilization for MT	Stabilizing hand placed on other hip to prevent rocking.
Vector of Force	Apply force at the ankle; attempt to push the leg back down to the table.

The quadriceps are essential to every aspect of movement. If your rectus femoris isn't firing, your entire kinetic chain will be off. You won't be able to stand, walk, run, lift or jump properly. Your body won't be able to bear load and the excess strain will go on your tendons, ligaments, joints and bones.

At only 44 years old, Tiger Woods claimed that in his 20s, running had destroyed his knees. That is an example of the long-term effect of putting plyometric load (e.g., body weight plus 50%) on the joints (ankles, knees, hips) using an athletic exercise (running) when the support musculature (in this case, rectus femoris) is not firing.

Full Muscle Testing Screen

For someone who merely enjoys athletic performance, a screen of the top two muscles listed above is an effective indicator of general muscle activation. For an advanced athlete, a full MT screen is recommended.

Plyometrics

To be able to MT athletic performance at any level it is necessary to understand plyometric exercises and their impact on the associated muscles and tendons.

An exercise is plyometric if you leave the ground and then absorb extra load when you return to it. You do this when you are running and jumping, which is the essence of athletic performance.

Your body already weighs 100% of what it weighs and when you factor in momentum and gravity with a plyometric, you can add an additional 50-60% on top of this. Let's use 50% as a nice round number and consider the following example:

If you weigh 100 lbs and can squat 100 lbs, it means you can squat 100% of your body weight. This factor is already well above average for many people but in a plyometric jump squat, your muscles are absorbing 150% of your weight on the way back down, so you would need to be able to squat 150 lbs to safely perform a plyometric.

To extend the example, someone who weighs:

125 lbs needs to be able to squat 187.5 lbs

150 lbs needs to be able to squat 225 lbs

200 lbs needs to be able to squat 300 lbs

250 lbs needs to be able to squat 375 lbs

Can you squat this much? A professional athlete usually can, an amateur athlete generally cannot and a non-athlete almost never can. But anyone can run and jump, so where is the extra load going? All the weight your muscles cannot absorb goes onto your tendons, which function like elastic bands. This is why the term that describes tendon functionality is elasticity. Elastin is actually a protein.

When you are young, you have naturally elastic tendons but as you age, particularly with a lack of conditioning, your tendons age. However, your body doesn't get any lighter, and as your tendons lose their ability to absorb load, the result is microtears (Pt3-Ch17).

The problem with microtears is that your conscious mind isn't able to register that they're happening. If we don't MT for it, they can become a full tear before we even know there is a problem.

Muscle Testing Athletic Motions

There is a simple way to bridge the gap between your conscious mind and what is happening at the level of the tendons: MT it.

If you want to identify whether your tendons can absorb the shock of a jump, perform a jump and within 3-5 seconds have someone MT the effect of that action on your nervous system.

When the physiological stress of any exercise is greater than your body's capacity to absorb it, the negative difference will show up as a weak MT. If it does, you have identified a motion or an exercise that you aren't ready for.

The solution then is to **measure** your form with a MT, **modify** it until it no longer MT weak and if need be, **manage** your capacity to perform that exercise by getting back to strength training (Pt3-Ch17) until you are strong enough to handle the excess load.

> **MT Protocol For Athletic Motions**
>
> 1. Start with a MT baseline.
> 2. Perform the activity, either one range of motion (ROM) or for a few seconds.
> 3. Then stop, and within 3-5 seconds, have someone MT you again. Compare.
>
> **A:** If still strong then good, but make sure you've done it right, this test is more often weak than strong.
> **B:** If weak, then you have identified an exercise or ROM that is detrimental. Try modifying it and retesting. If you can't find a ROM that MT strong, stop doing it until you get stronger.

Aspiring athletes who don't understand this principle are more likely to find out that they aren't ready for an exercise by injuring themselves.

However, the fascinating applications of this type of MT are to be found not in simply avoiding what you can't do but in modifying what you can do so that you can do it better.

This is the essence of athletic performance and for someone who is ready to exercise at this level, it is a game changer. It is common to experience a measurable increase in your athletic output once you use MT to ensure that your muscles are firing and that you are working within the range of load that they can support.

Applications

The information below is drawn from a 2-day course I used to teach called *BioEnhancement* which examines how to apply MT to enhance various sports and activities.

Running Whether for enjoyment, sports or marathons the essence of running is gait symmetry. Your running gait can be subdivided into four components: ankle flexion, stride length, thoracic rotation and arm swing. Very few athletes are able to pass a MT of their gait, it almost always tests weak but which of the four components is unbalanced? Each of these will need to be MT separately to identify which one is out of alignment. If you can get all four working together it can take tens of minutes off your marathon, for example.

Crossfit You will find that almost every crossfit exercise MT weak. Some of them are simply not biomechanically sound, being based on Olympic lifting, while others involve particularly aggressive plyometrics that require that the participant be able to lift as much as 175% of their body weight. For these reasons it is unsurprising that crossfit has one of the highest rates of injury of any sport.

Yoga Although the opposite of a plyometric, yoga is also a leading cause of sports injuries. In the same way that excess load from momentum can cause microtears, stretching a muscle too far can strain it. An advanced yoga posture can be MT the first few times to ensure the range of motion is within what the body can handle. A good yoga instructor will recognize this intuitively.

Golf One of the most popular performance enhancement exercises for golf is to rotate the upper body with load. This is done with a cable crossover machine or free weights. A MT of this activity will universally produce a weak response. The reason for this is that upper body rotation forces lower body rotation that stresses the spine. The lumbar vertebrae only rotate 3° to 4°, anything greater than that pinches the nerves. Rather counterintuitively, the best golf conditioning program involves doing a plank to protect yourself from rotation. A MT of the effect of rotation on the nervous system will confirm this. Your form on a golf swing can also be MT.

Further Reading on Athletic Performance

The Complete Muscle Testing Series: *Book 18 Muscle Testing for Athletic Performance* addresses 3 main topics.

Part 1 is a detailed analysis and breakdown of the walking and running gait cycle. Emphasis is on identifying and correcting gait imbalances. There is also a section on how to use athletic tape to temporarily reactivate the entire kinetic chain, which is appropriate for sports matches, competitions and marathons. This content is from days 2 and 3 of the 3-day VTS Level 1 course mentioned in Pt3-Ch17.

Part 2 is a reprint of the complete VTS Level 2 MT manual for the 100 most common muscles: their names, a picture of where to find them in the body and an outline of what range of motion they are MT in. It is relevant for every athlete, trainer, therapist, kinesiologist and teacher to master these details and when presented in a simple format, it is quite accessible.

Part 3 is a summary of all the organ-muscle relationships and contains a synthesis of which supplements can be used to support each organ for the purpose of muscle activation. This includes the complete VTS Level 3 and Bioenhancement course manuals.

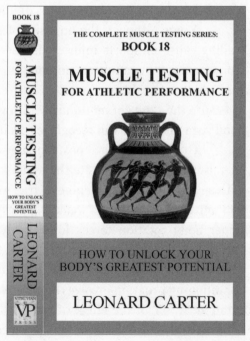

Attendance at these 4 courses used to cost $5000 when I was offering them. Book 18 shares this content in a condensed, accessible format.

THE HEALTH LADDER
A GUIDE TO SYMPTOMS AND THEIR ROOT CAUSES

CONDITION		RESOLUTION
7A		7B
6A		6B
5A		5B
4A		4B
3A		3B
2A		2B
1A		1B
0A		0B

5A. LOCATION

The regions of the body that manifest the stress from RUNGS 1A–4A, often below the awareness threshold.

5B. THERAPY

RUNG 5B Therapy is support-focused: vitamins, supplements, herbs and some manual treatments attempt to heal the Location (5A).

19

Muscle Testing

Your Hair, Skin, Teeth and Bones

What element from the periodic table do hair, skin, teeth and bones all have in common? If you're like most people you would guess calcium (Ca#20), but that's not the correct answer.

A MT analysis of each of these tissues indicates a clear pattern of deficiency: in men, strontium (Sr #38); in women, silicon (Si#14).

What is the relationship between strontium, silicon and these tissues? Why do men become deficient in the one and women in the other? Will supplementation resolve the problem? What are the other factors that underlie degeneration in these areas? Is it possible to repair our hair, heal wounds faster and without scars, rebuild (or at least protect) our teeth and solidify and strengthen our bones?

In the chapter below, we will explore the answers to these questions.

Tissue Minerals: Strontium and Silicon

While it is true that calcium is an essential ingredient in human tissue, it is very rare for it to register as deficient in a MT.

The consistent pattern is that men MT for needing strontium citrate and women for silicon citrate. This probably has something to do with sex hormones and sexual activity.

With men, strontium is a component of sperm production while with women, silicon is utilized as a natural internal lubricant. Regular or even periodic sexual activity then places increased demands for these two minerals on the body.

If sex were the only cause of the drain, the missing minerals might be made up in the diet, but this is where parasites enter the equation. At Rung 1A, a man will host roundworms. A particular sub-species of roundworm will excrete a 2A Bad Bacteria that requires the 3A Metal Toxicity strontium (Sr#38) as an essential ingredient in its cellular energy metabolism. Elemental strontium is toxic to the body but the body is full of the 5A nutritional mineral strontium citrate. These bacteria separate the strontium atom from its citrate molecule creating the paradox of deficiency in the nutritional form and toxicity in the elemental form.

Strontium citrate + 2A Bad Bacteria = Strontium #38 + citrate

When a man experiences the perfect storm of sexual activity plus a large worm excreting a toxic load of strontium loving 2A Bad Bacteria into his system, there are two levels to his strontium drain: whatever he doesn't expel sexually is eaten up by the bacteria and he runs chronically deficient. This deficiency is expressed in his hair, skin, teeth and bones over time. Usually the hair is the first to go. Strontium is a trace mineral and it is difficult to make up this loss from food alone.

With women, the concept is exactly the same but we can insert whipworm at Rung 1A, the 3A Metal Toxicity is silicon (Si#14) and the 5A deficiency is silicon citrate. The skin and hair will show symptoms and with age there will be a difficulty in producing internal lubricant.

Rung 1A must be treated to see progress in this area.

Hair

Healthy hair is the hallmark of a healthy body but what happens when hair breaks down? Whether the symptom is thinning or broken strands, split ends, loss of pigmentation or luster, or loss of the hair itself from minor to severe to baldness, changes in hair health are highly visible.

Which aspect of hair degeneration to prioritize may differ from one person to the next. Is the problem one of circulation, protein absorption, mineral metabolism or metal toxicity? Men's hair will MT for strontium, women's for silicon but these patterns may not improve from supplementation, which could provide the body with what it needs but could also worsen the symptom by providing the 2A Bad Bacteria with its favorite food.

The underlying factor is universally a parasite but knowing which parasite is directly causing the symptom can be a challenge, particularly when hair degeneration may be a more general tipping-point effect from multiple organisms. It is best not to assume that supplementation alone will help but instead, to MT and see.

The hair will MT for various 5B therapies: The B vitamins, omega 3, omega 6 and one or more amino acids. It might even respond to acupuncture. Just be careful not to feed the parasite causing these deficiencies too much of its favorite food or the symptom will worsen.

MT Protocol For Your Hair

1. Start with a baseline.
2. Gently pinch several dozen strands of hair and redo the MT (if there is no hair to be found, you might have answered your own question).

A: If the hair MT strong, you haven't found a problem.
B: If the hair MT weak, go to step 3 below.

3. Introduce a supplement against your bioelectric field and redo step 2.

A: If the supplement turns the (-) back to a (+), you MT for needing it.
B: If the supplement fails to turn the (-) back to a (+), there is no evidence that you need it.

266

Skin

If we think of skin as a cake that the body bakes it is obvious that multiple ingredients are needed. Deficiencies in these can be MT.

Beyond the distinction that men's skin needs strontium citrate and women's needs silicon citrate, the next most common ingredient for both genders is zinc citrate. Be careful of taking too much zinc, it causes nausea above 50mg.

Also try MT omega 3 and 6, and vitamin C. Various essential amino acids will MT at high doses. You would need a Supplement MT Kit to check this.

The most common application is to MT the skin for the ingredients outlined above. This can regenerate the appearance and potentially slow the signs of aging.

Another application is with a cut or some other skin injury. In the short term, until healing has taken place, any injured location will MT for needing extremely high quantities of the above ingredients. If these precise combinations and quantities are supplemented with up to 3x/day, it is actually possible to accelerate wound healing by a factor of four and to entirely avoid scarring, even in highly visible areas like the forehead. In these cases, a topical zinc cream is usually also required and can be MT for.

> **MT Protocol**
> **For Your Skin**
>
> 1. Start with a baseline.
> 2. Gently press the area of the skin and redo the MT.
>
> A: If the skin MT strong, you haven't found a problem.
> B: If the skin MT weak, go to step 3 below.
>
> 3. Introduce a supplement against your bioelectric field and redo step 2.
>
> A: If the supplement turns the (-) back to a (+), you MT for needing it.
> B: If the supplement fails to turn the (-) back to a (+), there is no evidence that you need it.

This information might be of particular interest to plastic surgeons who wish to minimize post operative scarring but applies equally in the home, which can be quite a rambunctious place between pets, children, toys and sharp kitchen knives.

Teeth

MT the teeth is very simple. The methodology entails touching a tooth and evaluating the effect of this on an indicator muscle.

In addition to the men's teeth MT for needing citrates of strontium and women's of silicon (usually from the horsetail plant), a mineral common to both genders is fluoride. This is well-known and fluoride treatments are a staple in dental offices. It is a partial myth that fluoride in toothpaste is bad for us. In fact, the causes of fluoride deficiency are not widely understood.

Fluoride is the nutritional form of fluorine (F#9). The body can make fluoride from fluorine.

Some 2A Bad Bacteria are fluorine-loving and will convert the fluoride in our teeth back to fluorine, causing tooth decay over time. These bacteria are hosted by a single-celled amoeba and these are in turn excreted into us by multi-celled parasites, usually filarial.

As the bacteria convert fluoride to fluorine, the body will appear to run deficient in fluoride and the tooth will rot. This has been the cause of great mystification to some dentist friends of mine who, not understanding parasite microbiology or its impact on the organic chemistry of fluoride uptake in enamel formation, are at a loss to explain chronic tooth decay in patients who brush regularly.

This does, however, explain why we understand that sugar consumption makes tooth decay worse. Sugar feeds and strengthens parasites.

**MT Protocol
For Your Teeth**

1. Start with a baseline.
2. With a clean fingertip, touch a tooth and redo the MT.

A: If the tooth MT strong, you haven't found a problem.

B: If the tooth produces a weak MT, go to step 3 below.

3. MT a supplement against your bioelectric field and redo step 2.

A: If the supplement turns the (-) back to a (+), you MT for needing it.

B: If the supplement fails to turn the (-) back to a (+), there is no evidence that you need it.

Bones

MT the bones presents more of a technical challenge than other areas. Not only is the MT itself more complex but interpreting the result is a multi-layered issue. We will explore both factors below.

On the surface, MT the skeletal system is a brilliant application. It could save months waiting for a bone densitometry test or could at least confirm that you need a more detailed scan. We can use MT information to help to design a targeted supplement program to accelerate bone healing. This also has diverse and extensive applications in analyzing and treating skeletal conditions like arthritis, osteoarthritis, rheumatoid arthritis and general osteoporosis.

However, the MT results should not be interpreted at face value. The bones will MT for the 6A Symptom, the 5B Nutritional Therapy, the 3A Metal Toxicity and the 2A Bad Bacteria. This is the pathology of a skeletal condition. But the 1A Parasite probably isn't in the bone itself. Thus, managing a skeletal condition at Rungs 3 through 6 seldom appears to produce the desired improvement.

MT Protocol For Your Bones

1. Start with a baseline.
2. With two hands, hold the forearm or lower leg and placing your thumbs together, produce a gentle pressure as if you were trying to bend a stick.
3. Within 3 seconds of this pressure, re-MT the indicator.

A: If the MT is strong, you haven't found a problem.
B: If the pressure produces a weak MT, go to step 4 below.

4. Introduce a supplement against the bioelectric field and redo steps 2 and 3.

A: If the supplement turns the (-) back to a (+), it is needed.
B: If the supplement fails to turn the (-) back to a (+), there is no evidence that it is needed.

In a 1A Parasite analysis, there is evidence that bone degeneration is associated with the parasites that are the hardest to eliminate, generally being in the filarial or tapeworm categories.

Further Reading on Hair, Skin, Teeth and Bones

In The Complete Muscle Testing Series: *Book 19 Muscle Testing Your Hair, Skin, Teeth and Bones* each of these areas is given systematic attention.

Part 1 is devoted to MT hair and includes the anatomy, mineral and amino acid makeup needed to draw conclusions about healthy hair formation and pigmentation, along with case studies.

Part 2 deals with the skin in detail, including the anatomy, supplementation, repair and case studies in resolving skin disorders like rosacea, eczema and psoriasis.

Part 3 covers teeth in detail, including tooth anatomy, remineralization and an analysis of single-celled parasite factors in tooth decay, along with case studies in dental repair.

Part 4 addresses bone and skeletal anatomy, including a detailed analysis of the various inflammatory, arthritic and degenerative conditions along with case studies in parasite factors and bone repair.

This material provides a context in which to understand how to look and be healthy throughout your life.

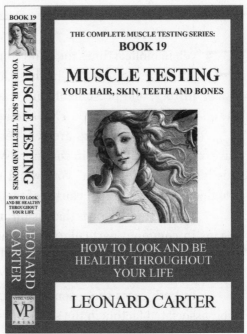

BOOK 19

THE COMPLETE MUSCLE TESTING SERIES:
BOOK 19

MUSCLE TESTING
YOUR HAIR, SKIN, TEETH AND BONES

HOW TO LOOK AND BE
HEALTHY THROUGHOUT
YOUR LIFE

LEONARD CARTER

MUSCLE TESTING
YOUR HAIR, SKIN, TEETH AND BONES

HOW TO LOOK
AND BE HEALTHY
THROUGHOUT
YOUR LIFE

LEONARD
CARTER

VITRUVIAN
VP
PRESS

THE HEALTH LADDER
A GUIDE TO SYMPTOMS AND THEIR ROOT CAUSES

CONDITION		RESOLUTION
7A		7B
6A		6B
5A		**5B**
4A		4B
3A		3B
2A		2B
1A		1B
0A		0B

5A. LOCATION

The regions of the body that manifest the stress from RUNGS 1A–4A, often below the awareness threshold.

5B. THERAPY

RUNG 5B Therapy is support-focused: vitamins, supplements, herbs and some manual treatments attempt to heal the Location (5A).

20

Muscle Testing
Your Vision and Hearing

E ven in biblical times the blind could not see and the deaf could not hear. Pathologies in these areas are as old as recorded history, and presumably much older. We know that Homer, the epic poet who composed *The Iliad* and *The Odyssey*, was blind.

The eyes and ears are two very different senses but they have one unrelated organ in common. Which organ would you guess this is? If you said "brain" you would be wrong, at least from the standpoint of MT the root causes of their respective imbalances.

The MT indication is that vision and hearing have the digestive organs in common, particularly the small intestine. With the eyes, the relationship is nutritional. With the ears, the relationship is bacterial.

In both cases these sense organs respond to fluctuations in their associated factors in the small intestine.

271

Muscle Testing Vision

Eye anatomy diagrams look relatively simple until we start examining some of the structural labels. By the time we need to learn what words like retina, cornea, choroid and macula actually represent, we're usually in line for an expensive eye operation or worse. The problem is that learning those names before they become an issue won't make any difference because they're all at Rung 7A: The Name.

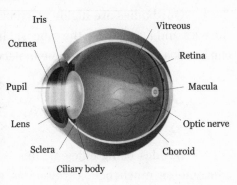

Here is some good news: we can skip the names if we learn one central principle about eye functionality. Once we have learned it, there is a single, simple MT to quantify it. The irony is that if we can master this one concept, we will have more control over how our eyes work than any specialist ever could.

The principle has to do not with the names of the eye structures but with something that is left off of the diagram: **fuel**.

If you think of your eye as a car it will be immediately obvious that the eye needs fuel. If it runs out of fuel it can't see anymore. That's simple enough.

Even more simple is the fact that most of the structural problems that arise with the eye (macular degeneration, retinal inflammation, conjunctivitis, cataracts and glaucoma) are often the secondary results of the eye having run low on fuel.

The primary fuel of the eye is the chemical retinol. Retinol interacts with proteins inside the eye to allow us to see light. The common name for retinol is vitamin A. Everybody knows this, but the role of retinol deficiency in eye degeneration and the effect that the digestive tract has on this is less widely known.

To understand this better we need to briefly examine the structure of the vitamin A molecule itself.

A single vitamin A molecule is just vitamin A, but if two of them become bonded together they form a more complex molecule called beta carotene.

Beta carotene is used by the body to manufacture its mucosal linings. This allows our lungs to absorb oxygen and our intestines to absorb food. We could almost think of beta carotene as fuel for the lungs and intestines. This directly relates to retinol.

Our bodies are highly efficient. Rather than use one fuel for the eyes and another for the mucosal lining, we have an enzyme that can break a single beta carotene molecule into two retinol molecules.

$$\text{A} \quad = \quad \text{Retinol (vitamin A)} \qquad \text{A} \quad = \quad \text{Beta Carotene}$$

Besides being efficient, this is a safety mechanism. We can consume as much beta carotene as we want. If we reach a toxic dose, the excess will spill over into our skin and we'll turn a shade of orange. But if we have too much retinol, it can cause liver and brain damage; to avoid this, our body only converts as much beta carotene into retinol as it needs. To extend the fuel metaphor, the body never pumps too much fuel into the eyes.

Our concern isn't with toxicity, it's with deficiency. How can someone living in the relative affluence of the 21st century, with access to basic nutrition, become so deficient in something they could get from taking a couple bites of a carrot? As always, parasites.

The concern isn't so much that parasites in the eye itself will feast on our retinol, though that is a possibility as filaria love the eye and so does toxocara. The issue is that parasites in our lungs and digestive tract will feast on those mucosal linings so that they can manufacture their own mucosal lining. When they do this, we run low on mucosal lining fuel or beta carotene.

Since the body recycles beta carotene for vitamin A, when our mucosal linings run low on fuel, our eyes run low on fuel. Frequently an onset of visual symptoms begins in the intestines.

While MT the intestines for 1A Parasites is the subject of other chapters, we are concerned here with the effect this has on our eyes and how to mitigate the damage. You could MT the eyes for parasites but your interpretation probably won't be accurate due to 2A Bad Bacteria from parasites in other regions flushing into the eyes.

It will be most efficient and accurate at this introductory level of analysis if you interpret a problem with your eyes as a deficiency in retinol. You can infer that the shortage is the secondary effect of a beta carotene drain in the intestines and you should conclude that supplementing the body with the missing fuel will provide support for your vision.

For this purpose you would MT the eyes but whatever the results of the test are, you would take that product orally in pill or food form. Your body will then deliver the fuel to where it needs to go, you won't need to think about that part.

Eye Supplements

There are various supplements we can MT on the eyes. Here are the top 3. Be sure to use quantity MT to confirm the dosage. Short-term therapeutic doses can be consumed up to 3x/day.

1. Beta Carotene
2. Lutein
3. Retinol—Vitamin A (watch out for toxicity)

Carrots work too. Less common products are lycopene, astaxanthin, zeaxanthin and alpha carotene. These are often difficult to find in supplement form, can be quite expensive and tend to be less effective on vision.

MT Protocol For Your Eyes

1. Start with a baseline.
2. Place a fingertip on your eyelid, keep the eye open, press gently into the eyeball. Redo the MT in this position.

A: If the MT is strong there is no problem. Try the other eye.
B: If the MT is weak, go to step 3 below.

3. Place a vision support supplement into your bio-electric field, redo step 2.

A: If the supplement fails to turn the (-) back to a (+), no evidence that you need it.
B: If the supplement turns the (-) back to a (+), MT for quantity, and bon appetit.

Muscle Testing for Vertigo

We associate the ear exclusively with hearing but interestingly enough the more common symptom to be experienced there by younger people is vertigo or dizziness.

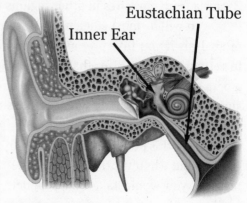
Inner Ear
Eustachian Tube

This has to do with 2A Bad Bacteria clogging either the eustachian tube or the vestibular system in the inner ear. When we examine an ear anatomy diagram, the regions of the ear look very tidy. However, they can become clogged with fluid, which is not tidy, in response to a 2A Bad Bacteria or a 4A Virus.

When this happens, it throws off our balance and proprioception. **Fluid causes vertigo**.

A MT of the soft tissue underneath the earlobe will indicate imbalances in these areas. In some cases, the 6A Symptom of dizziness can be managed at 3B Metal Detox (this would potentially starve the 4A Virus and the 2A Bad Bacteria of their food sources),

MT Protocol For Vertigo

1. Start with a baseline.
2. Place a fingertip in the soft area behind the ear lobe. Perform a MT while introducing soft pressure in this spot.

A: If the MT is strong, there is no problem. Try the other ear.

B: If the MT is weak, check for solutions at Rungs 2B, 3B, 4B and 5B.

or a 1A Parasite analysis can provide information about possible root causes. The emphasis here is on helping the body to drain the fluid that is causing the problem.

Muscle Testing Hearing

Hearing problems are generally divided into two categories: conductive and sensorineural. Conductive hearing loss usually stems from a self-explanatory obstruction. Fluid buildup in the eustachian tubes outlined in the previous section also falls under this group.

The sensorineural category is more complex. A MT can help here by providing information that may not otherwise be available.

The MT to assess hearing is quite simple. A short, percussive sound like the snapping of fingers is introduced next to the ear and a MT is performed within 3 to 5 seconds to evaluate whether this has provoked a weak neurological response. If it has, we have localized the problem and can now build on the negative baseline.

Quantifying sensorineural information using The Health Ladder can present challenges in interpretation but as a quick overview, Rungs 1-4 are relevant.

A Rung 4A Virus might show up. We could expect to identify a 3A Metal Toxicity, a 2A Bad Bacteria and a 1A Parasite but it will be difficult to assign causality to any of these, perhaps because a 5A Location (the stereocilia, for example) may be damaged. A MT would pick up the damage but not necessarily indicate the relevant ear structure, nor where the parasite was.

The point to bear in mind is that if a 2A Bad Bacteria or a 4A Virus are involved in hearing difficulties, they may show up in the ear because they originated from a parasite nearby but it is more likely that an organism large enough to cause a symptom at that scale would be located in the small or large intestines. These large organs have the best combination of available food and available space.

MT Protocol For Your Hearing

1. Start with a baseline.
2. Place your hand next to the ear and make a snapping sound with your fingers. Then quickly redo the MT.

A: If the sound fails to provoke a (-) MT, there is no evidence of a problem. Try the other ear.

B: If the sound provokes a (-) MT then you have a (-) baseline. Now you can build on this using various stimuli.

Further Reading on Vision and Hearing

The Complete Muscle Testing Series: *Book 20 Muscle Testing Your Vision and Hearing* is divided into 2 parts.

Part 1 looks at the history of blindness and deafness and cross references these symptoms with the likely parasite contributors to illuminate mankind's conflict with parasites throughout time. Both Homer and Milton, for example, were blind. Beethoven went deaf. It is interesting to speculate on what parasites they might have had.

Part 2, the eyes, explores the anatomy of vision from the eye structure to the occipital cortex. Various Health Ladder applications are examined, from 5B Therapies like supplementation to the effect of 2A Bad Bacteria on the eyes.

Part 3, hearing, examines the relationship between the ear structures and the auditory cortex. This is cross referenced with the physiology of lymphatic drainage pathways around the ears and the role of the ventricular system in the movement and processing of 2A Bad Bacteria.

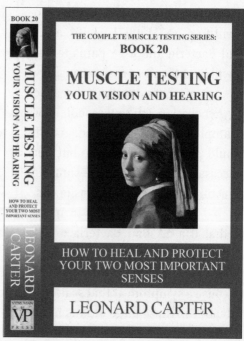

0A. THE VECTOR

All animals in nature are the primary or intermediate hosts to various species of Parasites (1A), many of which can infect humans.

0B. AWARENESS

Educate yourself. Start by reading *Experiments in Muscle Testing* by Leonard Carter. Then, apply what you learn.

THE HEALTH LADDER
A GUIDE TO SYMPTOMS AND THEIR ROOT CAUSES

CONDITION		RESOLUTION
7A		7B
6A		6B
5A		5B
4A		4B
3A		3B
2A		2B
1A		1B
0A		0B

21

Muscle Testing
For World Travelers

The world is such a wonderful place. Every country is full of a unique blend of reality with its own people, history, architecture, language, food, customs, art, geography, wildlife and climate. There are adventures to be had, experiences, relationships, romance, mystery, memories, relaxation and fun. And lots and lots of pictures to be taken. You may never look at these thousands of pictures again but they are yours, so now a little piece of the world is yours.

And sometimes you bring little pieces of the world back with you in your digestive tract and lymphatic system. Whether it was food poisoning, traveler's diarrhea, vomiting, fever, a skin rash or an insect bite, the fact is that going on a trip somewhere is the most common time for an adult to pick up a new species of parasite.

This subject is positioned at Rung 0 on The Health Ladder. Rung 0B Awareness of the 0A Vector is the only way to tour the globe without fear of parasites or food poisoning. Knowledge is power.

Top 10 Sources of Parasites During Travel

Here is a top 10 list of the most common ways you can pick up a parasite on a trip. Each of these is explored in detail below.

1. Airplane food
2. Water in foreign cities
3. Ice in your drinks
4. Bedbugs, Fleas, Lice and Ticks
5. Mosquitos
6. Fruit
7. Condiments and Sauces
8. Dairy and Cheese
9. Deli meats
10. Exotic animals

1. Airplane food

oB Awareness: Some people get sick before their plane has even left the runway. Not a great start to a trip. Any cheese, sauce, mayonnaise, salad dressing, milk or cream in your coffee, deli meats or syrup- or milk-based desserts are fair game for parasites.
Avoidance: Try to eat only those items from the menu that are both cooked and served hot.

2. Water in foreign cities

oB Awareness: Most countries have insufficient chlorination, old or dirty pipes, manure runoff from farmers' fields leaking into municipal water sources, reservoirs filled with bird, fish and rodent feces and no control over upstream contamination. A MT will indicate that virtually all tap water worldwide has parasite eggs in it. You're barely safer drinking bottled water. Many bottling companies use tap water and many street vendors who sell you brand name water simply fill brand name bottles with their own tap water. It's big business. Because you need 6-8 glasses a day of this stuff, every new bottle is a potential new problem. For more on this issue, see Pt3-Ch24 MT Your Water.

Avoidance: There are 4 ways you can safely get water into yourself.
1) MT every bottle, or at least spot check a few different bottles from the same brand at the same hotel. This is my primary strategy and it works very well. A single 1.5 liter bottle can last you the day if you're also drinking alcohol, so it's not as labor-intensive as it sounds.
2) When in doubt, drink beer. At 5-7% alcohol, parasites eggs can't survive and there is a high enough water content in beer to keep you hydrated. By contrast, wine and liquor will always be safe but the alcohol percentage in them is too high for you to stay hydrated.
3) Carbonation kills parasite eggs in 60 minutes, but be mindful of soda pop fountains that add corn syrup while pouring. The parasite eggs in the syrup-sweetened pop flavors are viable until they have soaked in the carbonation for a full 60 minutes.
4) Boiling works fine but you may not have access to boiled water when you're out on an excursion, and be mindful of your server pouring water that is no longer above the boiling point into a dirty cup. Also, once the water has fallen below 100°C/212°F (e.g., after it is used to steep coffee or tea), even if it still feels hot it won't be hot enough to kill the parasite eggs in milk or cream added after the fact.

3. Ice in your drinks
oB Awareness: Sometimes it's hard to remember that ice is frozen tap water, but it is. You should assume that all ice has parasite eggs in it. You might think that since you're putting the ice in alcohol or carbonation, that will make it safe but it won't. The ice would need to melt, become water and then sit in the alcohol or carbonation for 60 minutes. Now, I know what you're thinking, and you're right: this defeats the purpose of using ice. That's why ice is such a risk.
Avoidance: If you really want ice you can always MT it. Freezing doesn't affect the accuracy of a test, but good luck finding clean ice. If you can't find any, I suppose you can MT some water to make sure it's clean and make your own ice. That doesn't really work at a poolside resort when you want a piña colada, so your third choice is to take the risk and drink the parasite ice. There really are no simple solutions except to avoid ice.

4. Bedbugs, Fleas, Lice and Ticks

oB Awareness: Remember that all insects carry filaria. If you're bitten by one of the above creatures, the concern shouldn't be that you've picked up a 2A Bad Bacteria. If that was all you picked up it would be temporary. The real concern is that you've picked up a 1A Parasite from the filarial group. These can cause a chronic medical issue long after you're home. Review Pt3-Ch8 MT Parasite Vectors for more on this.
Avoidance: Your best way to avoid getting bitten by biting pests is to be careful in the quality of hotel you stay at. Check their online reviews. Then when you arrive, check your mattress under the sheets.

5. Mosquitos

oB Awareness: It is a misconception that getting bitten by the wrong mosquito will get you sick, whereas the right mosquito won't. There is no right mosquito. It is also a myth that only mosquitos in certain parts of the world carry filaria. Every single mosquito on the planet without exception carries filaria. It is true that some subspecies in some regions have particularly virulent strains, more on this below, but every single bite is a potential health risk.
Avoidance: The good news is that mosquito repellant works. Even better news is that you generally need to get bitten dozens of times for enough of the parasites to get into your lymphatic system that you can develop 6A Symptoms. Since everyone already has their own preexisting species of filaria acting as placeholders, the average adult can generally survive 1 or 2 bites (understood to be infecting you with a new species of filaria) without incident. Just be mindful of dozens of bites. That should stand out in your mind as potentially the most significant health event of your adult life because remember, filaria are the worst parasites you can get. They autopopulate over time.

6. Fruit

oB Awareness: Any waterborne parasite can make its way into fruit during the washing process. Some grocers even soak their fruit in water so it gets heavier, since they sell it by weight. In Asia, for the same sales benefit many street vendors will use a syringe to inject dirty tap water into the center of the fruit (watermelons, papaya, etc.).

It's not personal: A lot of them are poverty stricken, uneducated and happy to make an extra 10¢ on the sale. They don't understand that it could ruin your health for the next 40 years.

Peeling the fruit won't help. Once the water has soaked in through the thin skin of the fruit, it absorbs into the flesh and pulp by osmosis and carries the parasite eggs with it.

Avoidance: As stated, peeling won't help. Your only two choices are to MT each piece of fruit to confirm it's safe, or if you really want to eat something that MT weak, cook it. Just remember that a cooked fruit topping at a hotel might not have been cooked over the boiling point.

7. Condiments and Sauces
oB Awareness: See Pt3-Ch10 MT Your Food for more detail
Avoidance: MT, cook, avoid or take the risk.

8. Dairy and Cheese
oB Awareness: See Pt3-Ch10 MT Your Food
Avoidance: MT, cook, avoid or take the risk.

9. Deli meats
oB Awareness: See Pt3-Ch10 MT Your Food
Avoidance: MT, cook, avoid or take the risk.

10. Exotic animals
oB Awareness: As outlined in Pt3-Ch8 MT The Vector, all insects carry filaria. We can also get them from a jelly fish sting, snake bite or any other venomous creature. If you're bitten by an exotic animal, as with mosquitos and the other external parasites, watch for the onset of a 6A Symptom up to six months after the bite.

Avoidance: There's very little you can do since by definition getting bitten is accidental. Reactively speaking, you can at least try to MT the wound where you were bitten, and if that provokes a weak response, see if ivermectin turns the negative back to a positive. But if it does, how will you know if that's a new species of filaria or one you were already hosting? And then, can you find ivermectin at a nearby pharmacy? Is there a nearby pharmacy? Ideally, just don't get bitten.

Reactive Measures

Most people who pick up a parasite on a trip mistakenly assume they've only picked up a 2A Bad Bacteria. They take a 2B Antibiotic and call it a day. But 2B Antibiotics never kill 1A Parasites.

If the above precautionary measures don't work and you do get sick, there is a MT protocol to screen for newly acquired parasites.

We explored The Dosage Toxicity Problem in Pt3-Ch5. For whatever reason, this doesn't apply to a parasite you have just picked up. Newly acquired organisms all seem to MT for low doses of antiparasitic medications that are simple to find and safe to take.

You'll need access to these medications and you'll need to know what dosage to MT for. Refer to Pt3-Ch5 for more information.

Antiparasitic Medication Dosages for World Travelers

	Medication	Purpose	Quantity
1	Praziquantel 600mg	Treats fluke and tapeworm	2-33 pills
2	Mebendazole 100mg	Treats roundworm	1-6 pills
3	Albendazole 400mg	Treats whipworm/hookworm	1-4 pills
4	Ivermectin 6mg	Treats filaria	1-4 pills

Please be mindful of a few things:

1. This is not a recommendation to take these pills, that's between you and your doctor. But these are the doses to get MT for.

2. The MT Indicator point is the locus of the newly acquired symptom.

3. Number of times per day and number of days varies by medication.

4. If you find a protozoan (by MT for metronidazole), don't assume you have found the root cause. They live in the excretions of the multi-celled parasites you're already testing for above. If you're not getting a hit on any of the above doses and want to be thorough and check for protozoans, here are the testing ranges:

5	Metronidazole 200mg	Treats amoeba, giardia	2-4 pills
6	Nitazoxanide 500mg	Treats cryptosporidium	1-2 pills

Vacation Items to MT

Some things you might not have thought of MT are listed below. The lower your 1A Parasite burden is, the less reactive you will be to the 3A Metal Toxicity in these products.

1. Sunscreen: You'll be putting enough of it on that the chemicals and perfumes in it might cause a fair bit of reactivity, if you get one that disagrees with you. This will show up in a MT before you put it on.

2. Insect repellant: Same rationale as sunscreen above.

3. Alcohol: If you're still at a point where you react to many or most alcohols (because of the 3A Metal Toxicity in it that's feeding your 2A Bad Bacteria), you should be able to do some MT and see which one you don't react to. Then just stick to drinking that one.

4. Smoking products: The same as above goes for cigarettes and cigars.

Top 10 Misconceptions About Parasites and Travel

Here is a short list of misconceptions about parasites and travel that can get you in hot water:

1. Hot peppers have antiparasitic properties, and that eating them with, on, or in your food will somehow protect you. FALSE.

2. Coffee or tea are hot enough to kill parasite eggs in the milk or cream you add after the drink was poured. FALSE.

3. Alcohol kills the parasites in ice. FALSE.

4. Carbonation kills the parasites in ice. FALSE.

5. Proactively taking medicinal herbs like wormwood and black walnut will protect you from parasites. FALSE.

6. A food poisoning event is a bacterium, not a parasite. FALSE.

7. You got food poisoning because you or someone else didn't wash their hands. FALSE.

8. Staying in a 5-star resort will protect you from getting dietary or mosquito vectored parasites. FALSE.

9. When the symptom subsides, the parasite is gone. FALSE.

10. You can only get parasites on vacation, never at home. FALSE.

The Top 10 Worst Parasites

These are not only the top 10 worst things you can pick up on vacation, they are the top 10 worst parasites in the world.

If you're going to be globetrotting, you should know about these organisms in advance so that if you ever get one of them, you don't have to start combing through a microbiology textbook in a panic.

	Name	oA Vector	What is it? (Pathology)	Medication to MT for
1	**Loa Loa** (Medical Cond.: Loiasis)	Chrysops fly	A filaria that hatches in your eye and in one year, grows to a 10-inch long worm.	DEC, Albendazole, Ivermectin
2	**Guinea Worm** (Dracunculiasis)	Water flea	A meter long worm that takes a year to crawl through your leg and out your foot.	You just have to wait for it to crawl out
3	**River Blindness** (Onchocerciasis)	Black fly	A filarial worm from flies by rivers in Africa that causes blindness in 5% of cases.	Ivermectin. MT for dosage
4	**Flesh Eating Disease** (Leishmaniasis)	Sand fly	A single-celled parasite causing skin lesions and tissue necrosis.	Stibogluconate, Amphotericin B, Miltefosine
5	**Malaria** (Plasmodiasis)	Mosquito	A single-celled parasite that causes fever, chills, sweats and headaches.	Hydroxy-chloroquine
6	**Chagas** (American Trypanosomiasis)	Kissing bug	A single-celled parasite that can cause internal swelling and heart failure.	Benznidazole, Nifurtimox if caught early
7	**Viral Fevers** (Dengue, Yellow, Black Water)	Mosquito	Viruses causing severe fever and vomiting that come from some species of filaria.	No agreed-upon meds. Ivermectin?
8	**Sleeping Sickness** (Trypanosomiasis)	Tsetse fly	A single-celled parasite causing a sleep you might not wake up from.	Suramin, Benznidazole, Nifutimox
9	**Blood Fluke** (Schistosomiasis)	Snail in stream water	A microscopic fluke that penetrates your skin and lives in the bloodstream.	Praziquantel
10	**Elephantiasis** (Lymphatic Filariasis)	Mosquito	A filaria that autopopulates in the lymphatic system causing massive growths.	DEC (Diethyl-carbamazine), Ivermectin

Post-Travel Mentality

Whether you're happy to be home after a trip or sorry to be back, your health focus should be on the future.

If you have picked up a parasite on vacation and are immediately aware of symptoms, hopefully the information in this chapter will empower you to take appropriate action.

However, it is relatively uncommon to become symptomatic right away. The parasites you may have picked up need time to grow before they can get large enough to excrete enough 2A Bad Bacteria that you can finally, gradually develop a symptom. This can take six months and it is the same problem we observe with food poisoning events while at home. The episode comes and goes and you think nothing of it. Then, six months later when a symptom starts to develop, there is no evidence at that moment to get you thinking about a prior infection event. You need to be looking for it.

This is one of the problems with the autonomic nervous system being so inadequate at detecting parasites. Sometimes we have to wait until there are enough 2A Bad Bacteria to provoke a 6A Symptom and that can take time. If you're lucky, your preexisting parasites will act as placeholders and you will either not have sufficient room to pick up anything new or the new thing will not have sufficient room to grow.

If you're unlucky, you will get a symptom but only long after the fact. I met with one gentleman whose symptom was a sudden, momentary loss of memory. For a full minute he couldn't remember where he was or, terrifyingly, who he was. And every month the episodes were becoming more frequent.

Upon inquiry it turned out that he had spent two weeks living in the jungles of Borneo getting eaten alive by mosquitos, but that was eight months before our meeting and he never once suspected a connection between his trip and that symptom. This is a classic growth curve of a newly introduced species of filaria that over several months has autopopulated to the point where it is now causing a major symptom in the host.

Further Reading on Traveling

When you travel the world you are taking a trip into the planet's remote microbiological past. It is best to be as informed as possible.

The Complete Muscle Testing Series: *Book 21 Muscle Testing for World Travelers* provides a thorough analysis of the parasites we can pick up while traveling.

Part 1 is a detailed survey of all parasites and pathogenic bacteria and viruses around the world that are an infection risk for humans. It contains a complete list of everything you would need to know about getting any microscopic infections from travel, including the food forms they are commonly found in.

Part 2 is a summary of the insects and venomous animals you are likely to encounter on your journeys on land and water along with MT protocols for quantifying and managing the associated infections.

Part 3 is an encyclopedic parasite and health risk summary for every country of the world. For ease of reference it is organized alphabetically by country.

Woven together this is a complete account of all you would need to know to tour the globe without fear of parasites or food poisoning.

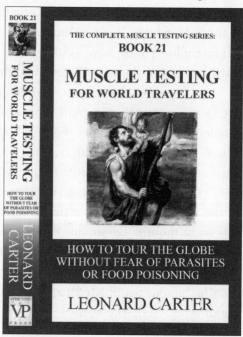

THE HEALTH LADDER
A GUIDE TO SYMPTOMS AND THEIR ROOT CAUSES

CONDITION		RESOLUTION
7A		7B
6A		6B
5A		5B
4A		4B
3A		3B
2A		2B
1A		**1B**
0A		0B

1B. FREQUENCY THERAPY

Eliminates all species of Parasites
(1A) from all locations. Clean,
quick, comprehensive and free
of side effects, it is **the future
of human healthcare.**

22

Muscle Testing

For Longevity

W ho doesn't want to live forever? I thought it was an obvious question until I started asking people. It turned out, almost nobody did.

The clarifying question of why not was revealing: "Well," many 70-year-olds would say, "I wouldn't want to be in this kind of pain for much longer."

There is an assumption that old age is characterized by physical decay which everyone has seen to some extent: high blood pressure, heart disease, swollen feet, digestive conditions, insomnia, bloating, weight gain, becoming crippled, erectile dysfunction, osteoporosis, arthritis, weakness and the loss of vision, hearing, taste, memory, mental acuity and energy not to mention hair. And pain, years of pain in the bones, skin, hands, feet, neck and back. Pain so bad you can taste it. And then fear. Fear of cancer or a heart attack, of leaving your spouse alone, of not being there for your kids, your grandkids, your pet. Fear that you can die at any moment and fear that you'll die a slow death, not remembering your own name.

Who can blame people for not wanting that to go on forever?

Longevity Studies

Any conversation about longevity has to be honest and very few of them are. Let's start with a summary of the dishonest longevity claims so we can see where the confusion lies.

Nanotechnology The expectation that mini robots will repair us. It's not going to happen, and if it does it won't be in the lifetime of anyone living in the 21st century, and if it is it won't be in the budget of anyone that doesn't also own their own rocket ship company.

Genetic Engineering It's not going to work on us because as long as we're still full of every parasite species in the biosphere, our genes are going to do what genes do. We need to address the 1A Parasite, not find a way to disable some gene for a 6A Symptom.

Super Foods They're great for the person selling the super food and for the parasite eating the super food. But I hope you have a strategy for dealing with the 2A Bad Bacteria that is excreted by the parasite because that's what's going to happen.

Healthy Habits This might put us in a category where we attain the same longevity as others in our group, but won't set us ahead of the pack and may not work at all due to 1A Parasites.

Blue Zones A great name for a book but a misguided way of thinking. It mistakenly assigns reaching an advanced age to the part of the world we live in without factoring in parasites from the local grazing animals, which are probably the real differentiating factors.

Longevity: A New Definition

An honest look at longevity more or less ignores the future and focuses on the present. The core question is very simple and practical: What can you do today to not die? Then when tomorrow comes, ask the same question. Then, continue asking that question every day until you run out of answers.

The most effective answer is to get your parasites out. Although you may get old eventually, this answer never will. Having no parasites is the essence of longevity.

The Problem with Good Advice

Assuming that longevity advice applies to you, without MT it against your current biology and parasite profile, probably won't go well.

Eat lots of protein But what if the parasites you host love protein and every time you eat it, your face and scalp get covered in a rash and you're in pain for a week? And maybe they don't like the amino acids in carbs, so maybe for you it's better to get your protein from carbs which causes fewer side effects in your case?

Drink coffee (Good because of its antioxidant properties.) But what if your brand of coffee is full of elemental selenium (Se #34) that's feeding the bacteria from the filaria in your cerebrospinal fluid that you got from God-knows-what insect bite over the years, so that by 10 a.m. you've got a headache, you're dizzy and you need to go back to bed? You might want to MT your coffee.

Exercise But what if you're in so much pain that you can't exercise, or what if you push through the pain (on the rationale of no pain, no gain) and hurt yourself and then you can't even walk?

Be positive But what if you're so full of 2A Bad Bacteria from parasites that their waste mimics your neurotransmitters and makes you feel miserable all day long? That's out of your control.

Do cardio But what if walking and running makes you feel like you want to die, gives you a migraine, puffs you up with inflammation and raises your blood pressure?

Take bone minerals But what if the whole reason you're deficient in bone minerals is that parasites and their bacteria ate them all, so when you supplement with more, you give your parasites more concentrated bioavailable minerals than they could have got from your diet in a month? In that case you'd feel significantly worse.

The problem with good advice is that you need to MT it to see if it applies to you, and the problem with MT is that something which MT positive on day 1 may not continue to MT that way after day 2. Day 1's mineral requirement could be day 3's toxicity. This is a common pattern and should not be overlooked or underestimated.

The Longevity Paradox

The result of the above information is that if you're healthy, you probably don't need a MT to tell you this. And paradoxically, if you're unhealthy enough to need to MT what's wrong, a MT alone probably won't help.

Humanity's traditional approach to longevity has been to allow the concept of survival of the fittest to take its toll, and to assign the rest to fate, karma, chance, destiny, luck or the will of God. Or perhaps to try the various approaches that help in some small way.

The human race has been around for a long time. We have a lot of longevity data. Realistically, if you want a different result than everyone else in history has had, you need to do something significantly different than anyone else in history has ever done.

The core of the matter is that the only way to live longer than you otherwise would have is to get your parasites out.

How Not to Die

The World Health Organization lists the top 10 causes of death in high-income countries. My commentary is added in parentheses.
1. **Heart disease** (parasites affecting the heart and circulatory system)
2. **Stroke** (longterm effect of bad bacteria over time)
3. **Alzheimer's and dementia** (bad bacteria inflaming the brain)
4. **Lung cancer** (parasites and bacteria in the intestines and lungs)
5. **COPD** (parasites and bacteria in the intestines and lungs)
6. **Lower respiratory infections** (parasites, bacteria and viruses)
7. **Colon and rectal cancers** (parasites and bacteria in the intestines)
8. **Diabetes** (parasites and bacteria in the intestines and pancreas)
9. **Kidney disease** (parasites in the intestines and kidneys)
10. **Breast cancer** (parasites and bacteria in the intestines and lungs)

Not dying of these conditions is relatively simple. Just get the parasites out that cause them. The longer you've had the parasites, the less benefit you will experience from their elimination since they can do irreparable damage, but don't underestimate the healing power of the human body...once you're off The Health Ladder.

Supplements to Sustain Life

Top 6 longevity supplements are the same as the top 6 supplements:

1. Beta Carotene A form of vitamin A to support all your mucosal linings (intestines, lungs, circulatory system, kidneys, eyes, mouth, etc.)

2. Vitamin B You should produce it in your intestines, or get it from your diet (mostly vitamins B 1, 2, 3, 5, 6, 7, 9, 12) but if you're full of parasites, their bacteria will cause a B deficiency in you.

3. Vitamin C It's water-soluble so you need it every day. It comes from fruit and vegetables but an elevated parasite load will increase your need for it, probably beyond the level you can consume.

4. Vitamin D This is the backbone of your immune system. You can get it from sun, dairy or meats but a high 2A Bad Bacteria load will result in an exaggerated need for it and some parasites can cause a negative reaction to it. This is the basis for an apparent allergy to the sun.

5. Essential fatty acids Whether omegas 3, 6, or 9, you need these to function but frustratingly, a parasite may be consuming so much of yours that supplementing with more makes you feel worse.

6. Essential proteins If you don't have enough of these you won't repair your cells. However, you are deficient to begin with because of parasites. Advanced forms of deficiency can result in food allergies.

As we can see, we need all these things to survive and they are the essential longevity supplements but the paradox of being deficient in them is that if a living organism in our body created that deficiency, consuming more may not help, or may even hinder us by feeding the parasite its favorite food. This is the **deficiency paradox**.

Before the parasites are eliminated, trying to force these nutrients into our bodies from expensive supplements probably won't do much good. After the parasites are eliminated, supplementation shouldn't be necessary, we should be able to get all these things from our diets.

Finding a good, parasite-free daily protein supplement may not be a bad idea but again, be wary of consuming protein in its root amino acid form if you're still full of parasites. A parasite will frequently be adapted to live off of a particular amino acid.

Longevity Super Foods

Where does that leave us with so-called super foods? You can MT them on yourself to see if they might help. The reason some of them may help is that they are condensed nutrient sources in a form that is more bioavailable to you and less bioavailable to a parasite. In this sense, super foods may represent a workaround to the deficiency paradox outlined above.

Top 10 List of Super Foods:

MT Protocol For Longevity Super Foods

1. Start with a baseline.
2. Find a (-) indicator point relevant to an organ you want to take the super food to support.
3. Building on that negative response, MT the super food to see if it returns the negative to a positive.

A: If a weak test plus the super food still MT weak, it's not super for you.
B: If a weak test plus the super food now MT strong, it looks like it will benefit that location. Go ahead and add it to your diet.

1. Blueberries Extremely high in vitamin C, beta carotene and lutein. This combination directly supports mucosal lining regeneration.

2. Dark green leafy vegetables (kale, spinach, chard, broccoli, seaweed) High in vitamins B, C, iron, minerals and carotenoids.

3. Lentils High in minerals and very protein-dense.

4. Tomatoes and Carrots Extremely high in beta carotene and lutein as well as many nutritional minerals needed for tissue repair.

5. Yogurt A nutritionally dense milk protein that has the added benefit of being rich in the acid-loving bacteria that help digestion.

6. Garlic, Onions, Ginger and Turmeric Rich in the sulfur minerals we need to survive and containing antibacterial and anti-inflammatory properties. This is why most traditional cuisines contain these foods.

7. Olive oil Made of oleic acid (omega 9) that your body can use to manufacture every other fat it needs except for omegas 3 and 6.

8. Salmon High in protein and essential omega 3 fatty acids.

9. Avocado A dense, full-spectrum fat, vitamin and mineral source.

10. Bran (from oat, wheat or rice) Nutritionally dense, high in fiber.

Products That May Shorten Your Lifespan...and Why

Sometimes getting the right thing into you isn't as important as avoiding the wrong thing. Many products contend for the title of least healthy, and you can MT these on yourself to see whether any of it applies to you.

Here is a top 10 list of the products least associated with longevity including explanations that might challenge some of your previous assumptions.

Top 10 List of Toxic Foods:

MT Protocol For Toxic Foods

1. Start with a baseline.
2. MT the product against your bioelectric field.

A: If the product MT strong it is okay for you.

B: If the product MT weak it is not okay for you.

You can clarify why it MT weak using the metal toxicity protocol.

Note: When MT tobacco, be sure to differentiate an unlit product from one that is lit. Combustion changes how products express themselves in a MT.

1. Tobacco The tobacco plant pulls up concentrated forms of 3A Metal Toxicity (such as cadmium, mercury, arsenic and lead) from the soil. You will find no better source of such a dense concoction of heavy metals. Inhaling this can result in a toxicity euphoria which may be why cigarettes are addictive, but if you have the wrong combination of 2A Bad Bacteria preexisting in your circulatory system, they will absorb the 3A Metals in tobacco and cause a more intense 6A Symptom.

Knowing this, and smoking anyway, and then suing tobacco companies when a 6A Symptom becomes the 7A Name lung cancer is highly unethical. The tobacco company was no more responsible for the cancer than your debit card was. There is some correlation with cost: cheap tobacco products will MT weak more frequently than expensive ones. Smokers know this intuitively and will settle upon a brand that agrees with them.

2. Alcohol Like tobacco, the grains and grapes that beer, wine and liquors are made from pull up unique combinations of 3A Metals from the soil. Alcohol itself is antiparasitic, as is the carbonation in beers so these are safest to drink when you're concerned about a water source and indeed, beer was a life saver in medieval Europe.

However, when an alcohol MT weak, which will frequently be the case, we can trace the negative response back to a 3A Metal Toxicity. Chronically exposing yourself to high concentrations of 3A Metals will only be an issue if you are high in 2A Bad Bacteria but that includes most of humanity. When these bacteria get their preferred metal source from some alcohol, they have a bit of a party and we call that drunkenness. So then how do we explain people who don't get drunk from alcohol? Or conversely how can some people feel intoxicated without having touched a drop? These variances are due to differing quantities of the 2A Bad Bacteria, or different types that prefer metals that only occur in specific products. You wouldn't know any of this without performing a MT analysis of your alcohols and cross-referencing it with a Periodic Table MT Kit but it is the case.

Blaming medical conditions on alcohol consumption probably misses the point. A person could derive the same toxicity profile from organic tea or coffee, or for that matter the grains themselves as from alcohol. It is perhaps the concentration of toxicity in a particular product, and our tendency to blame what is obvious that predisposes us to assign importance to the alcohol instead of understanding the relationship between the periodic table at 3A and the cloudy science of bacteriology at 2A.

3. Red Meat There is no MT that will tell you that red meat is clogging your arteries. The meat itself may MT weak but that will be traceable back to a 3A Metal Toxicity (e.g., arsenic or iron) or the amino acid profile of the meat which would be a Rung 5B analysis (e.g., the essential amino acid leucine). In the same way that supplementing with straight leucine might exaggerate a 6A Symptom caused by a leucine-loving parasite somewhere in your body, eating leucine-rich red meat might provoke a similar response. Such a response might indeed be the excretion of a bacteria that has a clogging effect on the arteries but I hope you understand that red meat isn't the only source of amino acids. You can get them from vegetables just as easily, and this actually does explain why some people react poorly to vegetables. Reactivity to meats is best understood at Rungs 3A or 5A and a MT analysis of red meat will probably indicate that it is no worse from a toxicity standpoint than poultry, legumes or nuts.

By contrast, the worst meat you can have is deli meat. It is rarely cooked properly and since we don't cook it either, assuming it is safe, it is not only a concentrated form of metal toxicities but also a lively source of parasite eggs. This means that deli meat not only contributes to existing (parasite) problems but creates new ones as evidenced by the numerous deli food recalls we periodically see in the news. You can MT this for yourself, the result will vary by product.

4. Sugar Most health authorities agree that sugar is poison for you but they generally don't agree on why. The reactivity to sugar actually has to do with the fact that parasites, being anaerobic organisms, breathe sugar like you and I breathe oxygen. Sugar is literally the breath of life for your parasites. When there is enough sugar in your blood stream they become much more metabolically active: they feed more and excrete more. So do their 2A Bad Bacteria. It's a bonanza. Some people can eat a high dose of sugar and almost immediately notice the corresponding flush of 2A Bad Bacteria into their blood stream.

This is why many people get immediately tired when they consume sugar and why sugar is understood to exacerbate almost every medical condition. A direct example of this is diabetes, which is often labelled sugar diabetes, though this is a misnomer since it confuses cause and effect. An indirect example would be hot flashes which only tend to happen six to eight hours after sugar is consumed.

Because parasites are so universal to the human condition, sugar tends to be widely experienced as a negative influence.

5. Saturated fat Interestingly, fried fats do not MT weak. Their negative influence probably has to do with secondary effects which upon further analysis would stem from some action of parasites or their bacteria on your circulatory system.

Summary of Super Foods and Toxic Foods

Understanding that these so-called toxic foods are toxic primarily because they make your 1A Parasites stronger and feed the 2A Bad Bacteria gives rise to a fascinating question: Would it be possible, or at least less harmful to consume these foods if your parasite count was down to zero?

The answer is yes. You could enjoy the fun of having tobacco, alcohol, red meat, sugar and deep fried foods without fear of dying, or at least not dying imminently, if your got your parasites out.

We've all heard of that grandfather who smoked and drank every day of his life and lived until he was 100. By contrast I'm sure every reader has heard of someone who ate organic, took their vitamins, went to sleep early, worked out, and died of a heart attack at 40. Outliers like these demonstrate the truth of what is being proposed here. Parasites take priority, diet is secondary to them and needing super foods at all, or reacting to toxic food forms, is a function of which subspecies of parasites we are hosting.

Without this vital piece of information, no conversation about longevity will actually directly apply to you. And as always, once your parasites are out, you've changed the rules of the game so completely that many of the former concerns are no longer relevant.

Supplements to Repair Damage

Repairing the damage of years of living with parasites will only be possible once they're out. Otherwise, you're not repairing anything, you're just feeding the parasites the very nutrients they love, and which they themselves have caused deficiencies in.

However, once the 1A Parasites and their 2A Bad Bacteria are out, there are targeted supplementation protocols that will help repair different areas of your body. To develop a better understanding of these, refer to the following chapters. To rebuild your:

Bones, see Pt3-Ch19	Vision, see Pt3-Ch20
Teeth, Hair and Skin, see Pt3-Ch19	Organ tissue, see Pt3-Ch2
Muscles, see Pt3-Ch17	Mind, see Pt3-Ch27

Further Reading on Longevity

The Complete Muscle Testing Series: *Book 22 Muscle Testing for Longevity* is an overview of the factors needed to promote maximal longevity.

Part 1 starts by exploring anecdotal accounts of the oldest people in history. It cross references this with what we know about the longest-living animals in the world and draws some useful conclusions.

Part 2 is a digest of the available information on super foods and longevity-specific foods from the nutrients that are in them to why we need them and how parasites cause deficiencies in them.

Part 3 explores ways that we can pursue longevity while hosting parasites, since this is the human condition.

Part 4 examines the concept of a post-parasite rebuilding regimen from diet to nutrition to exercise recommendations.

This information provides a roadmap for how to slow, halt and reverse the aging process.

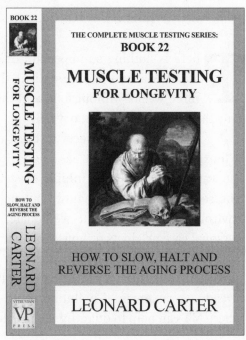

6A. SYMPTOM

The expression of RUNGS 1A–5A at a level that can be perceived or measured.

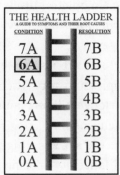

THE HEALTH LADDER
A GUIDE TO SYMPTOMS AND THEIR ROOT CAUSES

CONDITION	RESOLUTION
7A	7B
6A	6B
5A	5B
4A	4B
3A	3B
2A	2B
1A	1B
0A	0B

23
Muscle Testing
Breathing Conditions

There is nothing so important or easy to take for granted as air. It is a well-known statistic that the human body can go three weeks without food and three days without water but only three minutes without oxygen.

There are two aspects to breathing and in this section we will explore both: the first has to do with breathing conditions and the various factors that inhibit oxygen absorption in the lungs. The second, harder to quantify but no less important, deals with environmental toxins that we inhale, either from air pollution, personal care products or household chemical exposure.

If your lungs function normally the second category won't particularly matter to you but if you have a breathing condition already, environmental pollution could mean life or death. This is where MT can help to quantify the problem and the solution.

Muscle Testing the Lungs

Ordinarily, you would only be impelled to MT the lungs, one of the primary 5A Locations, if there were evidence of a breathing problem. If you need to do so, refer to Pt3-Ch2 for a reminder of the test point locations for lungs.

Assuming that you have identified a weak MT response to one or both lungs (they may exhibit different responses), the question is then how to interpret the weak response. Remember that a negative or weak MT alone signifies nothing of value. It is only when we can start with a strong baseline, find a weak response in the lungs and then build on the negative baseline that we can draw a conclusion about what is really going on.

Assuming this thought process, we can now proceed with a Health Ladder analysis of the various stimuli to assign importance to them.

MT Protocol For Your Lungs

1. Start with a baseline.
2. Touch a lung indicator area as referenced in Pt3-Ch2. Differentiate the right lung from the left.
3. While touching the indicator, redo the MT.

A: If either lung MT weak, go to step 4 below.
B: If neither lung MT weak, you have not found a problem.

4. Introduce various stimuli against the weak lung MT to see which one cancels it out.

Lungs and The Health Ladder

Rung 7A: The Name   Asthma
Rung 6A: Symptom   Shortness of breath, mucous, coughing
Rung 5A: Location   Lungs. Differentiate left from right
Rung 4A: Fungus/Virus Possibly, need to MT antifungals/virals
Rung 3A: Metal Toxicity Check for Hg, Al, Pb, As, Se, Fe
Rung 2A: Bad Bacteria Test for penicillin, doxycycline
Rung 1A: Parasites   Screen for whipworm, roundworm, fluke
Rung 0A: The Vector   Various food sources over time

Interpreting the Lungs

On the surface, a negative lung MT lacks meaning. Once we have turned the negative lung MT back to various positives using The Health Ladder, we reach an interpretation paradox that applies to MT many organs, but particularly to the lungs.

On the surface, since the lungs will MT for every 1A Parasite and 2A Bad Bacteria on the spectrum, it appears legitimate to assume the organisms are in the location being tested. And wouldn't it be wonderful if that were the case? Nobody would need to suffer from breathing conditions anymore: neither the symptom nor the uncertainty about the symptom would persist because now we could assume that all lung conditions were caused by parasites.

However, there is a problem with this assumption being accurate with respect to the lungs. It has to do with our circulatory systems. Any parasite anywhere in the body will excrete bacteria as it lives its daily life. As with our own daily excretions (urine, feces, etc.), parasite bacteria is extremely toxic. The human lymphatic and circulatory systems are designed to eliminate such toxicity via specific drainage pathways. One of these pathways is the lungs.

All 2A Bad Bacteria from parasites, as well as many parasite eggs (though they will not hatch in us, they can still create a mechanical obstruction), will potentially end up in or at least pass through the lungs in the process of their being flushed out of the body. Technically speaking, this means that the lungs could indicate MT evidence of a parasite that is located elsewhere.

This is in fact frequently the case. While the lungs can host quite a number of specific species, from meb 2 tissue roundworms to a variety of lung flukes, particularly praz 17 and 32, the most common location for a parasite that expresses itself in the lungs is in fact the digestive tract. Really, this is a window on why lung symptoms are so prevalent, but it is also a reminder of the sophistication of the body's lymphatic drainage pathways.

When an antiparasitic medication MT against the lungs, we should not assume that we have found the location of the parasite.

Supplementing for the Lungs

If the 1A Parasite has been eliminated, either from the lungs themselves or more commonly from the digestive tract where the larger worms (tapeworm, roundworm, etc.) will excrete enough 2A Bad Bacteria to cause a chronic lung condition, the 6A Symptom in the lungs should resolve almost spontaneously. The body should then heal itself by deriving nutrients from a healthy diet.

There are two scenarios where supplementation would be required: 1) If the parasite has just recently been eliminated and a short-term regimen of nutrients is called for to accelerate lung recovery. This would be particularly relevant in a case where there had been a prolonged lung condition resulting in tissue damage. 2) If the parasite has not yet been eliminated and a long-term regimen is needed to support the organ tissue to offset the chronic damage created at Rungs 1-4 on The Health Ladder.

If there is an ongoing parasite issue you will need to decide whether to try treatment or to manage it at Rung 1B Frequency Therapy, 2B Antibiotics, 3B Metal Detox or with 4B Antifungals/ Antiviral medication, but supplementation is a Rung 5B Therapy and would be the same whether the parasite was still in you or recently gone, since the lung tissue would respond to those nutrients whether they needed them for a week or a year.

There are 3 primary categories of nutrients that the lungs require for daily repair, and which they tend to MT for needing:

1. Fat-soluble vitamins Vitamin A, betacarotene or lutein. You will need to MT which one, what quantity and periodic re-tests will give you a picture of what kind of absorption is happening.

2. Water-soluble vitamins Primarily vitamin C, which often tests against mucosal membranes. This is probably why we mistakenly think vitamin C helps with a cold virus. MT for quantities up to 10,000 mg per dose but take that much at your own risk.

3. Amino acids These include collagen or NAC (n-acetyl cysteine or just cysteine). They help the lung tissue to repair itself but if the parasite is still alive, beware of feeding it its favorite food.

Avoiding Lung Metal Toxicity

While it is simple enough to state that a 3A Metal Toxicity will only stick to you when you're full of 2A Bad Bacteria from 1A Parasites, since everyone hosts multiple species of parasites we all need to contend with metals to some degree. When these are inhaled, they can stick to 2A Bad Bacteria in the lungs and create toxicity issues.

A healthy body can flush the lungs to eliminate nominal amounts of toxicity from inhalant forms. However, if a body is already overwhelmed by Rungs 1A-4A on The Health Ladder to such an extent that the 5A lungs develop a 6A Symptom, self-cleansing will be difficult and some form of intervention will be needed.

Eliminating inhalant forms of toxicity would require that you can identify them. There are obvious forms like car exhaust, air pollution and exposure to industrial chemicals that most people can move away from (in some cases this may literally require a change of address) but before you check the real estate listings in the next town over, consider the following sources of toxicity that you will carry with you in the moving truck:

Soaps, shampoos, hair products, makeup, makeup removers, shaving cream, deodorant, cologne, perfume, laundry detergent, fabric softener, dryer sheets, floor cleaners, air fresheners, synthetic fabrics, toothpaste, mouthwash, dish soap, laundry soap and off-gassing from your car, household wall paint, carpets and couch.

And then how about foods that you inhale the scent of? Tea, coffee, wine, beer, liquor, hot sauce, as well as smoke from tobacco and other products. The list is as endless as your diet.

The point isn't to be afraid of the world or try to avoid all of these things. It is to understand that toxicities are only sticking to the lungs because the lungs are full of 2A Bad Bacteria. Treating the bacteria directly with a 2B Antibiotic is seldom fully effective since it fails to address the 1A Parasite propagating more bacteria. If 1B Frequency Therapy isn't available to you, your best option is to treat a 3A Metal Toxicity with 3B Metal Detox.

It will be a lifestyle, but it could make a difference.

Muscle Testing Chart for the Lungs

To bring about an understanding of the lungs that is simple, practical and systematic, a synthesis of the information from multiple chapters is presented in chart form, specific to the lungs:

1A Parasite	2A Bad Bacteria	3A Metal Toxicity	3B Metal Detox
Roundworm	Mercury- or Cadmium-loving	Mercury (Hg#80) Cadmium (Cd#48)	Chlorella, Epsom Salt Bath, EDTA
Whipworm	Tin- or Lead- loving	Tin (Sn#50) Lead (Pb#82)	Activated Charcoal, Chlorella
Flukes	Aluminum- or Thallium-loving	Aluminum (Al#13) Thallium (Tl#81)	Spirulina
Flukes, Tapeworm	Arsenic-loving	Arsenic (As#33)	Wheat Grass
Protozoans	Copper- Silver- Gold-loving	Copper (Cu#29), Silver (Ag#47) Gold (Au#79)	Barley Grass
Filaria	Sulphur- Selenium-loving	Sulphur (S#16) Selenium (Se#34)	MSM

The binders listed above (chlorella, charcoal, spirulina, wheat grass, barley grass and MSM, as well as Epsom salts for external use or EDTA or DMSA by prescription) are generally easy to find. You would want to MT whether you needed them at all and at what quantity. Just remember that you only need 3B Detox because you've got 2A Bad Bacteria causing 3A Metal Toxicity to stick to you.

Managing the metals isn't a bad idea but it will be an ongoing project unless you intend to stop eating or breathing. Also, you should note that supplementing with the binders will eventually stop working if the underlying cause isn't eliminated.

Then, remember that expensive air filters might take additional stress off your lungs but won't change the fact that elements in their non-bioavailable form will continue to stick to you from various, often unpredictable inhalant sources as long as you continue to host 1A Parasites.

Really, the best way to breathe easy is to get your parasites out.

Further Reading on Breathing Conditions

The Complete Muscle Testing Series: *Book 23 Muscle Testing Breathing Conditions* examines in greater detail the practical functioning of the lungs and various breathing pathologies—how to understand them and how to fix them.

Part 1 covers advanced lung anatomy and the lymphatic drainage pathways that make the lungs the meeting point of various internal symptoms.

Part 2 assesses in detail the parasites that infect the lungs. When combined with an account of the bacteria from the lung-clogging intestinal parasites and cross-referenced with several major case studies about breathing conditions, it becomes apparent that parasitology holds the promise of a solution to many pulmonary medical conditions.

Part 3 analyzes the electrochemistry of air masks and filters that are becoming an essential need for people living in industrial cities around the world. This is focused at Rung 3B Metal Detox and involves an advanced airborne chelation technology under development at my company, Muscle Testing Labs.

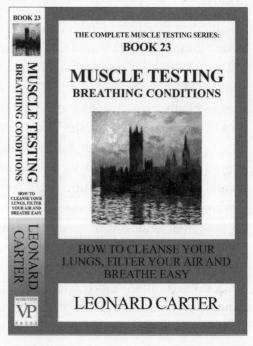

BOOK 23

THE COMPLETE MUSCLE TESTING SERIES:
BOOK 23

MUSCLE TESTING
BREATHING CONDITIONS

HOW TO CLEANSE YOUR
LUNGS, FILTER YOUR AIR AND
BREATHE EASY

LEONARD CARTER

MUSCLE TESTING
BREATHING CONDITIONS

HOW TO
CLEANSE YOUR
LUNGS, FILTER
YOUR AIR AND
BREATHE EASY

LEONARD
CARTER

VITRUVIAN
VP
PRESS

THE HEALTH LADDER
A GUIDE TO SYMPTOMS AND THEIR ROOT CAUSES

CONDITION		RESOLUTION
7A		7B
6A		6B
5A		5B
4A		4B
3A		3B
2A		2B
1A		1B
0A		0B

0A. THE VECTOR

All animals in nature are the primary or intermediate hosts to various species of Parasites (1A), many of which can infect humans.

24

Muscle Testing

Your Drinking Water

I t is simple enough to MT your drinking water. Just hold it against your abdomen and have someone perform a MT on you (and make sure it's not in a metal bottle). If it tests strong then drink your eight glasses a day and enjoy. But what if it MT weak?

As with a food that MT weak, there are two reasons that water will provoke a negative neurological response in a test.

First, and most often: it has parasites in it. Unlike the parasites that enter you via the food vector, parasites that live in and are transmitted by water tend to be specific to water. They cause acute symptoms, are difficult to eliminate and partly for these reasons, they are classified as waterborne parasites

Second, and less frequent: water will contain minerals or metals that can make us sick indirectly by feeding 2A Bad Bacteria that are propagated by a 1A Parasite we are hosting. This makes it possible for some people to actually be allergic to water.

In this section we will explore these two factors in detail.

Survey of Waterborne Parasites

As a reminder, the two main categories of parasites in the biosphere are single-celled (protozoans) and multi-celled (metazoans). The multi-celled are the worms we traditionally think of as parasites but single-celled organisms can also be parasitic and can cause much worse symptoms. Water is a vector for both categories of organisms.

In some cases, such as with fecal contamination of water due to manure or spring run-off over crop fields, you can pick up the same parasites that you would from any other food source.

But in other cases, certain parasites (either themselves or their eggs) are adapted to be spread primarily or even exclusively by water. These are called **waterborne parasites**.

The three most common waterborne parasites are presented below in chart form, along with their associated symptoms and the medication you would MT to identify them. Three others, including Naegleria Fowleri are added to show something unusual for contrast.

1A Parasite	Classification (single/multi)	**Medication to MT for**	6A Symptom
1. Giardia Lamblia (Beaver Fever)	Single-celled: Flagellate	Metronidazole 250mg	Greasy stools that float, frequent bowel evacuations
2. Entamoeba Histolytica (Amoeba)	Single-celled: Amoeba	Metronidazole 800mg	Traveler's diarrhea, stomach cramps
3. Crypto-sporidium (Crypto)	Single-celled: Apicomplexa	Nitazoxanide 500mg	Cramping, diarrhea, lasts 2-3 weeks
4. Guinea Worm (Dracunculiasis)	Multi-celled: Roundworm	No known medication	For a year the worm burrows down your leg, and you certainly feel it coming out
5. Blood Fluke (Schistosomiasis)	Multi-celled: Flatworm	Praziquantel 1200mg	Liver pain, cough, bloody diarrhea, fever
6. Naegleria Fowleri (Brain eating amoeba)	Single-celled: Amoeba	No known medication, doxycycline may help	Sudden onset of fever, you die in 24-48 hours as it quickly eats your brain

MT for Waterborne Parasites

In short, if someone is MT for needing one of the above medications, they may be hosting the corresponding organism. Formal laboratory diagnosis is highly specific but also expensive, time-consuming and subject to error and wait time. By then, the crisis is often over.

It is simpler to MT drinking water before you drink it, particularly if you plan to consume it regularly or if you have concerns about it. If it MT weak, and if one of the above medications cancels out the weak response, you can logically infer the presence of the organism associated with that medication. When performed accurately this is highly effective. If you don't have the medication, just remember The Golden Rule of MT: If it MT weak, avoid it.

MT Protocol For Water

1. Start with a baseline.
2. MT the water. Remember, you can't MT through metal.

A: If it MT positive, drink it.
B-1: If it MT negative, move to step 3 or try boiling it and retesting.
B-2: If it still MT negative after it was boiled, you have identified a 3A Metal Toxicity.

3. If you want to MT the water for parasites specifically, take the sample that MT negative (B-1 above) and place one of the antiparasitic medications next to it from the last page.
4. Redo the MT. The medication that cancels out the negative response will indicate which parasite you have identified.

Treating Your Water

If you have found a water sample that MT for parasites, you will need to treat it before you drink it. Parasite larvae or their eggs are eliminated from water by the following means:

1. Boiling Bring the water to a temperature above 100°C/212°F.

2. Carbonation Carbonate the water for at least 60 minutes.

3. Alcohol Bring the water to a level of 5% edible alcohol, wait 60 minutes.

4. Vinegar Add 10% vinegar to the water, wait at least 60 minutes.

5. Chlorination Too low and it won't work, too high and you can't drink it.

6. Sound It is possible to use an audible frequency to treat water.

Other Water Treatment Options

Additional techniques are also thought to be effective in eliminating parasites from water. Some work, some don't. The processes listed below should not be trusted without some form of MT verification.

1. Reverse osmosis This can work but performance varies between filters. If you need to drink reverse osmosis water, you should at least MT it once to ensure the equipment is working properly. CDC guidelines stipulate a filter size of 1 micron or less.
2. Charcoal filter Charcoal is effective in eliminating 3A Metal Toxicity, particularly in the 4-valence category (silicon, tin, lead). However, it does not have antiparasitic properties.
3. Survival straw Various claims state that it eliminates 99.999% of protozoans. Don't be surprised if the 0.001% show up in a MT. At millions per gulp, that means thousands are getting through.

Treating Yourself for Waterborne Parasites

On the surface, the pharmaceutical data seems promising:
Giardia responds to metronidazole 250mg 3x/day for 5 days.
Amoeba responds to metronidazole 800mg 3x/day for 10 days.
Cryptosporidium needs nitazoxanide 500mg 2x/day for 3 days.

However, the list of side effects doesn't sound encouraging. And then some medications don't work at all, or the symptoms return, or the parasite returns...from nowhere. What could be happening here?

There is an unappreciated principle about waterborne parasites that it is hard to find accurate information about: these organisms are so small and so specialized to the parasite world that once inside you, they may gravitate to your filarial and multi-celled parasites, infecting them and living inside them, parasitically. So your parasites have parasites too. Why wouldn't they, right?

This explains how severe cases of protozoan infections can sometimes kill previously immunocompromised individuals. What previous compromise have these individuals' immune systems made?

Parasites. Every animal on the planet, including us, hosts multi-celled parasites, and every multi-celled parasite hosts single-celled parasites. The problem this presents is that medications tailored to treat us for our single-celled parasites were not designed to treat our multi-celled parasites for their single-celled parasites.

We might assume that if we got treated for our multi-celled parasites first that would solve the problem and it would, if a comprehensive treatment were available. However, The Dosage Toxicity Problem makes a full pharmaceutical treatment regimen unsafe.

This is why everyone will MT for some small quantity of single-celled waterborne parasites (e.g., some negative indicator on every person will be cancelled out by metronidazole 250mg or 800mg).

This explains where these organisms are coming back from when they appear to come back from nowhere. To put things in perspective, most bottled water sold by most big companies will both 1) MT weak and 2) Be cancelled out when MT against metronidazole, confirming the presence of waterborne parasites. Not only is the average person unaware of this but government regulatory agencies don't even police it at this level of scrutiny.

In humans and in bottled water, waterborne parasites are treated with the same mentality as metal toxicity. There is a minimum acceptable level below which nobody cares and above which certain agencies are legally required to take action.

The only people that are forced to care about this issue are those who have such a high preexisting parasite burden that any additional exposure to single-celled protozoans tips their immune system, causing medical-level reactions that draw accusations of sensationalism and hypochondria from outside observers.

Two technologies would revolutionize the waterborne parasite problem if they were available: 1) A sound technology that could clear water of any parasitic invaders and 2) A 1B Frequency Therapy that could treat the human host for multi-celled and single-celled organisms, bypassing the limitations of dosage toxicity and the inadequate chemical FQ delivery systems of the current medications.

Metal Toxicity in Drinking Water

If drinking water provokes a negative MT response even after it has been boiled, carbonated, soaked in alcohol, marinated in vinegar, chlorinated, treated with sound, run through a reverse osmosis filter and shaken, not stirred, then the only remaining possibility is some toxin in the water, most likely a 3A Metal Toxicity.

Most of these can be filtered out, which is why filtered water looks cleaner and tastes better. However, some questions arise. Don't some minerals belong in drinking water? What is the difference between a rock mineral and a nutritional mineral? Doesn't the body use these minerals to survive?

Bioavailable Versus Non-Bioavailable Minerals

When applied to health, the term mineral is a bit of a misnomer. Technically, mineral is a geologist's term for different types of rocks. You can't metabolize or digest rocks because they are in a form that is not bioavailable to us.

Using calcium as an example, it exists in nature as chalk or calcite minerals. Chemists will then break these down to extract pure calcium (Ca#20). We can't digest either chalk or pure calcium. For it to change into a bioavailable form that we can digest, a plant needs to pull that calcium up out of the ground and add a nutritional molecule (amino acid) onto it such as citric acid. When bonded to calcium (Ca#20), citrate (C6H8O7) turns calcium into calcium citrate. This is a form that your body can digest and use for cellular metabolism.

If you imagine a screwdriver with no head, only a shaft, it obviously wouldn't fit into any screw. It's just a piece of metal. Then when you add on the head it can fit a particular screw. Different heads will then fit different screws. The head of the screwdriver is the amino acid that makes elements from the periodic table bioavailable to us by changing them into a form that we can absorb and use in our cells.

You can't metabolize calcium (Ca#20) because you're not a spinach plant, though there are some minor exceptions to this.

Bioavailable Mineral Forms

Nature is highly efficient: there are multiple forms of the same root element. Using Magnesium (Mg#12) as an example, we cannot digest its elemental form but it is bioavailable in other forms:

Nutritionally Magnesium citrate, -glycinate, -bisglycinate, -malate, -carbonate, -gluconate. There are others.

Topically Magnesium sulfate (i.e., Epsom salts)

Inert Magnesium stearate (used as a filler in vitamin capsules)

There is some evidence that we can absorb nonbioavailable forms of minerals from water (such as calcium, magnesium, silicon, etc.) but they would probably translate into bone mineral forms, via enzymes in the digestive tract or possibly in the bones themselves, that can take some minerals and tack on an amino acid in the same way a spinach plant does, though probably not anything as advanced as a citrate molecule. These would more likely end up as carbonate or malate molecules.

The more practical question is whether there is too much of the mineral in your water, or whether too much of it is sticking to you. Remember that elemental calcium or magnesium in your water would tend to stick to you if you had too many 2A Bad Bacteria coming from too high a burden of 1A Parasites.

Unlike our bodies, which are selective about which minerals they will absorb, 2A Bad Bacteria absorb precisely the elemental forms of the minerals that are toxic to us. Your concern, then, isn't whether you're getting too many minerals from your water but whether your 2A Bad Bacteria are. There is a scenario where a high enough bacterial load will render you reactive to the minerals in water. This can even create a situation where a person gets sick or bloated from drinking mineral water and feels that they are allergic to it. A MT analysis in such cases reveals an underlying reactivity to the element in the water, which is traceable through the bacteria back to the parasite.

So as always, the conversation comes back to parasites. Simply enough, we can MT our water for minerals. If there is a problem, try filtering the water and retesting it or choose a different water source.

Further Reading on Drinking Water

An expanded form of this information is available in The Complete Muscle Testing Series: *Book 24 Muscle Testing Your Drinking Water*. This book is divided into 3 parts:

Part 1 includes a complete list and analysis of waterborne parasites found around the world with the MT protocols for identifying them.

Part 2 looks at water metal toxicity in more detail, particularly with respect to the means by which nonbioavailable forms of dissolved minerals are metabolized by the body.

Part 3 analyzes the extent to which it is possible to use sound frequencies to kill parasites in water, something that could have an uplifting effect on parts of the world subject to high levels of fecal water contamination.

This is one of the technologies being developed at my company, Muscle Testing Labs.

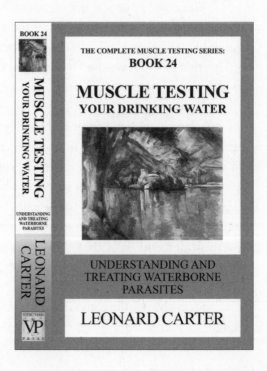

6A. SYMPTOM

The expression of RUNGS 1A–5A at a level that can be perceived or measured.

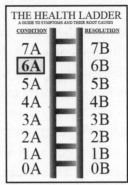

THE HEALTH LADDER
A GUIDE TO SYMPTOMS AND THEIR ROOT CAUSES

CONDITION	RESOLUTION
7A	7B
6A	6B
5A	5B
4A	4B
3A	3B
2A	2B
1A	1B
0A	0B

25

Muscle Testing
Your Sleep

S leep is the great equalizer. Whether we are rich or poor, wise or foolish, kind or wicked when we are asleep we are on our own. Whether we have a good sleep or a bad sleep, sweet dreams or nightmares, our sleep is intrinsically linked to our health.

Interestingly enough, the quality of our sleep and our dreams appears to be connected but there is no known MT that allows us to analyze dreams. You'd have to read Freud or Jung for that. However, there is a MT that can analyze sleep.

We can't MT sleep when we're awake because at that time it is only an idea. And we can't MT what's going on during sleep because we would need to wake up to do it, thus no longer being asleep. What we need is an indicator of sleep that we can MT while awake and there is one: the pineal gland, which is part of the endocrine (hormonal) system. But the pineal gland is buried deep inside the brain so how can we MT it?

Muscle Testing the Pineal Gland

As with other brain structures like the hippocampus and amygdala, it isn't possible to MT the pineal gland using touch as this will not differentiate it from the adjacent brain structures, nor would touch get in deep enough to activate it electromagnetically.

There is a very simple workaround that you can do at home or anywhere else. Start with a baseline MT, then close your eyes and retest.

A simple blink wouldn't work for this purpose, the eyes must be kept closed. This probably has something to do with the fact that when the eyes

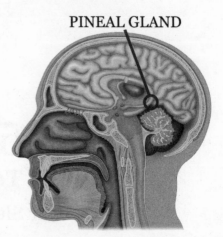

PINEAL GLAND

are closed for long periods of time (i.e., during your night's sleep), the pineal gland excretes the hormone melatonin which propagates a cascading set of reactions around the brain. This must be ingrained in the neuronal system to the level of a reflex for the closing of the eyes in a waking state to be sufficient to provoke the same physiological response as an actual episode of sleep.

If the MT indeed provokes a weak response, we have confirmed that there is a problem but not yet what it is. We must now build on this to identify the nature of the problem.

MT ▭ MT

MT Protocol For
The Pineal Gland

1. Start with a baseline.
2. Close your eyes and keeping them closed, have someone MT you.

A: If the MT is strong, good.
B: If the MT is weak, you have identified an imbalance in the pineal gland.

You can build on this MT by observing which MT stimulus cancels out the weak response.

MT ▭ MT

Categorizing Pineal Imbalances

Sleep imbalances fall into various symptomatic categories. The most common are not being able to get to sleep, waking up in the middle of the night or waking up too early in the morning. It doesn't matter which applies to you as they all have the same root cause: the pineal gland isn't functioning properly and you don't need a MT to know it is happening. You know it because you're wide awake.

The extreme form of these is full insomnia which is Ancient Greek for "not sleeping" and this encapsulates the problem. If you are not sleeping in your native language, translating that into Ancient Greek and pretending it explains things is entirely unhelpful.

This is where a Health Ladder analysis of the various layers to sleep becomes indispensable.

Insomnia and The Health Ladder

Rung 7A: The Name   Insomnia

Rung 6A: Symptom   Various forms of sleeplessness

Rung 5A: Location   Pineal gland is the best MT indicator

Rung 4A: Fungus/Virus You may MT for antifungals or antivirals

Rung 3A: Metal Toxicity Most common are Hg, Al, Tl, Pb, As

Rung 2A: Bad Bacteria   Always

Rung 1A: Parasites   Various organisms, need to MT them

Rung 0A: The Vector   Various food sources over time

On the surface there appears to be unusual complexity to identifying which parasite is at the root of a sleep imbalance. In a clinical setting, every parasite the subject hosts will potentially express itself in the pineal test, so how can we assign blame to one organism? Or is it more of a build up of organisms causing a tipping point effect?

Perhaps the best way to get to the root of this question is to examine the actual biological pathway between the 1A Parasite and the 6A Symptom of sleeplessness. It would be very rare for an actual parasite to be in or near the pineal gland so how is a parasite physically causing sleep issues?

Parasites and Sleep: The Connection

As we explored in the analysis of breathing conditions (Pt3-Ch23), the primary pathways by which a parasite causes symptoms in the body are the circulatory and lymphatic systems.

Simply put, the 1A Parasite is wherever it is, but when it excretes waste, that waste in the form of 2A Bad Bacteria is circulated elsewhere. The body is trying to get it out but there is often no direct evacuation pathway so the waste must travel the entire length of the body before it can be excreted.

That process of circulation can take the 2A Bad Bacteria to the lungs, where it will cause a breathing condition, but it doesn't necessarily or only travel through the lungs. It can circulate elsewhere. As part of this process of circulation, it often if not always gets into the cerebrospinal fluid that fills the spinal column and that the brain is suspended in and nourished by.

The cerebrospinal fluid (CSF) acts as a direct pathway between the 1A Parasite, its 2A Bad Bacteria and your brain. The CSF is part of what is called **the ventricular system**. The ventricles of the brain are a set of interconnected cavities that produce and filter the CSF.

VENTRICULAR SYSTEM

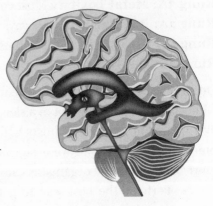

Seen in the diagram to the right, if the brain were rocks underground, the ventricular system would be caves in the rocks and the CSF would be water flowing through the caves.

When a parasite excretes enough 2A Bad Bacteria to overwhelm our circulatory and lymphatic systems' basic cleansing abilities, the additional material will spill over into the CSF and affect sleep, among other things.

A Personal Example

On a personal level, there was a lifetime history of sleep issues. In childhood there was the inability to fall asleep, sometimes until 6 o'clock the next morning. I filled the time by reading detective novels. In later years this evolved into waking up at various times of the night.

It was not helpful to be assured by different practitioners that the time of waking corresponded with some meridian chart, so that if it was 1 a.m. to 3 a.m., that wasn't a sleep problem at all but a liver problem, whereas if it was 3 a.m to 5 a.m, that was lungs. Nobody could satisfactorily explain why this was.

Sleep Meridian Chart

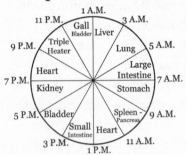

A couple fruitless years were spent taking liver and lung support supplements before it became clear that the underlying assumptions were false, since they were rooted in the misconception that the 5A Location was the source of its own 6A Symptom. This is a primary limitation in all alternative medicine.

Sleep only improved when, over the years, I had the experience of eliminating my 1A Parasites one species at a time. They were targeted in order from the easiest to kill to the hardest. I can attest that throughout that time I had poor sleep but that it improved progressively. It was only when I eradicated the last of my parasites that finally, a deep and perfect sleep became the norm. This also ended years of sleep apnea (snoring), which many people are told causes insomnia. My feedback is that both insomnia and snoring are caused by the same underlying issue: 2A Bad Bacteria that has clogged the CSF in the ventricular system and is inflaming the sinuses.

My interpretation of what I experienced is that two factors are present with insomnia: 1) Many microfilarial parasites can cause a tipping point 2) Large parasites always play a dominant role.

This is consistent with clinical findings in other people.

Managing the Pineal Gland

As with all the other conditions outlined in this book, if our 1A Parasites are eliminated we won't need to think about the symptoms. If they remain, we won't be able to think about anything else.

Managing the pineal gland is only necessary if our parasites remain. Should that be the case, there are a few rungs where we can take effective action: Rungs 3B, 5B and 6B.

Rung 3B Metal Detox We can determine which binder cancels out the weak pineal MT. Our choices are magnesium citrate, boron glycinate, activated charcoal, MSM, or the greens binders. These will potentially minimize the symptom, though not eliminate the root cause of it.

Rung 5B Therapy There are numerous things we can try. Using nutritional therapy, we can MT the pineal gland for melatonin, which is a popular and well-known sleep aid. There are also anti-inflammatory products like omega 3 fish oil or curcumin (very condensed turmeric). Using manual therapy, we might find that regular chiropractic adjustments help, or lymphatic drainage massage, or craniosacral therapy, all of which facilitate the movement of the CSF throughout the ventricular system, which may assist in washing out the 2A Bad Bacteria from the 1A Parasites.

Rung 6B Treatment A number of highly effective pharmaceuticals have been designed to assist in sleep. Generally termed sleeping pills, these may help but remember that action at Rung 6B does not treat the root cause which may emerge as a different symptom over time.

It would be convenient if the 1A Parasites could be treated with antiparasitic medication, and you're welcome to try this. You might get lucky but you will eventually run up against The Dosage Toxicity Problem with pharmaceuticals. Since the hardest-to-kill parasites tend to cause sleep issues, and since they tend to MT for dosages higher than it is safe to take, sometimes in the thousands of pills, drugs aren't consistently an option.

Really, it would be simplest if everyone in the world had access to an effective form of 1B Frequency Therapy.

Further Reading on Muscle Testing Sleep

The Complete Muscle Testing Series: *Book 25 Muscle Testing Your Sleep* is divided into 3 parts.

Part 1 surveys the physiology of sleep from the phases (light, deep, REM) to the ventricular system, the pineal gland and the neurochemistry of what happens while we are sleeping. This is intended to be a general summary of all the information available about sleep physiology and is the basis for understanding upon which the subsequent information is founded.

Part 2 evaluates in detail the impact of parasites and their bacteria on the ventricular system and the sleep cycles. Emphasis is placed on using a MT analysis to manage pineal gland imbalances.

Part 3 embarks on a somewhat fanciful journey into dreams and the impact that parasites have on them. This analysis draws largely from historical and biographical accounts of the famous scientists, writers, artists and composers and paints a picture of how parasites might have made a contribution, whether positive or negative, to human consciousness over time.

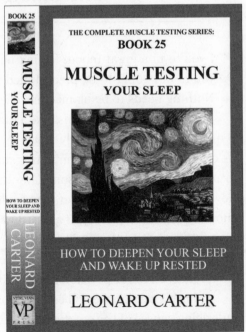

6A. SYMPTOM

The expression of RUNGS 1A–5A at a level that can be perceived or measured.

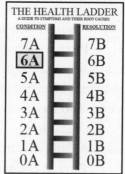

THE HEALTH LADDER
A GUIDE TO SYMPTOMS AND THEIR ROOT CAUSES

CONDITION		RESOLUTION
7A		7B
6A		6B
5A		5B
4A		4B
3A		3B
2A		2B
1A		1B
0A		0B

26

Muscle Testing

The Emotions

I f you're in a great mood, feeling happy, centered and peaceful, you're not going to be preoccupied with why that is happening. Nothing needs to be blamed and there is nothing to MT.

It is when our emotions take a turn for the worse that we start to question them, particularly when the negativity seems to have a life of its own. Telling a person in this state that they should be more positive is a bit like telling someone who is trapped in debt that if they just worked a little harder they could be a billionaire. A positive emotional outlook can be just as hard to reach as a billion dollars.

Are negative emotions yours or are you just tuning into them? Are they caused by brain chemistry, gut chemistry or parasites? How about foods, stress or psychological coping mechanisms?

In this section we will explore how to use MT to quantify the underlying causes of the emotions.

Muscle Testing the Emotions

On the surface, MT the emotions seems conclusive: a negative emotion provokes a weak response.

But this is a superficial level of interpretation. It completely misses the point to conclude that the emotion is bad for you, or your own fault.

All we have found with an emotion that provokes a weak MT is a negative baseline to build on.

To assign meaning to the negative baseline we must use The Health Ladder to quantify the information we're interested in.

This is the best pathway to letting go of self blame and guilt.

> **MT Protocol For The Emotions**
>
> 1. Start with a baseline.
> 2. Provoke the emotion by holding it in mind for 10 seconds.
> 3. Then get MT during this.
>
> **A:** If MT is still strong, good. No evidence of physiological stress.
> **B:** If MT is weaker than the baseline, you can infer that running synaptic electricity through the emotional cortex is causing physiological stress.
>
> When you have identified an emotional trigger for B, that is your new baseline. Now explore it by MT various stimuli against it to see which one turns the (-) back to a (+).

The Health Ladder and the Emotions

A MT analysis will reveal unique data for each person. For example:

Rung 7A: The Name Anger
Rung 6A: Symptom Feeling irritable, everything sets you off
Rung 5A: Location Amygdala **at 5B:** MT for omega 6
Rung 4A: Fungus/Virus MT for fluconazole or valacyclovir
Rung 3A: Metal Toxicity Lead (Pb#82)
Rung 2A: Bad Bacteria Penicillin
Rung 1A: Parasites MT for albendazole
Rung 0A: The Vector Probably something from long ago

Yes, this person has an emotion, and yes it can be named. But is the name causing the symptom? Is the symptom causing itself? If there is clearly whipworm and lead toxicity caught up in the emotion, could the parasite and the metal play a bigger role in the emotion than we suspect?

The Neurobiology of Emotions

Emotions are complex, multifaceted things. They are thought to arise in the limbic system of the brain but there isn't complete agreement among neuroscientists on the models. Are neuropeptides cause or effect? And how about the soul? Or facial muscles?

There are measurable factors to an emotion:

1. The Brain Structure A number of regions in the brain, such as the **amygdala**, **hippocampus** and **hypothalamus** are all associated with the emotions. Some process emotions, others send a message to the pituitary gland to release hormones and neuropeptides.

2. Neuropeptides Proteins found in some brain regions that may also circulate throughout the body as in *Molecules of Emotion* (Pert, 1997).

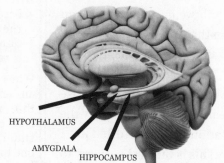

HYPOTHALAMUS

AMYGDALA

HIPPOCAMPUS

3. Neurotransmitters Specific proteins (serotonin, dopamine, GABA) found between synapses that facilitate nerve signal communication.

4. Triggers These can be circumstantial, psychological, foods, smells or parasite bacteria. Even a facial expression can provoke an emotion.

5. Karma Who knows, right? Maybe this is what you're going through because you're meant to go through it. Hawkins says that this is valid.

Here's an idea for establishing causality: 1) Karma = 2) Trigger = 3) brain structure = 4) neuropeptide = 5) neurotransmitter = 6) your prefrontal cortex/conscious mind becomes aware of an emotion.

It sounds reasonable and works with or without karma.

The question is what link in this chain are we MT when we MT an emotion? The most likely answer is that we are MT whatever has physiological priority from a bioelectromagnetic perspective.

323

The Vagus Nerve and Enteroendocrine Cells

There are 12 main wires in your brain, called the 12 cranial nerves. Of these, 10 stay inside the head (eyes, ears, nose, face, etc.), the 11th goes down the spinal column and the 12th, the **vagus nerve**, goes to the gut, your stomach and intestines.

If you've ever had a gut feeling, it got to your brain via the vagus nerve and this is one of the pathways we're interested in for errant emotions that don't belong in the brain.

The vagus nerve picks up signals from the gut such as the vomiting response and acid reflux.

ENTEROENDOCRINE CELLS

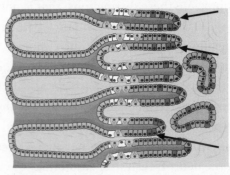

Some of the signal receptors and generators in the lining of the intestines are specialized cells called **enteroendocrine cells**. These cells are able to send messages back to the brain via the vagus nerve about what they sense in the intestinal environment. In fact there is an entire network of neurons in the gut, about 1% as many as the brain itself has, that may contribute to this process of information gathering and relaying. Our intestines really do have a mind of their own.

The enteroendocrine cells can pick up chemical messages from various sources: foods, your good bacteria, 1A Parasites, 2A Bad Bacteria, and 3A Metal Toxicity. When something is wrong, they generate a signal that something is wrong.

Unfortunately that signal isn't conveyed to the prefrontal cortex where we could process it consciously and know exactly what went wrong. We have no idea what went wrong. More often than not, we don't even know that something did go wrong.

This is why we need MT. At the very least, the vagus nerve signal does provoke the stress response. This can be MT and built on.

Serotonin Pathways

There are layers to understanding how a parasite can cause us to experience an emotion.

At Rung 1A, we have large parasites (roundworms and flatworms) and smaller parasites (filaria and microfilaria), each of which host single-celled parasites (protozoans). All of these excrete their own combinations of 2A Bad Bacteria. It would be interesting to quantify which parasites excrete which bacteria but because the average person lacks a sufficient grasp of the field of bacteriology to appreciate these distinctions, that is not the focus here.

One way or the other, at Rung 2A, Bad Bacteria are being constantly excreted into our systems. If these are in the digestive tract, they will probably register with the enteroendocrine cells.

Some of these bacteria act at the Rung 5A Location where they create a deficiency in or inhibit the function of the amino acid tryptophan. If bacteria cause a local or widespread tryptophan deficiency, the cascading metabolic effect of this will be a deficiency in the neurotransmitter serotonin.

Serotonin is involved in regulating mood, appetite, digestion, sleep, memory, and sexual desire. We have a scenario here where a 1A Parasite via its 2A Bad Bacteria is shutting down sexual desire or appetite, or causing a bad mood. This wouldn't make sense at 7A.

Nobody in a bad mood thinks, "Hmm, it must be a parasite excreting a bacteria that is inhibiting my tryptophan absorption and resulting in serotonin deficiency, that's clearly why I am in a bad mood." But that may be exactly what is happening.

Then multiply for every species of parasite we host, every type of bacteria they excrete, every amino acid there is and every neurotransmitter this can have an effect on for every day of your entire life and you have a profile for your emotional imbalances.

This is not your fault. Yet how are you supposed to piece this together? Only a detailed MT analysis of the precise amino acids, neurotransmitters, bacteria and parasites, combined with a knowledge of how to interpret these factors would lead to understanding.

Top 5 Emotional Imbalances

If you are having a genuinely terrible day your emotions are probably a healthy response to the circumstances. Trauma is real and serious. We don't need a MT to tell us that we've been bitten by a snake.

It is when emotions have a life of their own that we should start putting thought into whether something internal is causing them. Here are 5 chronic negative emotional states that are probably caused by a parasite. It's something to think about.

1. Anger
2. Sadness and Melancholy
3. Depression
4. Fear and Anxiety
5. Apathy, Lack of motivation

A Health Ladder analysis reveals interesting data about these emotions.

Top 10 Psychiatric Conditions

Whether the condition is major or minor, it is a valid line of inquiry to see if the psychopathology resolves or even just improves when a comprehensive 1B antiparasitic treatment has been administered.

1. Depression (severe)
2. General Anxiety Disorder
3. Obsessive Compulsive Disorder
4. Schizophrenia
5. Bipolar disorder
6. Autism (severe)
7. PTSD
8. Addiction
9. Alcoholism
10. Eating Disorders

For practitioners interested in doing more work in this field, look for microfilaria in the cerebrospinal fluid - you'll find it. The pathology could be the result of an unusual, unique species of filaria or it could simply be that the host has hit a tipping point of species. Since microfilaria autopopulate, symptoms often worsen over time.

This is why these conditions are exacerbated when the patient eats sugar, especially refined sugar. Parasites breathe sugar like you and I breathe oxygen. Some of them also like dairy and gluten.

In the right hands this information could uplift millions of people around the world who suffer from mental illness.

Freedom from the Emotions

Certainly, a comprehensive 1B Frequency Therapy would be ideal.

But only when we understand that chronic negative emotions are the physical indicators of the cascading effects of 2A Bad Bacteria from 1A Parasites stimulating 5A neurotransmitters to misfire in our guts and our brains can we be mentally free.

First, free from guilt. It means that we are not at fault for our chronic negative emotions. With maturity, honesty and spiritual awareness this fact becomes more obvious. It is sometimes also necessary to overcome the decades of self-help spirituality from the 20th century that told us we had emotional blockages, had manifested past trauma in our tissues, had the wrong color schemes in our houses, the wrong coping mechanisms in our minds and that we had failed to forgive others and ourselves. Guilt, guilt, guilt.

By imposing a Health Ladder interpretation on the emotions it becomes immediately clear that we can experience them but are not at fault for them. The fault only arises when we take possession of a negative emotion, personalize it and get a payoff from it.

What follows second is freedom from negative emotion itself. While it is ideal if the parasite can be eliminated, the knowledge that the emotion is not ours is often sufficient in itself to free us from bondage to the state of mind the emotion engenders.

The fact is that emotions spontaneously arise from The Field of consciousness itself. They aren't ours, we just tune into them, like radio stations. With a progressive letting go of our attachment to emotions, there comes an inner silence. Within the silence is happiness, and within the happiness there is rejoicing. This state of mind is an embodiment of a verse from the gospel of Luke: 2:14. *Glory to God in the highest, and on earth peace, good will toward men.*

It is possible in this way with intention, devotion and a lot of letting go to transition from being at the mercy of negative emotions to being a source of peace and kindness that radiates back out into the world, blending with the general psyche of mankind and perhaps, uplifting it a little. Imagine that.

Further Reading on Muscle Testing the Emotions

In The Complete Muscle Testing Series: *Book 26 Muscle Testing the Emotions* we consider the impact of MT evidence on each of the major negative emotional states as well as some distinct psychiatric profiles.

Part 1 delves into the neurobiology of emotions from the neurotransmitters, proteins, enzymes, hormones and nutrients that fuel our feelings to the brain structures we perceive them with.

Part 2 probes the murky sciences of neurobacteriology and neuroparasitology to draw some practical, causal conclusions about the impact of parasites on our emotional states.

Part 3 organizes a decade of clinical notes into the top 50 emotional pathologies from anxiety, anger and depression to addiction, bipolar disorder and schizophrenia. This section includes a line of commentary on emotional states as they relate to David Hawkins' *Map of Consciousness*.

This information offers a unique window on the largely unexplored world of parasites and their effect on the emotions.

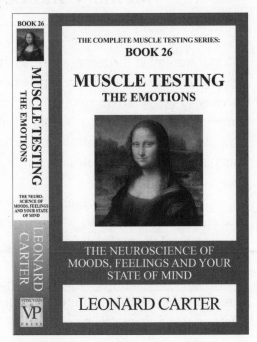

THE COMPLETE MUSCLE TESTING SERIES:
BOOK 26

MUSCLE TESTING
THE EMOTIONS

THE NEUROSCIENCE OF MOODS, FEELINGS AND YOUR STATE OF MIND

LEONARD CARTER

5A. LOCATION

The regions of the body that manifest the stress from RUNGS 1A–4A, often below the awareness threshold.

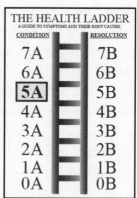

THE HEALTH LADDER	
A GUIDE TO SYMPTOMS AND THEIR ROOT CAUSES	
CONDITION	RESOLUTION
7A	7B
6A	6B
5A	5B
4A	4B
3A	3B
2A	2B
1A	1B
0A	0B

27

Muscle Testing
Memory and Cognition

I still remember the teenage thrill I felt when I learned of memory and cognition enhancing supplements. "Wow!" I thought. "A way to get smarter...from a pill." And they all had such great names: royal jelly, ginkgo biloba, pycnogenol, bacopa monnieri, phosphatidylserine. I went out and paid good money for some of them and took twice the dosage recommended on the bottle...and then nothing happened.

Years later when I was able to cross reference an understanding of neurobiology with the MT indicators for the hippocampus (memory) and the prefrontal cortex (cognition), I finally understood why the supplements hadn't worked, and couldn't have worked.

To share in this understanding, we need to come to an agreement on what constitutes the term works and the obvious question that follows: Works on what?

Muscle Testing Memory

Memory functionality is generally thought to be localized in the hippocampus, a structure found at the geographic center of the brain.

The challenge with MT any brain structure is that unlike the soft tissue of the digestive tract, we can't palpate it. Since the basis for a MT working is generally that the proximity of the human hand provokes a bioelectric response in the target area, there is neither a way to accurately touch-test the hippocampus, nor to touch it in isolation from other brain structures.

HIPPOCAMPUS

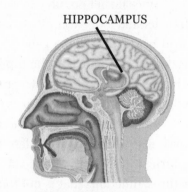

However, there is an alternate way to MT it. By utilizing our memory for some recollection, we are firing synapses that innervate that specific area. If we can clear the mind and then consciously and only exercise the memory, this will produce a physiological response that is relative only to the hippocampus.

If there is some imbalance in that region it will provoke the system-wide stress response and MT weak.

By MT the effect of this process we can not only identify whether some problem is happening but then also quantify what it is.

MT Protocol For The Hippocampus

1. Start with a baseline.
2. Use your memory to try to recollect something. Maintain this attempt for 10 seconds.
3. Then have someone MT you during or immediately after.

A: If response is strong, good. No evidence of stress.

B: If the comparative MT is weaker than the original baseline, you can infer that running synaptic electricity through the hippocampus is causing an unknown physiological stress.

Memory Treatments

For those who desire more specifics, it is fair to acknowledge that neurobiologists generally understand memory to be a function of four main areas: primarily the hippocampus, but also the amygdala, the cerebellum and the prefrontal cortex.

Since it isn't possible to accurately MT any of these areas, it is both easier and more accurate to use the memory test outlined above. We will proceed with the generalization that any memory problem indicates an imbalance in the hippocampus, which is understood to be a placeholder for all four structures. If there is a problem in any of these structures it will show up as the priority in the MT.

The technique of MT the use of the memory as a practical exercise also allows us to isolate the short-term memory from the long-term memory as there can be a problem with one of these structures/functions that is not found in the other.

Once we can isolate a weak response with a MT, this answers the question of "Works on what?" The objective is now to identify what stimulus will cancel out the weak MT response.

The various memory supplements listed above are positioned conceptually at Rung 5B: Therapy. If introducing one of them into the bioelectric field cancels out the weak MT response, we can infer that it will help in some way but this brings us to the core question: What constitutes the term "works"?

Since we understand that a 6A Symptom (failing memory) is happening in a 5A Location (the hippocampus) that will by definition have a 3A Metal Toxicity (clogging effect) sticking there because a 2A Bad Bacteria (causing inflammation) is coming from a 1A Parasite (that may or may not be nearby), the action of memory supplements becomes clear:

Herbal memory supplements like bacopa, pycnogenol and ginkgo tend to have a binding effect at 3B Metal Detox. This is confirmed by analyzing their action on element samples. Pycnogenol has a 4-valence binding action like charcoal, ginkgo has a 2-valence action like magnesium and bacopa is 1-valence like potassium.

We can see now based on the architecture of this issue why these supplements would appear to work on some people and not others, or sometimes work and other times not work at all. We can imagine a scenario where someone had a toxic burden of hookworm or whipworm that they had perhaps acquired from a product grown in manure (the 0A Vector); where these organisms were excreting a 2A Bad Bacteria that was lead-loving (the 3A Metal Toxicity); where they would MT for elevated levels of lead that would show up in a blood or hair metal analysis and that would be exacerbated by the lead already in their tap water; and where the bacteria and lead had clogged the cerebrospinal fluid over time. Memory functionality in the hippocampus would deteriorate as a result of this. If they screened for memory supplements, they would MT for pycnogenol because of the 4-valence relationship between pycnogenol and lead, and if they supplemented with it, they might feel a mild clearing effect on their mind. However, it wouldn't cure anything because the parasite, the bacteria and the lead would still be in them.

This process of equating the 1A Parasite with the 2A Bacteria, the 3A Metal Toxicity and the 5A Location is relevant if we are looking for an effective 5B Therapy like a memory supplement, but it's a band-aid solution. We can now see why Alzheimer's research has been stalled for 50 years. Not only is the research not focused on finding a Rung 3B binder for the aluminum that everyone knows is associated with Alzheimer's, but it's generally not even looking for a 5B memory supplement, let alone the 1A Parasite causing the condition. Instead, the focus is on a 6B Treatment, preferably one that could be monetized via a pricey medical patent.

The solution to memory issues requires reducing the problem to Rung 1B: Frequency Therapy. A MT of the hippocampus cross-referenced with antiparasitic medications will indicate that a 1A Parasite is always at the root of the 6A Symptom if we test a high enough dose.

It is remarkable to see how much the memory clears when 1A Parasites are no longer causing chronic 2A Bad Bacterial pollution.

Muscle Testing Cognition

Compared with memory, cognitive functioning is more complex. The brain region generally responsible for this is the prefrontal cortex (PFC), which is an area that blankets a number of different, smaller structures that encompass learning, planning, decision making, governing the emotions with logic and even the personality.

PREFRONTAL CORTEX

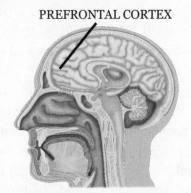

As with the hippocampus, we can't palpate or touch the PFC. Although part of it is nearer to the surface of the skull, how do we know we're not MT something else like the scalp itself?

As with memory, the most accurate way of MT the PFC is to clear your mind and consciously introduce the brain function you want to evaluate (note: this is very different from Truth Testing).

An example of something to explore would be mathematical reasoning: have someone MT you while you are thinking through a calculation. If this provokes a weak response you have found a problem to build on. Another thing to MT would be your reading speed, which might have to do with the logical processing of the ideas, or might indicate something in the occipital lobe at the back of the brain.

It doesn't actually matter what structure you're MT per se, just that you can find a weak MT response to build on.

MT Protocol For The Prefrontal Cortex

1. Start with a baseline.
2. Engage in some function of the PFC such as mathematical reasoning, logic or decision making. Maintain this for 10 sec.
3. Then have someone MT you during or immediately after the exercise.

A: If strong response, good. No evidence of stress.

B: If the comparative MT is weak, you can infer that something is interfering with you running synaptic electricity through this brain region.

Cognitive Treatments

Unlike memory, which can be more unidimensional, cognitive imbalances tend to involve a pronounced nutrient deficiency.

At Rung 5B we can MT various amino acids to see which one cancels out the weak response produced by the PFC activity listed above (math, logic, etc.). It would be common to find a need for phosphatidylserine (PS), lecithin (vitamin B4), GABA (a neurotransmitter) and other more targeted proteins like uridine. Just be cautious of over-supplementing with these products before you have addressed the underlying 1A Parasite and 2A Bacteria. Remember that there is a deficiency in these nutrients for a reason, and that the parasite/bacteria combo has caused this deficiency.

Paradoxically, supplementing with the thing we're deficient in will feed the parasite/bacteria its favorite food, making it stronger. At this level of specificity, it could be assumed that the organism causing the deficiency is local (e.g., somewhere in the brain region itself, or in the associated cerebrospinal fluid) but it could as easily be located elsewhere (such as sinuses, esophagus, lungs or the digestive tract). This is necessary to understand so that when MT for the parasite, we use the correct indicator, but if a comprehensive 1B Frequency Therapy were available, it would address all locations simultaneously.

There will be a period following the elimination of the parasite when it is still appropriate to supplement with the amino acids while the brain heals itself and regrows any damaged synaptic connections, but dosage should be MT weekly and tapered down once the product has soaked in. Eventually the brain should be able to get everything it needs from a balanced diet without requiring supplementation.

This is a special area of interest in my case. In my teens I was able to read three books a day and I averaged two a day for years. In my 20s and 30s I lost the ability to process printed information and only regained that capacity in my 40s once I had eliminated the specific parasites causing that symptom, which in my case were filaria.

Don't let anyone tell you that cognitive degeneration is a function of aging. It is a function of parasites.

Other Neurological Indicators

In a clinical setting it is interesting to make neurobiology an area of particular focus. There are a number of indicator points around the brain that can be MT, but remember that the technique of isolating the area using a targeted thought pattern will always be more precise than trying to localize the brain structure using touch.

Below are a few examples of some common neurological symptoms. Just remember that this knowledge is abstract and useless unless we can use MT to build on the negative baseline.

Neurological Indicators to Be Muscle Tested		
Common Symptom	Brain Structure	How to Provoke the Location
1	Speech impairment	Broca's Region	Engage in speech
2	Headaches	Can be anywhere	Generally works to touch the symptomatic area
3	Brain fog	PFC	Try to think clearly
4	Dizziness	Cerebrospinal fluid pressure	Press behind one of the ears, touch works for this
5	Poor concentration	PFC	Try concentrating

Parasites in the Brain

It is a misconception that parasites don't cross the blood/brain barrier. They usually wash into a particular brain region as a microscopic egg. Some hatch, some don't. Even an encysted egg in a particular brain region can cause serious harm, and disconcertingly, some brain tumors will have a living worm at their center.

The brain is subject to the same categories of parasites as every other body region and this can be quantified with the five main antiparasitic medications. If you want to MT these medications against neurological locations, you should understand that the brain frequently MT for higher than average doses of the medications.

Most important, don't make it too complex. More often than not, what MT/looks like a parasite in the brain is simply 2A Bad Bacteria that has washed there from a parasite in the digestive tract.

Further Reading on Memory and Cognition

A more detailed account of this information is found in The Complete Muscle Testing Series: *Book 27 Muscle Testing Memory and Cognition.*

Part 1 investigates the ways that parasites and their bacteria can influence brain physiology from passive contamination of the cerebrospinal fluid in the ventricular system to active invasion and cyst formation. This is considered in reference to the states of mind, prioritizing mental over emotional, found in David Hawkins' *Map of Consciousness.*

Part 2 demystifies the neurobiology of how we think and what we think with, giving special attention to measurable factors like amino acids, essential fatty acids, vitamins and minerals, and how these up-regulate functioning of the neurotransmitters.

Part 3 presents the data from the clinic notes on 50 neurological disorders in areas like Alzheimer's, dementia, epilepsy, amnesia and hallucinations, ranging from mildly symptomatic to severe cases.

This book offers a unique perspective on the impact of parasites on memory and cognition. It is a roadmap for how to think faster, remember more and maintain mental clarity.

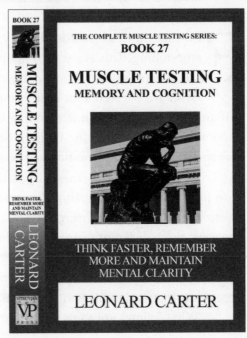

0B. AWARENESS

Educate yourself. Start by reading *Experiments in Muscle Testing* by Leonard Carter. Then, apply what you learn.

28

Muscle Testing
Collected Case Files

From the dawn of recorded history, learning has been based on storytelling. This is a way to humanize information, making it relevant and giving it memory tags to help recall it at a later date.

We have covered a lot of information spanning a number of different subject areas. Understanding is to be found in integrating these topics, not considering them in isolation. Sometimes the best way to relate to this information is through a story.

At a clinical level, the story is the case file. A collection of case files would be interesting if it could help to demonstrate the relationships between the rungs on The Health Ladder, and illustrate the ways these different factors can influence someone's experience of a health condition.

Presented in this way, the information can seem more accessible, more relatable and more real.

What follows are a few such examples.

Severe Anaphylaxis to Dairy

Personal: When I met A., he was a 28-year-old father, married and living in central Alberta. A pastor's son, he had moved to Alberta from the maritime provinces for the industrial boom. He worked as a laborer, met a girl, fell in love, got married and had a daughter. Everything was going well except that he had a severe dairy allergy. We met because he was referred by a friend who felt that her celiac disease had been resolved as a result of my advice.

Pathology: When he was accidentally exposed to dairy, which happened about 2x/month, he experienced immediate, extreme bloating, stomach pain and chills, followed in about 15 minutes by gassiness, diarrhea and then days of constipation. He was losing weight, felt exhausted all the time, and when these episodes happened he needed to take 3-4 days off work to recover. This wasn't laziness. With the digestive symptoms, exhaustion and resulting chills, he simply couldn't do his job until the symptoms had settled down. He was told that this was a dairy allergy, that it was autoimmune, that there was nothing he could do about it beyond avoidance, so he lived in fear of dairy, couldn't eat out, had to make a fuss about the food at parties and missed work for several days a month.

Findings: Using the Confirmation Triangle, we found that A. MT for praz 18 as the likely cause of his dairy allergy. This was probably a stomach/intestinal fluke. In the week following our assessment, he told me that his doctor wouldn't agree to write him a prescription, but that he had taken matters into his own hands: One of his friends was about to take a vacation in Mexico and they had agreed to bring back the pills for him. Within a month of our conversation, he had taken praz 18. We retested after this and dairy failed to provoke a negative neurological response, meaning it looked like he could safely eat it.

Result: He ate it, and was fine. This blew his mind. It meant that he could stop thinking about dairy, stop needing time off work, stop getting sick, stop losing weight and start feeling normal again.

Follow up: When someone has a dairy allergy eliminated, it is important that they understand the dairy paradox: consuming more dairy will lead to getting more parasites from dairy, and some of these can cause another dairy allergy. But they may cause it indirectly.

There is a scenario where a newly acquired parasite can agitate one we are already hosting, and that this combination of the two organisms is the factor that we experience as an allergic state.

An interesting event in A's case might shed some light on this. I had started experimenting with 1B Frequency Therapy using electromagnetic waveforms to try to replicate the chemical FQs of the antiparasitic medications, and he thought it was a cool idea, so periodically he would come over and we would try out my latest numbers. He felt that a milder form of the dairy allergy had gradually returned and that these experimental treatments would provide a reset.

On one of these visits he was late and we were rushed. I did a quick MT and found alb 4, which was hookworm or whipworm. We did a FQ treatment, it looked like it had worked on alb 4 and he left.

The next morning I received a text from him. Around 11 p.m. the night before he had begun to experience unusual stomach cramps. A trip to the bathroom had led to a 2-hour adventure on the toilet and in that time he had passed a 4-foot tapeworm.

I had never even suspected a tapeworm in him. At the time my bias was to assume that praz 2 indicated tapeworm, and he had MT clear for praz up to 66 pills. This episode had two results. The first was that even though he continued to consume dairy, and presumably get parasites from it, he no longer felt his old dairy allergy symptoms. This reinforced my growing theory that something in the background such as a tapeworm was likely to keep a person on edge, immunologically, and make them likely to develop an allergy.

The second result was that I changed gears in my clinical focus and started MT for the tapeworms I wasn't finding in other people. It turned out that praz didn't stop at 66, it went up above 100,000 pills. Knowing to look for flatworms this far above the safe level, using the pills as parasite placeholders in the testing, was a game changer.

25 Years of Asthma

Personal: F. was 50 years old, divorced and a single mother of two boys. Having become free from the abusive relationship that was her former marriage, she was able, through hard work and dedication, to create a stable life for her sons, maintain a job and care for her aging mother. This was more difficult than it should have been because she hadn't been able to breathe properly for 25 years.

Pathology: Having been diagnosed with asthma in high school, breathing difficulties followed her throughout her life so that she couldn't climb stairs without huffing and puffing. There was the need for an inhaler 4x/day. Activity was limited, exercise was impossible.

Findings: F. had every parasite I could find at the time, so it was hard to know what was causing what. Most notably, her stomach MT for meb 1 (roundworm) and her lungs MT for praz 17 (lung fluke). The severity of the symptoms indicated the likelihood that the praz 17 in the lungs was representative of multiple organisms but I couldn't be sure. We used her 4x/day need for the inhaler as a baseline to judge progress. She made the decision to talk to her doctor about taking rounds of mebendazole and praziquantel. Her doctor supported her taking meb 1 because at 1 pill, it was a low dose supported by a standard medical textbook. However, the doctor wouldn't sign off on praz 17 since his textbook was based on the misconception that praziquantel should be prescribed by body weight, and her body weight only indicated praz 11. But the MT indication was that praz 11 wouldn't be sufficient to work on the praz 17 in her lungs.

Result: She decided to take the meb 1 first, since that was what she could get a prescription for. This was of course between her and her doctor but I wanted to see her be able to breathe so we kept in touch on the issue. She took the meb 1 and to her horror (or delight, I couldn't quite tell which) she passed a toilet full of ascaris lumbricoides, the human common roundworm, which is frequently indicated by meb 1. It is thinner than a pen and about 8 inches long.

She passed about 15 of them.

This reduced her need for an inhaler from 4x/day to 1x/ day, which was interesting because it showed that even though the roundworm wasn't in her lungs, it was still excreting a bacterium that was in part washing out through the lungs and contributing to a significant portion of her lung symptoms.

By actually seeing the worms in the toilet, she was able to merge her understanding of meb 1 as an abstract idea with meb 1 as an actual organism. This led her to wonder 2 things: 1) If meb 1 was a real thing, could praz 17 also be real? and 2) If eliminating meb 1 improved her breathing so that she only needed an inhaler once a day now, could eliminating praz 17 get her fixed up the rest of the way?

Her doctor wouldn't sign off on this. The stool test had showed no evidence of lung flukes and there was a liability concern about prescribing a medication for which there was no paper trail.

In her own words, F. didn't give a damn about a paper trail. She just wanted to breathe and she couldn't figure out why, in a country with supposedly the best medical system in the world, she couldn't get a prescription for a basic antiparasitic medication.

She eventually had to get the praz in Mexico. The timing lined up with a girls' weekend away so she bought it at a pharmacy somewhere near the resort and took it when she got back to Canada. This time she didn't see anything in the toilet because you don't see a lung fluke in a bowel movement. But it worked fine. A retest of her lungs confirmed that I could no longer find praz 17. After that, she could breathe without an inhaler. She was cured to her satisfaction.

Follow up: We have kept in touch. There were no subsequent breathing issues. As far as she is concerned, her asthma is a thing of the past. She keeps a backup inhaler but it has expired by now. She recognizes that the 7A Name of asthma served its purpose at the time. But now she also knows that a combination of roundworm and lung fluke were the 1A Parasites that excreted the 2A Bad Bacteria that was causing her lungs, the 5A Location, to become 6A Symptomatic. Rung 7 is only permanently resolved at Rung 1.

12 Years of Celiac Disease

Personal: E. was a retired grandmother of a wonderful family. Eventually I met almost all of them. She taught a class at the local Christian private school and with her husband, had an active social life, having dinners with other retired couples 2-3x/week. She was positive and kind and I could see why she was in high demand as a dinner companion. It was always a challenge for her to meet in restaurants because she had celiac disease, so she preferred to host people at her house. Her close friends would have her over and carefully prepare gluten free meals, and at home, she needed a special toaster so she didn't get sick from the crumbs in the family's gluten toaster. She had heard that I had helped someone else with a gluten allergy and had driven from two hours away to talk to me about it.

Pathology: E. had developed digestive issues 25 years earlier that were diagnosed as IBS. Then, 12 years previous to our meeting she developed celiac disease. Within an hour of exposure to gluten, her stomach would start burning and bloating. This was followed by days of diarrhea, bloating and gassiness. This was accompanied by discharge from the ears, congestion and general body-wide achiness.

Findings: Using the Confirmation Triangle, it was apparent that she exhibited the standard pattern of gluten MT against stomach for praz 11.

She expressed an interest in trying out the 1B Frequency Therapy I was in the process of developing, and by this time I was having success with praz 11 so I agreed to try. It took 4 hours to calibrate the electrical FQ to produce a correspondence with praz 11. Then, because her reactivity was only expected to commence an hour after eating gluten, she needed to eat some and we had to wait to see whether it would translate into the desired outcome.

I stepped over to the adjacent donut store and bought her a chocolate donut. We MT this and the neurological indication was that there would be no negative reaction. This was the first piece of gluten she would have deliberately eaten in 12 years, not to mention the first chocolate donut. She ate it.

Everyone who goes through this process has the same cute reaction: fear, trepidation, and then they take the plunge, they eat the food. Then more fear, then disbelief, then shock. Nothing happens. They spend a few moments processing that nothing has happened. They have broken through an invisible barrier: the barrier of fear. Some people cry. It is a special experience to be with people in that moment of their awareness–of their realization of Truth. Now that I have seen it a thousand times, I know that they will get through it but in E.'s case we weren't sure. I sat with her and we waited.

There was no immediate response and a MT confirmed that her body wasn't undergoing any negative reaction to the gluten. Since we needed to wait an hour to be sure, she went out for lunch and we arranged to retest at the 2-hour mark. As soon as she left, she decided that it was indeed going to be fine and she ordered a gluten pizza lunch (I had not recommended this). She enjoyed every bite.

Result: At the 2-hour retest, she still MT clear for gluten and was an hour overdue for the horrible symptoms she had been accustomed to. This confirmed to our mutual satisfaction that we had eliminated the organisms causing the reactivity. She was in disbelief but happy. The funny thing was, she was happy when she had come in. It is a wonderful thing to see someone move from a happy state of completeness to a happy state of completeness, yet somehow be changed in the process. It is one of the wonders of consciousness.

Follow up: E. has been eating gluten every day since then without incident. We have met again but more often it is because she has brought in one of her grandchildren for an appointment. I have heard stories from her and from her friends about the disbelief, the shock when she goes out for dinner now and orders a meal full of glorious gluten and eats it from start to finish. This is complex for people to process because we don't live in a world where anyone is ever cured of anything. Her friends leave those dinners wondering if healing is possible after all.

Further Reading on the Collected Case Files

Unlike the notes that Carl Jung published in his case files on psychopathologies, I have not made it a habit to record details about people's personal lives in my clinic files. But these details are what make the story real and reveal the significance, and my personal memory of these events is precise and extensive.

While particular symptomatic cases may be of academic or clinical interest, the fact is, these are stories about real people's lives. They were mothers, fathers, farmers, business owners, children, students, pet owners—human beings with feelings, thoughts and fears. And with symptoms.

While observing all the necessary confidentiality, I feel a duty to convey the significance of the case files because the love that these people had for life, and the kindness that I felt for them seems to be the truth of the matter.

It may not be possible to convey unconditional lovingness (Hawkins cal. 540) in this format but in The Complete Muscle Testing Series: *Book 28 Muscle Testing Collected Case Files*, I have tried.

In this way, perhaps the stories, the joy of existence and the revelation that it is possible to be free from illness will not fade unrecorded into the sands of time.

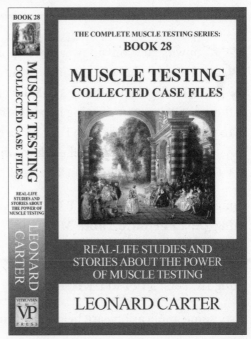

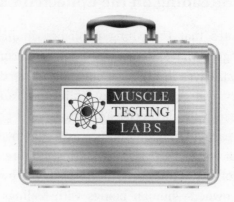

29

The Complete
Muscle Testing Guide

Knowledge is only power if we apply it. Each of the preceding chapters contain specifics about which indicator points to MT and which products to MT against them. What is missing is the practical matter of being in possession of those products. What is required is an organized MT Kit for personal use.

In this chapter we will explore which products are needed in MT Kits for different rungs on The Health Ladder:

Rung 5B: a **Supplement MT Kit**
Rung 3A: a **Periodic Table MT Kit**
Rung 2B: a **Bacteriology MT Kit**
Rung 1B: a **Parasite MT Kit**
Rung 1B: Pets: a **Pet MT Kit**

Also, some applications are below: a list of foods to MT at home.

Supplement Muscle Testing Kit (Rung 5B)

If you really want to understand nutrients and supplements, it's not enough to know what they do. Technically, it doesn't matter what they do, it only matters whether we need them or not.

To identify this, you will need to MT a sample of the supplement against the indicator point and that depends upon having access to the product in question. It is helpful to have all the things you wish to MT organized in a kit like the one in the image below.

Depending on how much detail you want to go into with your analysis, there are about 90 things you might want to have in this kit. These include all 9 essential B vitamins, vitamins C, D, E and K, several forms of A (A itself, beta carotene, lutein, etc.), omega 3 and 6, the main 20 nutritional minerals, the 9 essential amino acids, at least 18 non-essential amino acids and 5-10 digestive enzymes. There could be another 20-30 supplements you're personally interested in.

Beware of companies that sell MT Kits made of water vials that they claim have the essence of the supplement in them. There are a number of things that can go wrong with this. If they're even imprinted correctly, which is doubtful, the vial is unlikely to retain its electromagnetic signature once it has been touched by your hand. These products do great harm to the science of MT by negatively affecting trust in the scientific nature of the field as a whole.

By contrast, having access to bottles with actual 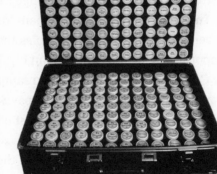 pills in them makes quantity testing possible which is essential to understanding the nuances of MT.

Be sure to only MT with real products, not **watery replicas**.

The Ideal Muscle Testing Kit

There are 6 challenges to overcome in assembling a home kit.

1. Kit size The standard number of pills in a retail bottle is 100-200. One or two bottles of pills are manageable but 90 bottles are not. Besides tracking them all down and ensuring you have quality products, you would need a large suitcase to cart them around. Then you would spend half your time searching for the right bottle.

2. Accessibility This is solved by taking 5-10 sample pills and placing them in smaller pill bottles designed for MT purposes. But then to keep track of what product was in which bottle you would need to write on them with a marker. It would smudge and/or look like a third grader had made them.

3. A Nice finish It would take about two full days to graphically design some nice-looking labels, and then a week or so to custom-order sticker labels that both fit with your graphic design and fit on your sample bottles. Things to consider are how the sticker label surface wears over time and whether the glue holds against the plastic. But then you've got 90 little bottles rattling around in a box and you still can't find any of them.

4. A Nice case Finding a nice-looking case to house your sample bottles is generally easy, they range from $50-$300.

5. Inserts Custom-making a foam insert that fits your carrying case is very time consuming. The holes that the bottles fit into and more important, slide easily in and out of, should be placed symmetrically.

6. Cost To be in possession of 10 sample pills of strontium citrate, for example, you would still have to pay $30-50 for a good quality bottle of 100-200 pills. At an average cost of $30 per bottle, you would pay $2700 for 90 products. Your final cost of the test bottles, the sticker labels, the time for graphic design, the trial and error of printing the labels on the stickers so the design is centered, the cost of the foam, the time to layout where the bottle insert holes should be in the foam, the time to cut out the holes and then to assemble all of this as a finished product would be around $3500 and 60 to 80 hours.

Periodic Table Muscle Testing Kit (Rung 3A, 3B)

If you want to learn the language of organic chemistry at Rung 3A Metal Toxicity, you will need your own Periodic Table MT Kit. Because you will only require small sample sizes, a complete kit of pure element samples can be assembled for between $1000-$2000 depending on its quality. Some elements are more expensive than others (e.g., gold vs aluminum). As with the ideal MT Kit outlined above, the hard part (whether in cost or time) is assembling a set of containers to house the element samples and finding a James Bond style briefcase to keep them in. Too bad you couldn't have Q-branch make one up for you. Here's the one I use at Muscle Testing Labs, I made it by hand when I first started doing work in biochemistry.

In particular with the elements, it is helpful to have them color coded by valence electron instead of proton as that is how they are MT.

I originally assembled all of the non-radioactive elements (#1-83 minus #43 and #61) and then added in a geiger counter to scan for everything radioactive (#43, #61 and #84+). It was an interesting project but unless you're a nuclear physicist you probably don't need a geiger counter. The only radioactivity I ever found was ambient radiation in the air, of which there is a surprisingly large amount.

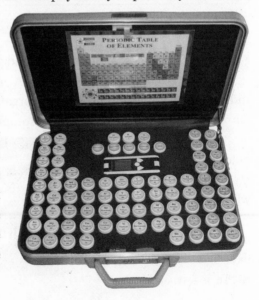

I used to custom make these kits for my students because it was impossible to find one with nice finishings that was made for daily use and none of them were color coded by valence electron.

Bacteriology Muscle Testing Kit (Rung 2A, 2B)

MT Kits that are specialized in these areas are of great interest to doctors and medical researchers as they have the potential to change how we look at microbiology, bacteriology and immunology. Imagine the efficiency of knowing in seconds the right pill to take or prescribe.

It is a cautionary note, however, to members of the general public that many things can and will go wrong if you try to self-medicate with prescription pharmaceuticals. This is not recommended.

The information that follows is intended for specialists only.

Bacteria The following medications are representative of the top 10 categories of 2B Antibiotics essential to any Bacteriology MT Kit:

Top 10 Antibiotic Categories			
1	Penicillin, Amoxycillin	6	Azithromycin, Clarithromycin, Erythromycin
2	Tetracycline, Doxycycline	7	Trimethoprim-Sulfamethoxazole
3	Cefotaxime	8	Gentamicin
4	Ciprofloxacin, Levofloxacin, Moxifloxacin	9	Dalbavancin, Oritavancin, Vancomycin
5	Clindamycin, Lincomycin	10	Imipenem/Cilastatin

Buddy's Muscle Testing Kit

A Pet MT Kit is focused on Rungs 1B and 3B of The Health Ladder.

At 1B you will need the main medications that treat and indicate parasites in animals. If those organisms cannot be eliminated, emphasis shifts to managing the symptoms.

The 3B Metal Detox binders for pets are barley grass, chlorella, spirulina, wheat grass and MSM.

Pet antiparasitic medications are similar to those for people. The exception to this is fenbendazole.

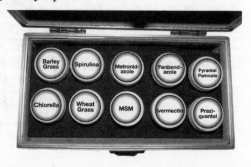

Parasite Muscle Testing Kit (Rung 1B-medication)

A Parasite MT Kit is essential at every stage of your interest in parasitology. You can use antiparasitic medications to confirm the presence of parasite eggs in foods that MT weak (the egg in the food appears to MT for the same quantity of pills as the hatched organism in your body). The kit is also invaluable at home or when traveling to know which parasite you have picked up in a food poisoning event.

How to acquire these pills varies from one country to another. They are over-the-counter in India and Thailand, for example, but are only sold by prescription (and at 40x the cost) in the U.S. and Canada.

Just be mindful of the legal issues surrounding buying and traveling with prescription medications in some countries.

Suggested Quantities of Antiparasitic Meds to MT	
Praziquantel 600mg x 33 pills	Pyrantel Pamoate 125mg x 10 pills
Mebendazole 100mg x 50 pills	Metronidazole 200mg x 10 pills
Albendazole 400mg x 30 pills	Nitazoxanide 500mg x 4 pills
Ivermectin 12mg x 20 pills	Hydroxychloroquine 200mg x 2 pills

Muscle Testing for Frequencies (Rung 1B)

There are numerous parasite zappers on the market but none of them meets our MT requirements. Their output frequency fails to MT against any target location. A MT will confirm this. Since most of them are preprogrammed and not adjustable they are not otherwise useful.

Because this science is based on a combination of waveform physics, a type of nonlinear mathematics I had to develop and some other applications not currently in use, it wouldn't be fair to pretend that this was a simple field to play around in.

You're welcome to, of course. You will need a digital function generator. They cost between $500 and $5000. There are thousands of interdependent variables and your guideline to know if you're on the right track will be that unlike the zappers for sale around the world, your FQ should actually MT against the target 5A Location.

Application: Foods to Muscle Test

Here is a list of foods you can MT at home if you want to screen for parasite eggs in your diet. These are common parasite sources.

Dairy Products	Condiments	Raw Meat
milk	ketchup, mustard, relish	all deli meats
butter	barbecue sauces	(bologna, pepperoni, etc.)
cream	hot sauces	all sushi
sour cream	salad dressings	mussels and oysters
cheese	soy sauce	smoked salmon
cottage cheese	mayonnaise	salmon locks
yogurt	processed cheeses slices	all fish sauces
ice cream	hollandaise sauce	all fish eggs (roe, caviar)
whipped cream	jam, jelly	rare beef
whey protein	peanut butter	beef jerky
Syrups	**Oils**	**Other**
corn syrup	canola oil	nuts: Look for the warning "was processed in a facility that also processed peanuts": peanuts are grown in manure and are not well washed
pancake syrup	soy oil	
maple (corn syrup added)	grape seed oil	
fruit syrups	olive oil	
These tend to MT weak because corn syrup was added	These tend to MT weak because canola oil was added but this is seldom stated on the ingredients	dates, figs
		flour (wheat, corn, etc). It is difficult to wash the manure off of flour.
Spices	**Snacks**	**Fruit and Vegetables**
black pepper	chips (flavoring)	figs (due to the thin skin)
herbs	gummy candies	papaya (thin skin)
powdered spices	donuts (topping or filling)	apples (infrequently)
Any spice that touched the soil during growing or harvesting	check any snack where flavoring was added after it was cooked	lettuce
		For any vegetable that has soil on it, washing usually works

Remember that if you already have a normal parasite load, the bacteria from your existing organisms will protect you from eggs from these new species hatching, so you may be immune to this diet.

The Complete Muscle Testing Guide

For information on how to order the MT Kits outlined above, refer to our website:

www.muscletesting.com/kits

Note that some kits may not be available in some countries due to health regulations.

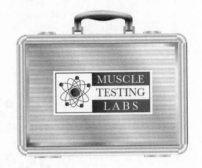

The Complete Muscle Testing Series: *Book 29 The Complete Muscle Testing Guide* is a collection of all the MT outlined in the preceding 28 books, along with some supplemental tests. It also contains a series of lists of things to MT that might not otherwise be obvious to check for with explanations of some of the variables that come up when using the MT Kits.

This is a compendium of MT for daily use.

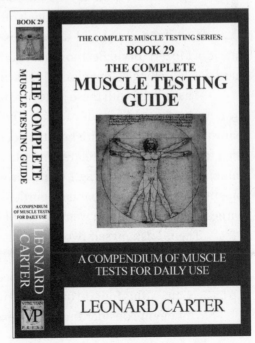

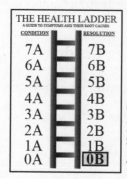

THE HEALTH LADDER
A GUIDE TO SYMPTOMS AND THEIR ROOT CAUSES

CONDITION	RESOLUTION
7A	7B
6A	6B
5A	5B
4A	4B
3A	3B
2A	2B
1A	1B
0A	0B

0B. AWARENESS

Educate yourself. Start by
reading *Experiments in Muscle
Testing* by Leonard Carter.
Then, apply what you learn.

30

Muscle Testing
Perspectives on History

It is a pastime of mine to read the poets, writers and philosophers of Western history, to flip through folios of painters and sculptors and study the lives and discoveries of the great scientists. The music of Mozart, Bach, Beethoven, Vivaldi, Chopin and Rachmaninov has been a lifelong companion. It calls me back to a time long past.

I have lived with these historical figures since I was young and by now they are old friends of mine. The more I learn about MT and parasites, the more I realize how the conditions they all suffered and died from were parasite-related. And because they are old friends of mine, I find myself wishing I could have helped them. I study their biographies, watch their parasite burdens magnify over the years and witness when their health went downhill for the final plunge.

Then, I ask myself two questions: 1) What parasites would I find if I could go back in time and MT them? and 2) If I could have helped them, how might history have been different? I have written up an account of this for 200 of my favorite people. Here are a couple.

You might consider this a MT perspective on history.

W. A. Mozart (1756 - 1791)

Age at death: 35   **Hawkins Cal**: 540

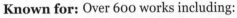

Known for: Over 600 works including:
23 piano concertos, 41 symphonies,
22 operas, 17 piano sonatas, 12 violin concertos,
15 masses incl. the famous *Requiem mass*
Greatest composer in history

Cause of death: Dropsy (swelling), pain and vomiting

Commentary: At 15, I discovered Mozart and a new world opened up to me. But digital music didn't exist and CDs, just invented, were expensive or hard to find so I would ride my bike to the local library and sign out Mozart records. The record box set of the complete piano concertos and symphonies of Mozart weighs about 30 lbs and I happily lugged every pound of it across town in my backpack. I had to ride back with it every 3 weeks to sign it out again.

Mozart by age 15 was already one of the most famous musicians in Europe, having written 12 symphonies, 4 piano concertos, 16 violin sonatas, 4 masses, 2 oratorios, 2 kyries and 5 full-scale operas. He composed many of these in his head and wrote them out with a quill pen.

Notable Medical Conditions: Smallpox, bronchitis/pneumonia, rheumatism. Also typhoid fever and gum disease.

Most common parasite to cause dropsy and vomiting:
Anyone who vomits has ingested a large number of parasites from a dietary source. Flukes, roundworms, a tapeworm or even whipworm would do it. As the larvae emerge from their eggs, they excrete a 2A Bad Bacteria that begins to modify the host's microbiome. This is experienced as nausea and triggers the vomiting response

These bacteria then flush throughout the circulatory system and agitate other parasites such as filaria, and their bacteria. This causes the swelling that is experienced as dropsy, but the dropsy is secondary.

The physiology of dropsy: Dropsy was a common medical diagnosis as far back as ancient Greece when it was called *hudrops*, from *hudor* (Ancient Greek for water). The limbs appear to fill up with water because the white blood cells are cleaning up a massive attack of filaria and their bacteria in the lymphatic system.

But what stirred them up? Short of a trip to the tropics, which Mozart did not take before his death, it would not have been a new species. The most likely cause of this immunological explosion was that he had picked up some new, aggressive species of flatworm or roundworm from a random meal somewhere. Upon ingestion, the new larvae emerged from their eggs and commenced a full-scale bacterial war against all the existing parasite species in his body, which would have been the parasite version of kicking a hornet's nest. We can infer Mozart's parasite profile from his lifelong symptoms: pneumonia was probably lung fluke, rheumatism is from filaria and the time he got typhoid fever would have been when he picked it up, probably from a mosquito. This ultimately provoked the symptom of dropsy.

What final parasite put him over the edge? Intestinal flukes? A tapeworm? Whatever it was, it upset his immune system so badly that it killed him, unless you believe that he was poisoned by Salieri.

What we lost If Mozart had lived another 35 years, to age 70, what might he have accomplished? Another 600 compositions? More? How many piano concertos, symphonies, operas and masses are lost to the mists of time? There is so much love in the world and there is a particular kind of radiance, almost unbearable, that arises when you listen to Mozart. The mind, the heart and the soul all want more of it, but in Mozart's case this was not to be.

His requiem mass for the dead is one of the greatest celebrations of life in music history.

Signature:

René Descartes (1596 - 1650)

Age at death: 53   **Hawkins Cal:** 490

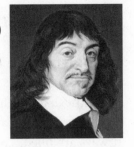

Known for: *Cogito, ergo sum*: I think, therefore I am
Cartesian (analytical) Geometry
Considered the father of modern philosophy

Cause of death: Pneumonia after early morning horseback riding

Commentary: When I was 16, and learned that *cogito, ergo sum* was Latin for "I think, therefore I am," it cemented my decision to study both Latin and philosophy at university. I acquired the philosophical works of Descartes and by 17 had read them all...and understood next to nothing.

We think of Descartes as a philosopher and mathematician but he was actually one of the great polymaths of history. He had a sufficient understanding of cosmology, math, physics, metaphysics, biology, Latin and swordsmanship to write books about them. The Western world lost one of its greatest minds but I gained a hero. What was not to love? Descartes was infamous for sleeping in until noon and at 17, so was I.

Notable Medical Conditions: Surprisingly few. He was healthy enough to become a soldier and continued horseback riding and fencing (that he even wrote a treatise on, now lost) throughout his life. He appears to have had a blend of parasites that left him relatively immune to medical complaints and symptoms.

Most common parasites to cause pneumonia:

1. **Intestinal parasites** A new roundworm, hookworm or a tapeworm could lead to bacteria being excreted through the lungs.

2. **Lung parasites** A lung fluke or a roundworm that hatched in the lung tissue could have done it. Their constant bacteria as they fed and grew would have wiped out the good lung bacteria in Descartes' lungs, leading to a cough that worsened daily. The oA Vector isn't too hard to imagine. He was tutoring at a castle that month. Darned castle food gets you every time. It was probably the oysters.

The physiology of pneumonia The word comes from the Ancient Greek. *Pneuma* has to do with wind. The accumulation of the 2A Bad Bacteria from an overload of 1A Parasites leads to elevated levels of bacteria throughout the body. The lungs are one of the main lymphatic detox pathways. As bacteria flushes out, this is experienced as phlegm, a cough or a cold. When it becomes severe, the pneuma or airways are filled. This is called pneumonia.

But how could Descartes go from perfectly healthy to dead from parasite bacteria in a single week? He must have picked up something really unusual. Some new species of tapeworm might do it, or a massive load of flukes or roundworms from a really unlucky meal. It is notable, though, that there were no symptoms of vomiting that we would associate with the acquisition of a new intestinal parasite so this must have been a species that directly affected the lungs.

Descartes did not receive a blood letting, as if that would have helped, because his physicians couldn't agree about whether to give his condition the 7A Name of pneumonia or instead to call it peri-pneumonia, which apparently did not require a blood letting.

Thus ended one of the greatest minds of history.

———————————◦⊂——————————

What we lost In the 33 years of his adult life, Descartes invented Cartesian geometry, rational philosophy and a modern perspective on cosmology. His works are still required reading in Western philosophy departments. Most notable were the two proofs he put forward on how to use reason to justify the existence of God, something that academics today might do well to spend some time reviewing.

What could he have accomplished if he had lived even another 30 years? I estimate that he would have influenced the subsequent development of Western philosophy more toward theism, which would have had an incalculably positive effect on Europe.

In pace requiescat, René.

Signature:

Further Reading on Historical Figures

As far as I know, my analysis of the probable parasites that led to the deaths of the greatest minds of history is unique.

If this is an area of interest, and you would like to read more, feel free to check out The Complete Muscle Testing Series: *Book 30 Muscle Testing Perspectives on History.*

In Book 30 there are 200 profiles, each with a 2-page outline as seen above. Mozart and Descartes were two of my favorites, and two of the most tragic deaths, but the real tragedy was who I had to leave out of this chapter:

Artists: Michelangelo, DaVinci, Raphael, Renoir, Turner, Constable and others.

Composers: Bach, Brahms, Beethoven, Bizet and that's just from "B."

Poets: Milton, Wordsworth, Coleridge, Blake, Tennyson, Frost, Keats and Yeats.

Writers: Dickens, Dostoyevsky, Poe, Hugo, Doyle, Joyce, Tolstoy, Hemingway, London.

Philosophers: Aristotle, Aquinas, Spinoza, Leibniz, Schopenhauer and Nietzsche.

Scientists: Copernicus, Newton, Darwin, Einstein, Lister, Pasteur, Semmelweis.

Psychoanalysts: Freud, Jung

We also find accounts of the lives of explorers, sages and mathematicians—too many to list here.

My old friends.

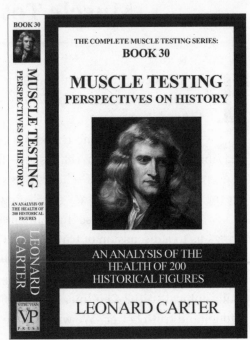

THE COMPLETE MUSCLE TESTING SERIES:
BOOK 30

MUSCLE TESTING
PERSPECTIVES ON HISTORY

AN ANALYSIS OF THE
HEALTH OF 200
HISTORICAL FIGURES

LEONARD CARTER

```
THE HEALTH LADDER
A GUIDE TO SYMPTOMS AND THEIR ROOT CAUSES
CONDITION          RESOLUTION
  7A                  7B
  6A                  6B
  5A                  5B
  4A                  4B
  3A                  3B
  2A                  2B
  1A                  1B
  0A                 [0B]
```

0B. AWARENESS

Educate yourself. Start by reading *Experiments in Muscle Testing* by Leonard Carter. Then, apply what you learn.

31

The Philosophy of
Muscle Testing

T he essence of MT is truth. When we perform a MT outlined in this book, we seek to identify some truth about the thing being tested.

Even when someone chooses a type of MT that is virtually guaranteed to give an incorrect answer—finger pulling, body swaying or even Truth Testing itself—the truth is still foremost in their minds, except that in these cases they are fleeing from it for some reason.

A matter that is so fundamentally about truth inevitably brings us to a discussion of truth itself. This has classically been the domain of religion and philosophy.

What is truth? Is there a difference between religious and philosophical truth? Can linear, scientific MT somehow help us to understand truth better? We will explore these questions now.

Religion Versus Philosophy

Religion is the organized form of spirituality. **Spirituality** describes the calibration range of 500-1000 and is contextualized by Hawkins as being concerned with The Field of reality that is nonlinear.

While the low 500s (cal. 500-539, Lovingness) involve a movement out of linearity and into nonlinearity as a general world view, the higher 500s (cal. 540-599, Unconditional Love, Joy) are experienced as inner joy that arises from each moment of existence. By cal. 575 it becomes difficult to function in society and "the world one sees is illuminated by the exquisite beauty and perfection of creation" (Hawkins, *Transcending the Levels of Consciousness*, p.255, 2006). This is the domain of the saint and the mystic.

A movement into cal. 600 and beyond involves Enlightenment and a progressive letting go of the self. The great sages and spiritual teachers of history have all taken this path. Some interesting calibrations in this range are Confucius 590, Lao Tzu 610, Meister Eckhart 705, Plotinus 730, Dōgen 740 and Huang Po 960.

In some cases, we have a record of these journeys in consciousness but the radical subjectivity of spiritual awareness is such that it must be experienced to be understood. When you cannot experience it but want to understand it anyway, that's philosophy.

Philosophy was originally designed to help describe truth using linear reason (cal. 400s). While it is best to remember that the sign pointing at the Moon is not the Moon, it is essential that humanity should have an agreed upon linear way of thinking when talking about truth and for this reason, **philosophy** is very important.

However, **the problem of philosophy** is that it can be and is used to justify falsehood. Because philosophy is trusted, false philosophical assertions become a trojan horse in the citadel of truth.

The truth is absolute, so this orchestration of falsehood has come to be represented by the term relativism, which seeks to justify itself by proposing that the truth is only true relative to how you look at it. Hawkins calls this the wolf in sheep's clothing (cal. 120).

Truth in History

To understand what some philosophers have spent centuries trying to destroy, we should examine what others took millennia to create.

Philosophy had a troubled start. **Socrates** (c.470-399 BC, cal. 540) devoted the better part of his life in Ancient Greece to pointing out to the pre-Socratic philosophers that they didn't know what they were talking about. That we now label them pre-Socratic tells us how right he was, and that the Athenians voted to have him executed (by hemlock) on the charge of corrupting the city's youth shows us how much some of them hated him for it.

The life of Socrates is represented in a series of dialogues by his leading student, **Plato** (c.428-347 BC, cal. 485). These stand out as one of the finest literary and philosophical achievements in human history, though what are probably Plato's own thoughts about society in his *Republic* were a disappointing precursor to the evils of 20th century communist totalitarianism (Plato, *Republic*, Books 5-6, 375 BC).

The brightest light in the history of philosophy was **Aristotle** (385-323 BC, cal. 498). He invented modern logic as well as the scientific approaches to the fields of ethics, politics, rhetoric, biology, zoology, physics, metaphysics, psychology and literary criticism. The essence of Aristotle is summed up in the crisp assertion that A is A, a clean articulation of linear truth and the basis of modern science.

Eight hundred years after Aristotle, **St. Augustine of Hippo** (354-430 AD, cal. 550) brought a new current into philosophy. In his *Confessions* (Augustine, 400 AD) he demonstrated a pathway to transcending linear reason by moving into nonlinear lovingness. The strength of his vision was a factor in the success of Christianity.

St. Thomas Aquinas (1225-1274 AD, cal. 570) was then finally able to reintegrate Aristotelian logic for a society that had become much more spiritual, ushering in the modern philosophical age.

The legacy of these five thinkers has been to present mankind with a brilliant articulation of reason in the cal. 400s, a clear pathway to the nonlinear truth inherent in the cal. 500s and an undying glimpse of the power and beauty of classical civilization.

Falsehood in History

Kant (1724-1804): The key to spreading falsehood is to mask it in impenetrable language and Kant was a master of this. An example is seen in his subversion of the golden rule, which originally states "Do unto others as you would have them do unto you." Kant retitled it the fancy-sounding **categorical imperative** and rephrased it as "don't do unto others as you would not have them do unto you."

Linguistically this sounds the same until we consider what purpose the extra negatives serve. Simply put, they take love out of the equation. We can understand the horror of this idea more clearly if we try to say I love you in Kantian language: "I don't not love you..." If you ever want to see what a soul looks like that is completely devoid of love, sit down and read the 1200 pages of Kant's *Critique of Pure Reason*, *Critique of Practical Reason* and *Critique of Judgement*. These works could aptly be renamed *An Attack on Reality* Vol. 1-3 and none of their meaning would be lost.

Hegel (1770-1831): We have some insight, then, into what kind of person Hegel must have been to pick up the pages of Kant and find a deep, validating truth in them.

Fundamentally uncomfortable with the logic of Aristotle, Hegel developed a tangled system of historical analysis using what he called triads: thesis, antithesis and synthesis, otherwise described as the concrete, the abstract and the absolute. This sounds reasonable enough but in application it was expressed as a random idea plus a random idea equals a random idea, with no accountability to actual logic.

This absurdity reaches its height in his book *The Science of Logic* (Hegel, 1816) which would have set the reader's expectations more clearly if it had been titled *The Philosophy of Opinion*.

The ultimate expression of Hegel's philosophy is found in the now famous **Hegelian Dialectic** which was one of the earliest ways of saying your thoughts create your reality. This is an anthem to relativism. If your thoughts create your reality then the truth can be whatever you want it to be and there is no accountability to morality.

Marx (1818-1883): What we get when we combine a complete lack of love (Kant) with a complete lack of logic (Hegel) is the philosophy of Marxism and unsurprisingly, Marx was a devoted Hegelian.

Marx (cal. 135) expanded the Hegelian dialectic to something he called **Dialectical Materialism**. If Hegel's dialectic was a fancy way of saying your thoughts create your reality, dialectical materialism was a fancy way of saying your thoughts about someone else's possessions make them your possessions because you want them.

This idea was popular with an impoverished class of serfs in Russia in the early 1900s, and Marx's ideas were put into bloody effect by these serfs, led by Lenin (cal. 70) and later Stalin (cal. 90).

There was an evolution from hating love to hating logic to hating property rights to hating all authority in general, namely truth. From this "arises the dualistic victim/perpetrator paranoid distortion that is then projected onto society" (Hawkins, *Truth vs Falsehood*, p.203). The result of Marxism was 150 million murders in the 20th century.

Frankfurt School: At the height of all this death it was temporarily unpopular to be associated with Marx so a group of the most evil intellectuals in America and Europe renamed themselves from the School of Marxist Sociology to the Frankfurt School.

Chief among these was **Herbert Marcuse** (1898-1979, cal. 150), an ex-CIA agent turned radical leftist philosophy professor who synthesized the essence of Marxism into the tenets of modern relativism: that all truths are arbitrary and relative, as are language, definition and meaning. The structure of society is fantasized to be repressive as justification for the aim of **Deconstructionism**, the actual name of a philosophical movement with the stated goal of anarchy, atheism and replacing love, family and morality with control by the state. Society should then be reconstructed where there are no (or infinite) genders, no morality, sexual limitations or truth. In short, absolutism (cal. 650) should be replaced by relativism (cal. 125-190).

If this doesn't sound familiar, you haven't been watching the news since 1990. This is why Dennis Prager of Prager U, a great voice of reason in our time, states that the Left destroys everything it touches.

From There to Here

Critics of the above characterizations will object that this is an oversimplification of the works of these philosophers, that they have each written thousands of pages of text and that we couldn't hope to understand them at such a superficial level.

I will thank such critics in advance for seeing the point so clearly. Love and truth are extraordinarily simple. There is no complexity to them whatsoever. A hug requires no explanation. Kindness and compassion are obvious. There is more truth in the wagging tail of a dog (cal. 500) than on a single page of a single one of these morally corrupt intellectuals' books.

When we contrast the consciousness calibrations of the philosophers of the 20th century with the great philosophers of history it is easy to see how Hawkins explains that the modern university has fallen from its former glory in the high 400s down to a catastrophic 180, a full 20 points below the critical threshold of cal. 200 that differentiates truth from life-threatening falsehood.

Consciousness Calibrations of the Philosophers			
Marx cal. 135	Lyotard cal. 185	Socrates cal. 540	Aquinas cal. 570
Marcuse cal. 150	Popper cal. 185	Plato cal. 485	Berkeley cal. 470
Kristeva cal. 150	Foucault cal. 190	Aristotle cal. 498	Descartes cal. 490
Derrida cal. 170	Husserl cal. 195	Aurelius cal. 445	Spinoza cal. 480
Lacan cal. 180	Sartre cal. 200	Augustine cal. 550	J.S. Mill cal. 465
(Reassembled from *Reality, Spirituality and Modern Man*, Hawkins, 2008).			

One could imagine sitting in a modern day philosophy classroom where the teacher was speaking glowingly of Kant, lovingly of Hegel, longingly of Marx with callous disregard for the 150 million souls of the 20th century dead from communism; where the curriculum was steeped in the vile falsehood of the Frankfurt school, deconstructionism and Habermas the anarchist (cal. 100).

In such a lecture as this it would be natural to feel that you had become lost and fallen into darkness. In this quicksand of relativism the light of reason would only be a gleam in the cold distance. You might find yourself longing for the warm simplicity of someone stating that A is A. How do we get back to that truth?

Realizing Truth

A society waking up from such insane chaos doesn't need yet another philosopher, it needs a clinical psychologist. It is unsurprising, then, that a new prophet of truth was to be found in the person of Canadian psychology professor Jordan Peterson. His book *12 Rules for Life* (Peterson, 2018) is notably subtitled "*An Antidote to Chaos.*"

Peterson became an overnight international phenomenon for his no-nonsense approach to politics and spirituality at a time when Western society was starving for both. In his writing and video lectures, he talks of love and joy as readily as reason and in speaking out against the great evils of Marxism, communism and moral relativism he has naturally become an inspiration for a world that is ready for the truth. In fact, his Rule #8 is **Tell the truth**.

Muscle Testing and Truth

Truth isn't relative to what we perceive, it is an absolute that we realize. It is our choice to realize it but also our responsibility. One doesn't have to be religious to be spiritual or for that matter, spiritual to understand the basics, which Hawkins once summed up as "Follow the 10 commandments and avoid the 7 deadly sins" (Hawkins, lectures).

One of the benefits of engaging in MT as a means of enhancing our awareness of reality is that it reinforces the supremacy of absolutism as a world view. The constant reminder that things MT strong and not-strong, true and not-true ultimately brings us back to an awareness that there is an absolute reality outside of our own egos.

This is one path to humility. It is also a reminder of the peril of ego-based self delusion that in a small way is seen in false types of MT such as finger-pulling, body swaying and Self Testing.

After inheriting 400 years' worth of dogma, indoctrination, obfuscation, endless sentences leading nowhere, deliberate confusion, lying, dissembling and cloaking falsehood in fancy terminology, we can remind ourselves that we can experience truth in any moment by accurately performing a MT. It really is that simple.

Further Reading on Philosophy

Most of the histories of Western philosophy available today were written by academics who had a pronounced leftist agenda. Indeed, many of these were atheists and relativists who wouldn't know the Truth if it bit them.

What is needed is a history of philosophy where the agenda is the truth. The Complete Muscle Testing Series: *Book 31 The Philosophy of Muscle Testing* is written with this at heart. This analysis is particularly interested in truth that calibrates above 500, meaning one of the great truths of history not a simple, transitory linear truth.

First, it is presented from the perspective of absolutism as outlined in the above chapter and in a way that is consistent with the teachings of David Hawkins.

Second, the belief systems of each philosopher are considered according to their Hawkins consciousness calibration, whenever that information is available.

This two-factor analysis is applied to every major Western philosopher in historical order, about 100 in all. They are evaluated based on how their assertions compare with absolute reality.

In the spirit of St. Thomas Aquinas' *Summa Theologica*, this book is a *Summa Philosophica* for the 21st century.

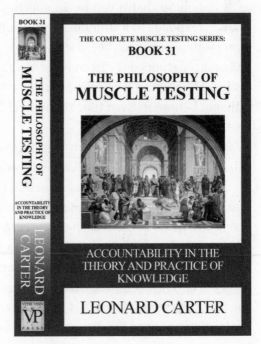

```
THE HEALTH LADDER
A GUIDE TO SYMPTOMS AND THEIR ROOT CAUSES

CONDITION          RESOLUTION

  7A                  7B
  6A                  6B
  5A                  5B
  4A                  4B
  3A                  3B
  2A                  2B
  1A                  1B
  0A                 [0B]
```

0B. AWARENESS

Educate yourself. Start by
reading *Experiments in Muscle
Testing* by Leonard Carter.
Then, apply what you learn.

32

The Logic of
Muscle Testing

The most common objection to MT is that someone will not believe that it can be an effective indicator of how the body responds to a stimulus. This would be understandable if they were watching a video because a weak response looks like the patient has simply stopped trying to resist the tester's pressure. However, it is just as common for someone to have MT performed on them and still not believe it. Even though they feel the difference in strength, it is simply unbelievable.

Since it is not logical to deny the reality of a sensation that we directly perceive, we have identified a **contradiction**.

Contradictions tell us something about how we understand reality. Either one of our premises is wrong or our conclusion is wrong. Logic allows us to use reason to dissect a seeming contradiction like this and find out which of these is the case.

In an absolute reality there are no contradictions, only misconceptions. Learning what our misconceptions are not only tells us about ourselves, it teaches us about reality and this is invaluable in leading us out of the desert and into the truth.

Isolating Premises

A **premise** is an idea that we assume to be true. This is not to be confused with a **conclusion**, though it often is. A conclusion is the logical assumption that we make based on our premises. The process of linking premises together to form a conclusion is called making an **argument**. This is not the same as being confrontational, an argument in logic is a proposition with premises and a conclusion.

The process of consciously articulating our premises is a habit of mind that may need to be learned, it may not come naturally. A week-long reading of Aristotle's six treatises on logic, the *Organon*, is recommended for this purpose. These six books should be the cornerstone of every educational curriculum in the world.

Let us isolate the premises from the proposition that MT is an effective indicator of how the body responds to a stimulus.

The premises in this argument are that:

A. The body has a bioelectric field.

B. The bioelectric field extends 3-5 inches beyond the skin.

C. The bioelectric field responds to changes in electric charge.

D. Changes to the bioelectric field's charge can come from within the body or from without, due to the uniform diffusion of electricity.

E. Internal or external stimuli can affect the charge of the field.

F. The muscles, depending upon electric charges to communicate, can be responsive to changes in the body's overall electric charge.

G. The muscles are sufficiently responsive to produce perceptible changes in strength relative to changes in the body's electric charge.

H. The motor skill of MT is assumed to be performed effectively.

I. The patient is physically capable of producing a strong MT.

J. The tester is capable of differentiating strong and weak responses.

K. A single stimulus is being introduced in a controlled fashion so that only one variable is brought under consideration.

L. A binary logical thought process is used to evaluate the MT.

We can see that there are at least 12 relatively sophisticated premises acting as the basis for the conclusion that MT is an effective indicator of how the body responds to a stimulus.

Truth Tables

When we organize our premises onto a chart and assign them a value, this is called a **truth table**. In a truth table, T stands for true and F stands for false. We are looking for an argument that is true.

A truth table incorporating the above 12 variables would take up more space than we have on this page, but we can reduce that argument to its 3 pivotal premises: A, C and G.

A summation of the logical proposition here is that if A and C and G are true, then it must be true that MT is an effective indicator of how the body responds to a stimulus. To clarify, A and C and G must all be true simultaneously for the conclusion to be true.

We can see in the first line of the truth table below that this is the case and it has consequences on the argument that follows: we are welcome to question premises A, C or G. But if we accept them as true, we do not have the luxury

Truth Table for A + C + G = Conclusion			
A	**C**	**G**	**Conclusion (A+C+G)**
T	T	T	T
T	F	F	F
F	T	F	F
F	F	T	F
T	T	F	F
F	T	T	F
T	F	T	F
F	F	F	F

of disputing the conclusion. This is how truth tables work and how reality works.

And then, if we choose to dispute premise A or C or G this is not a conversation about whether we believe in MT, like it, find it comprehensible, convenient or socially acceptable; it is a discussion about biophysics, biology, neurology or biomechanics.

These are conversations that we as a society can have. Perhaps we should be having them. But it is not acceptable to dispute a conclusion despite its validity. This goes against the basic structure of logic and that is not reason, it is **ego**. Perhaps it is ego that we should really be having a conversation about.

Ego in Logic

It is uncommon to encounter a page on ego in a text about truth-functional logic but this is an oversight by the authors of those texts.

Ego enters into every argument in the form of an **agenda**. It is natural to want to win an argument (even a logical one) so it is standard to choose premises that support one's preferred conclusion. This is why academic and medical studies are so notoriously biased and why this body of work deliberately excludes all of them.

We should think for ourselves. That's the point of MT.

"But have they done studies???" someone will ask.

This is a question I have encountered again and again over the decades with respect to the scientific legitimacy of MT.

The "but" clarifies that the questioner doesn't like the conclusion, that they're already looking for a way to contradict it. The "they" is a plea to authority: any authority as long as it supports what they already believe to be true. The emotion used to express the word "studies" is the most revealing. The questioner feels that something not studied is simply not safe.

Why is this? We're all in it together. We all stand to benefit if these conclusions about parasites and MT are true. Nobody loses here, we all win. But ego loses, doesn't it?

We have believed in the philosophy of diagnosis for 2400 years. Diagnosis is based in ego. There is a lot of history here, a lot of unconscious bias. The way out of this is to learn to orbit our opinions around the information we find in the bioelectric field. This requires humility and letting go of the ego payoff of being the originators of every thought in our minds. The pathway is to learn how to MT, learn how to evaluate the propositions made in this book and ascertain for yourself whether some or all of them are correct.

These proposals are logical and scientific but your willingness to try the experiments in MT outlined here and to evaluate whether they are scientifically reproducible is a function of ego.

Logic is a tool but our egos are the material that we work with. Ultimately, being logical requires letting go of the ego.

Logic in Practice: Example 1

A central argument in this body of work is that antiparasitic medications can be MT against negative indicator points on the body to confirm the presence of parasites in that location.

The essential premises in that proposition are that:

A. Antiparasitic medications have a specific electromagnetic relationship with the parasites they are tailored to treat.

B. An organ that hosts a parasite will MT weak when provoked.

C. The body's bioelectric field is capable of passing through a plastic bottle to contact the antiparasitic medication inside it.

D. The body's bioelectric field will pick up a positive or negative charge from any medication it comes into contact with.

E. A negative organ MT can be turned back to a positive when the cause of any negative charge is cancelled out by something that has an electromagnetic relationship with it.

Each of these premises is a sophisticated idea. Nobody said MT was simple. However, a simple way to express this proposition in logic is that if A & B & C & D & E are all true at the same time, then it must be true that antiparasitic medications can be MT against negative indicator points on the body to confirm the presence of parasites in that location.

Anyone who disputes this conclusion can now isolate which premise they disagree with. Invariably, given a sufficient knowledge of physics, biology, pharmacology, parasitology, neurology and biomechanics, the above premises can be understood to be accurate.

It is at this stage that ego might enter into the picture, but it shouldn't need to. The logic of MT is the logic of Spock. We don't need Vulcan ears or green blood but we must evaluate our premises according to science, we should organize them in truth tables for clarity and we must draw the conclusions that logic obligates us to.

Formal **truth-functional logic** enables us to think for ourselves and avoids the converse which is thinking other people's thoughts, living in fear, indulging in ego and being lost in a desert.

Logic in Practice: Example 2

There are 4 additional facts that support the proposition that MT a dosage of antiparasitic medication like praz 11 against a negative organ test location is an accurate indicator of the presence of a parasite:
1) Praz 11 is the agreed-upon dosage used by doctors 2) After someone takes praz 11, it is the case that they no longer MT for needing it 3) After taking praz 11, it is common to observe flukes in the next day's bowel movement 4) When the flukes that praz 11 treats come out in the toilet, if retrieved, washed and analyzed in a MT, the weak response they produce is in fact cancelled out by precisely 11 pills of praziquantel (not praz 10, not praz 12).

The most popular question with parasites is that of whether there are effective alternatives to medications. We can MT praz 11 as a reality check for any alternative therapy we want to try.

If an organ location MT for praz 11 before we introduce the alternative therapy, and then we introduce the therapy, and then the organ location no longer MT for praz 11 afterwards, we can assume that the alternative therapy was just as effective as taking praz 11.

Logical Analysis of the Effectiveness of an Antiparasitic Treatment		
	Alternative Treatment	Does the location still MT for praz 11 afterward?
1	Herbal remedies: black walnut, wormwood	Yes, still tests
2	Rife Frequency	Yes, still tests
3	Hulda Clark Parasite Zapper	Yes, still tests
4	Taking actual praz, but less than praz 11	Yes, still tests

We can see from this analysis that these alternatives are not effective at bringing about a state where praz 11 no longer MT against a location. From this we must conclude that they have not worked.

Very often, someone will conclude that a treatment has worked simply because they feel a little better. This is not logical. Logic only allows us to conclude that a treatment has worked when, after introducing it, we can no longer find praz 11, for example.

Further Reading on Logic

The arguments presented above are condensed and abbreviated. It is important for a greater cultural understanding and discussion of these issues that they be expanded. Each premise of each argument needs to be spelled out for all to see, as well as similar write-ups for every other aspect, controversial and otherwise in the MT arena.

The Complete Muscle Testing Series: *Book 32 The Logic of Muscle Testing* does just that.

First, we cover the basics of truth-functional logic, both clarifying the necessary terms and using practical examples to develop familiarity with this rather abstract but vital way of thinking.

Then, we explore the logical arguments behind every aspect of MT, from bioelectric field functionality, product testing and Surrogate Testing to the advanced conclusions that have to do with parasitology, quantity testing, bioelectrodynamics and advanced mathematics.

This provides a thorough and accessible survey of advanced logic and of the science of bioelectrodynamics upon which MT is founded.

Book 32 provides clear thinking for complex issues.

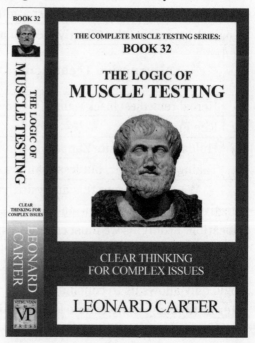

BOOK 32

THE COMPLETE MUSCLE TESTING SERIES:
BOOK 32

THE LOGIC OF
MUSCLE TESTING

THE LOGIC OF MUSCLE TESTING

CLEAR THINKING FOR COMPLEX ISSUES

CLEAR THINKING
FOR COMPLEX ISSUES

LEONARD CARTER

LEONARD CARTER

VITRUVIAN
VP
PRESS

THE HEALTH LADDER
A GUIDE TO SYMPTOMS AND THEIR ROOT CAUSES

CONDITION	RESOLUTION
7A	7B
6A	6B
5A	5B
4A	4B
3A	3B
2A	2B
1A	1B
0A	0B

0B. AWARENESS

Educate yourself. Start by reading *Experiments in Muscle Testing* by Leonard Carter. Then, apply what you learn.

33

The Politics of
Muscle Testing

If the philosophy of MT has to do with the clash of paradigms between truth (absolutism) and falsehood (relativism) in the approach to reality, the politics of MT has to do with tradition versus change.

The fact is, we're all in this together. The most stubborn resistors of change are still subject to the multi-layered problems represented by the 8 rungs on The Health Ladder. The question is not whether we all wish to be free from these factors but how, and therein lies the problem: What information is considered valid and what to do about it are intrinsically political issues.

Where there is a lack of consensus on these matters there will be political conflict.

Conservative Versus Liberal

The classical political spectrum spanning the conservative and liberal viewpoints can be seen as a tug-of-war between rival motivations about how society should operate. The conservative perspective wishes to maintain (i.e., conserve) the existing order of things and the liberal perspective seeks freedom (i.e., liberty) from this traditionalism.

The far-right end of the spectrum tends to result in brutal, repressive, religious totalitarianism (e.g., the Spanish inquisition, puritanism, the Salem witch trials and numerous modern-day regimes in the Middle East, North Africa and South East Asia) while the far-left quickly descends into vicious, murderous, atheistic totalitarianism (e.g., every communist and socialist society in history including the Soviet Union, Cambodia, Viet Nam, Venezuela, Cuba and China). It is interesting to note that Hawkins placed both the far right and the far left at cal. 80. To put that in perspective, Hitler was at cal. 40. The far right and the far left are not far off from this evil.

Those of us who live in the free world are free from the political extremes outlined above, but we are not free from the tug-of-war of conservatism versus liberalism and the paradox of political freedom is that we may not want to be. What the political right conserves is generally what is best, and what has been proven to be in everyone's best interest over time. What liberalism seeks to liberate from are the limiting factors in the traditional ways of doing things.

When a dynamic tension between conservatives and liberals is found, society can flourish, although a center/right-leaning society tends to be the most stable over time, and to allow for the most flourishing. The Canadian Prime Minister Stephen Harper articulated this quite well in his book *Right Here, Right Now* (Harper, 2018).

Given this perspective on the tension between right and left in a free society, we can see where MT is positioned. The traditional medical philosophy of diagnosis has been conserved until now since over time it has represented the most effective health model. A competing philosophy based on interpreting the bioelectric field (i.e., MT) necessarily desires liberty from the established paradigm.

It is apparent that the milieu of a conservative-liberal political system is optimal for society in allowing new ideas and approaches such as MT to flourish and integrate themselves sociologically.

The Health Ladder as a concept, with MT the bioelectric field as its basis and 1B Frequency Therapy as its fulfillment, will probably start at center-left on the spectrum. Then very quickly as people recognize that it is here, that it is real and that it is worth conserving it will move to center-right and with The Health Ladder will become the new medical orthodoxy, replacing the previous philosophy of diagnosis as the new most effective health model available.

This is an illustration of the way that society changes over time to accommodate itself to new technology and as outlined, a culture that embraces the center-right and center-left approach to politics is best positioned to take advantage of such new information

Resistance

It is a characteristic of the conservators of the traditional, accepted viewpoint to fiercely resist change. When a certain type of person has power, whether political, financial or administrative, they will endeavor to exert influence to resist change in proportion to their ability.

A basic amount of **resistance to change** is natural but when conservatism becomes a pathology then irrationally, there is a desire to conserve the old even when it is clearly inferior to the new. With courage and time, change can be embraced and understood to be safe.

Likewise, it is the characteristic of those that desire liberation from tradition to support change, to be open minded about a new idea and more enthusiastic about trying it on for size. Without this open mindedness, new ideas cannot make their way into our culture.

We need liberal values up to a point, but when liberalism becomes a pathology then irrationally, liberation is sought even from the liberating idea. With maturity it is recognized that things of true value, once they are introduced, need to be conserved. This recognition comes with experience, which is why many people embrace liberalism when they are young and conservatism when they are older.

Change

Once the reality of the factors outlined in this book becomes widely accepted, a certain amount of **change** will be called for almost immediately. Inevitably, this will come from the bottom-up, so to speak, from individuals in the general public upward to the corporations and health regulatory agencies whose role it is to respond to the public need, though they sometimes forget this.

Using David Hawkins' critical point analysis, here are some recommendations of the top 4 most efficient things society can do politically about the information contained in this body of work.

1. Redefine pasteurization It is a fact that the general public believes that the term pasteurization implies that something has been boiled to a safe temperature (i.e., 100°C/212°F). It is equally a fact that the food processing industry that deals with dairy products and crop-based oils, syrups and sauces does not use that temperature as a guideline. Instead, 88°C/190°F is more standard.

Farmers aren't any more responsible for this than the cow. It needs to be, can be and should be mandated at the level of the manufacturing and production facilities. It is a simple matter to define pasteurization as a required minimum temperature of 100°C/212°F for a minimum of 15 seconds. The general public shouldn't even need to think about this, it should be happening automatically.

2. Redefine raw Most, if not all, health regulatory agencies perpetuate the myth that both freezing and smoking can render raw meat safe.

Freezing generally applies to sashimi (raw fish). It is believed that raw fish is safe if it is frozen sufficiently. This simply doesn't line up with the evidence where there appear to be parasite eggs in the flesh that are alive and well after exposure to those temperatures.

Smoking applies to deli meats. These are almost consistently raw at their center, and are either preserved with chemicals to smell smoked (i.e., liquid smoke) or are exposed to actual smoke but not at temperatures or durations that bring the center to the boiling point.

377

The result is that all sushi and deli meat contain biologically viable eggs from every species of parasite that the animal hosted.

One solution is to cook the raw meat, another is an international mandate that a 1B Frequency Therapy be used on all raw meat to render it parasite egg free. There is a way for that to work, and it would solve all of the above problems. Before any of these solutions can be discussed however, let alone adopted, it needs to become clear that a solution is needed, and this will require that we redefine, or clarify, our understanding of what constitutes rawness.

3. Redefine illness Instead of the current diagnostic model, where the name of a condition is on some level presumed to cause it, we need to switch to The Health Ladder model of interpretation.

Ideally, a patient would be given a tailored Health Ladder profile: This is your 7A Name which summarizes your 6A Symptom, it is happening in this 5A Location where you are experiencing this 4A Virus that is feeding on this 3A Metal Toxicity that is sticking to you because of this 2A Bad Bacteria that is of course coming from this 1A Parasite. There is a chance that you got it from this 0A Vector.

Such an 8-layered approach to illness would recontextualize the symptom, clarify what treatment format was most appropriate and free the sufferer from the limitations of the diagnostic tradition.

4. Redefine treatment Once 1B Frequency Therapy is proven to effectively and comprehensively resolve admissible medical conditions, it will make sense in most cases to define an effective medical treatment as one where all parasites are eliminated.

This redefinition of what constitutes a treatment will allow for the establishment of a new set of minimum expectations that should include the consistent survival and recovery of the patient.

Once the symptomatic patient is out of the state of crisis, it will finally be time to adopt an appropriate long-term diet and exercise program consistent with their lifestyle and goals. Our healthcare system can and should then move from reactive symptom management to proactive wellness management.

Responsibility

The implementation of the above changes will allow us to stop presuming that medical conditions are caused by the names that summarize them so that focus can move to the root causes of illness.

Since there is no chemical solution to The Dosage Toxicity Problem, it is clear that as a society we need to transition from the use of chemical FQs to electrical FQs in treating medical conditions. That is the essence of the concept of 1B Frequency Therapy.

When this transition happens, we will be living in a world where it is possible at least to be completely free from illness. Just imagine that. This evolution in technological awareness will meet the criteria where we are entitled to consider ourselves to be living in a stage of civilization thought of as **Space Age Medicine.**

The pathway to Space Age Medicine is predominantly political. The great civilizations of history, the Egyptian, Vedic, classical Greek and Roman, the Renaissance European, Victorian and early American were not simple times where glorious achievements were handed around on silver platters to passive citizens. They were challenging times. People struggled, fought and died for those accomplishments.

In the same way, if we want to live in the era of Space Age Medicine we will need to struggle and fight for it. The pathway forward is to learn how to understand and apply MT so that together we can create a civilization founded on an understanding of bioelectricity.

This entails personal responsibility: to use the content in this book as a reference manual instead of as passive entertainment; to apply MT in your daily life; to learn how to reproduce the experiments in MT outlined here so that you can be an authority rather than simply an opinion holder; to refrain from using Truth Testing and false types of MT; to adapt your thinking about health to The Health Ladder model; to motivate other people to use MT and to read this book so that we can begin a societal dialogue about these ideas; to take personal and political action to bring this truth to the world.

Nobody is going to hand Space Age Medicine to us. We need to want it and work for it. Only then will we value it and deserve it.

Further Reading on Politics

Since truth in society is political, the use of MT is intrinsically a political issue. We now understand that the philosophical conflict between absolutism and relativism is really one of truth versus falsehood. The politics of MT has to do with how we agree to implement truth in society.

The Complete Muscle Testing Series: *Book 33 The Politics of Muscle Testing* is a summary of a few decades of notes that I've collected on politics and absolutism. It is organized into 3 main parts:

Part 1 is an analysis of how different political systems throughout history have oriented themselves around absolute truth. This is extrapolated from a few hundred original texts in history and political philosophy. It is consistent with Hawkins' view of history and politics as found in his book *Reality, Spirituality and Modern Man* (Hawkins, 2008).

Part 2 covers the ways that MT can uplift our current health dialogue by prioritizing truth over opinion. It explores the politics of things like how to MT for a virus, and how 1B Frequency Therapy could fit into the modern interconnected medical system.

Part 3 contains a series of predictions about the impact of MT on a future society.

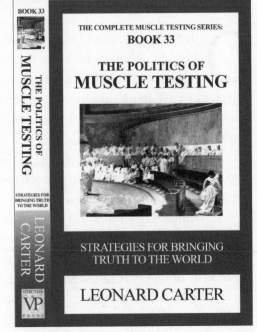

```
THE HEALTH LADDER
A GUIDE TO SYMPTOMS AND THEIR ROOT CAUSES
CONDITION          RESOLUTION
  7A                  7B
  6A                  6B
  5A                  5B
  4A                  4B
  3A                  3B
  2A                  2B
  1A                 [1B]
  0A                  0B
```

1B. FREQUENCY THERAPY

Eliminates all species of Parasites (1A) from all locations. Clean, quick, comprehensive and free of side effects, it is **the future of human healthcare.**

34

The New Science of
Muscle Testing

O ur journey began in a metaphorical desert of health. It has been the human condition to live in this desert because the mind isn't wired to know the inner workings of the body and the psyche isn't able to differentiate truth from falsehood by thinking about it. The only choice we are left with is to decide who to follow to find the truth.

Our awareness of the desert is linear. We can only perceive and act on what is available to our senses and our senses tell us that the desert goes on forever. That's what got us lost in the first place.

What we need to know to get out of the desert is nonlinear: the truth. Once we recognize the truth we can head in the right linear direction and start walking. But sifting the truth from all the million unknowns of reality is not something the linear mind is capable of.

This requires an understanding of how to recognize nonlinear reality. It requires a new science.

42

In the sci-fi classic *The Hitchhiker's Guide to the Galaxy* by Douglas Adams (1979) we find an amusing scenario that encapsulates the problem of nonlinearity in modern science.

A pan-dimensional civilization wants to know the answer to the great question of life, the universe and everything. To find this answer, they build a supercomputer called Deep Thought. After running a seven and a half million year program, Deep Thought finally comes up with the answer: 42. This is mystifying and it reveals that nobody knows what the actual question was.

We find a similar problem in quantifying nonlinearity. The simple definition of nonlinearity is that the change of input does not match the change of output. In short, the answer might as well be 42 as anything else because in a nonlinear system there are too many factors to be able to know how to predict what any answer will be.

The standard solution is to match up a linear process that approximates the nonlinear system. This is called **linearization**. Imagine A.I. imitating human speech in 2020 and you'll get the idea.

But how do we know what linear process to select for the approximation of a nonlinear system? This depends on what nonlinear system we're talking about and is the domain of chaos theory.

Examples of nonlinear systems are the weather, solar magnetic surface cycles, the fluctuation of animal populations, fluid dynamics, gravitational waves, human health and of course, life itself.

The problem with the nonlinearity of human health is that we don't have a linear model we can use as an approximation. Like the pan-dimensional beings in *The Hitchhiker's Guide*, we don't actually know what the question is and there are too many factors to account for: moment to moment changes in nutrient absorption, hydration, temperature, circulation, bacterial load, lymphatic response, cellular repair, sodium-potassium pump ion cycling, neuropeptide and hormone levels all make guessing impossible and then differences in age, weight, gender, genetics and nutrition make it unthinkable. And then how does the soul fit into it? 42 is as good a guess as any other.

The Great Question of Life...

To be able to have a discussion about what constitutes the answer to the question of health, we need to be clear on what the question is.

We are not concerned here with what the frequency (FQ) of human life is but of parasite life. The Health Ladder makes it clear that the best strategy for rebalancing health involves killing a 1A Parasite and to do this, we need to know what FQ parasites die at.

Recognizing that a parasite is alive, the technical problem becomes clear: The FQ needs to be harmless to the human host but lethal to the parasite within. We need to run a FQ through two life forms but only kill one of them. The specific question is at what FQ does parasite life die that human life doesn't?

The best way to think of a FQ killing a parasite is to recall the example of a sound wave shattering a wine glass, though technically what is happening is much more complex. This leads to 3 problems and each requires a solution:

1. Terminal Frequency It is an inconvenient fact that an almost infinite number of FQs will demonstrate a MT correspondence with the parasite indicator but only a few will actually kill the organism. MT is the guideline but the desired outcome of a **terminal FQ** can only be achieved after years of hard experimentation in thousands of hours of trials. Then the real problems show up.

2. Nonlinearity The assumption until now has been linear, namely that if only we could find the right FQ it would be terminal to the parasite. This fails to take into account that the organism is alive which makes it a nonlinear system just like its human host.

A parasite can die at its terminal FQ but in each new moment of time the terminal FQ needed to kill it is different because unlike a wine glass, a life form is in a constant state of bio-fluctuation. It is changing. What was the correct FQ in one moment will not be the correct FQ moments later because it is a different time. Rife didn't understand this. It is one of several reasons why his numbers don't work.

The problem of nonlinearity in life then has to do with navigating the dynamic unpredictability of each new moment. If we try using linear math to arrive at a terminal FQ for a parasite, we find that the linear FQ de-syncs and stops working a few minutes into every experiment. A MT will confirm that this has happened.

We not only need to find which FQ is terminal to parasite life, we also need to find a way to navigate the dynamicity of that FQ needing to be different every few upcoming minutes. This principle is arguably the core mathematical problem of chaos theory.

In arriving at the solution to the problem I tried using some of the available forms of mathematics: combinatorics, topology, set theory and nonlinear finite dimensional analysis. For the record, none of them worked because they are each fancy forms of linearization. What was needed was a math form founded on nonlinear terms. Such a mathematics—**infinite nonlinear dynamics**—does exist but it is not developed in a way that is useful for biological systems. It was easier to solve the problem in isolation from any previous work in the field. This required the creation of a new form of mathematics. There isn't space to explain it here but it does provide an elegant resolution to a central problem and without it I couldn't have moved forward.

When this solution is applied to **the problem of infinite dynamicity** in a biological nonlinear system, we can derive an electrical FQ that is also a terminal FQ that is able to remain synced to a parasite until its death. This now leads us to the biggest of the 3 problems.

3. Delivery Mechanism The FQ we have arrived at still needs to be delivered to the parasite. This is a complex, counterintuitive problem because these organisms exist at unique wavelengths in the body.

The answer to this enigma required the creation of a branch of chemical engineering that we might call **bioelectrochemical engineering** as it entails the development of a novel means of delivering the FQ to the parasite via a **delivery mechanism**.

Although this field is linear, it is notable that every alteration to the delivery mechanism changes the root nonlinear FQ needed, requiring incremental modulation within the above described math form.

499 and 500: The Great Scientific Divide

It is an oversimplification to think of reason (Hawkins cal. 400-499) as the extent of what is knowable, and the nonlinearity of the 500s as the unknowable, spiritual realm. This is not exactly the case.

Information is still accessible at and above cal. 500. The problem with nonlinearity is that more information is available than linear reason alone can process. A scientist trained to think in the 400s is not necessarily also capable of grappling with this volume or type of content because nonlinear thinking has not traditionally been part of the scientific method. This might explain why the scientific establishment is inclined to use a defeatist term like chaos to describe a branch of mathematics, chaos theory (cal. 455), that on the surface at least we are supposed to be trying to make sense of.

The solution to the problem of infinite dynamicity that seems impossible at cal. 455 becomes apparent in the 500s. This is because in the 400s, the extreme dependency on reason leads the thinker to feel obligated to be the author of every thought. In the 500s an awareness that truth is a quality of The Field of reality replaces the need to be the personal author of that truth. A letting go of ownership creates the open mindedness to recognize the truth that is already there. This, once realized, can be contextualized back in the 400s as linear scientific fact but to someone limited to the 400s it will not be immediately apparent where the realization came from.

The reaction of the world might be to label this genius but that isn't accurate. The great geniuses of history all calibrated in the 490s: Aristotle (498), Descartes (490), Newton (499) and Einstein (499). By contrast, thinkers who were able to transition into the nonlinearity of the 500s as a way of being are either unknown today: William of Ockham (535), Eric Hoffer (505); or known for things other than scientific achievement: Jung (520), Bach (530), Socrates (540).

Scientists and academics can easily share in the perspective that truth is fundamentally nonlinear. It is to be found in classical music, paintings, poetry and religion. Some call that inspiration, some might call it spirituality. Hawkins called the low 500s Lovingness.

The New Science of Muscle Testing

When we apply the motor skill of MT to a scientifically structured experiment in MT and use logic to interpret the data we can derive from the binary neurological responses an image of absolute reality as it applies to our health.

At a practical level this provides us with information about our health that we have not previously had access to because of the nervous system disconnect between our senses and our conscious minds. This enables the understanding that The Health Ladder is a more accurate theoretical model than the Ancient Greek philosophy of diagnosis that has served us with mixed results for the last 2400 years.

If these were the only benefits of MT, they alone would justify its incorporation in the healthcare system, the educational system and the human psyche as the next logical step in the evolution of human health awareness.

However, there is a more fundamental benefit of MT. By acting as a baseline for absolute reality it provides us with a feedback loop that we can use to solve a core problem in chaos theory: the problem of infinite dynamicity. This enables us to do the historically impossible—to create a system of mathematics that can be used to derive numbers that can act as the terminal frequency for infinitely dynamical targets such as parasites. This allows us to kill them, solve The Dosage Toxicity Problem in pharmacology and restore health.

When we expand from this particular mathematical solution to more general applications in chaos theory it opens up the likelihood of solving problems in other areas of chaos such as fluid dynamics and turbulence in the Navier-Stokes equations. In this way MT finds itself at the center of the most advanced mathematics of the 21st century.

Truth exists in the nonlinear field of awareness and is available to the scientific mind for recontextualization in linear reality. By consistently using MT as a benchmark for conceptualization, mentation and experiment design it is possible to get so far out of the desert of uncertainty that we find ourselves in a new scientific landscape, that of Space Age Medicine.

Further Reading on the New Science of Muscle Testing

The idea that technology can get us out of the desert of health is based on the principle that physics, math and electromagnetism can be used to kill parasites. This is dependent upon specific solutions to problems within chaos theory.

We have touched on a technology that contains three components. The first is an application in waveform physics that makes it possible to produce a frequency that can kill a parasite. This is outlined in *Book 6: Muscle Testing Healing Frequencies*. The next, involving the delivery mechanism for this frequency is outlined in *Book 7: Muscle Testing Healing Compounds*.

The final component, nonlinearity, is the topic of The Complete Muscle Testing Series: *Book 34 The New Science of Muscle Testing*. In this book I outline the new form of mathematics that I have developed that solves the problem of adapting a finite frequency to the infinite randomness of a living organism.

The New Science of Muscle Testing introduces a divergent way of thinking from pervious linear norms. It makes possible a set of applications in healthcare that can change the world.

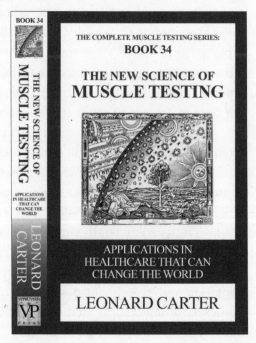

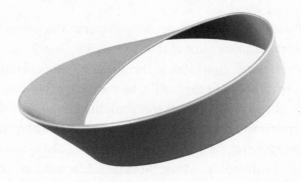

35

Muscle Testing

The Nonlinear Domain

U
ntil now we have explored the primary application of MT
which is in the linear domain that is logical, measurable
and scientifically reproducible. To attempt to quantify the
nonlinear domain we must now examine the modality of Truth
Testing.

What is the basis in physics for Truth Testing? Can it work?
If it does work, where is the truth coming from? Does it work for
everyone or only some people? When performed accurately, what
can Truth Testing tell us?

These questions will be explored below, along with a section
summarizing some of the Truth Testing data derived by David
Hawkins in the areas of spirituality, cosmology, astrophysics and
climatology.

The Physics of Truth Testing

To understand Truth Testing we must examine the physics of how thoughts work. Is a thought a real thing and if so, how?

As the mind generates a thought, the thought takes on a temporary existence in linear reality, measurable in femtoteslas (one of the smallest units of electromagnetism). Imagine an invisible hand making a splash in an invisible pool of water. But when the splash hits you, you get wet for real. Real electrons at the quantum level are displaced by the splash a thought makes. Electrons are physically scattered in this mini tidal wave of reality created by consciousness.

In spirituality and consciousness studies this is called a **carrier wave**. It can be perceived when sitting in the presence of an advanced spiritual teacher. It can also be measured during a MT. The movement of electrons takes place at a field strength that is sufficient to have a biomechanical impact on muscle firing.

The polarity of the muscle, which communicates electrically by sending signals along its nerve axon, can be switched from (-) to (+) or from (+) to (-) in response to incoming electrons that are propelled by the carrier wave of a thought. A MT of anyone near the thought field will potentially exhibit strong or weak responses to this stimulus.

But how should we interpret this responsiveness? At the simple level of binary mathematics, it appears to be merely a biomechanical accounting system. But in actual accounting, your bank account would have a very different meaning if it was at +20,000 versus -20,000. In a similar way, do positive or negative MT responses to thoughts carry meaning beyond the face value polarity?

This is the essence of the question about Truth Testing. Hawkins says they do. He states that the MT "is a general response of consciousness itself to the energy of a substance or a statement" (Hawkins, *Transcending the Levels of Consciousness*, p. 373, 2006).

Experience says they don't. If you've ever tried Truth Testing you will have experienced a disconnect between the result of the Truth Test and the reality of the situation. So a thought is real and truth is real but can Truth Testing work for non-enlightened beings?

Can Truth Testing Work?

So that we are clear on an effective protocol to identify the success or failure of Truth Testing, the following experiment in MT is proposed:

Set up a random number generator on a computer to select a number from 1 to 100. Without looking at the result, with a testing partner, Truth Test what the number is. Then, check. If Truth Testing works for you, your answer should be correct 100 times out of 100.

Anything less than 100 correct answers is a problem because in a controlled experiment like this we can check our accuracy but the whole point of using Truth Testing is to find an answer when there is no other means of confirming that information. Even if our Truth Testing results were 90% accurate, how could we know which responses were in the 90% versus which were in the 10%? We couldn't, so we can't trust the process.

To address the obvious cases where Truth Testing does not work, Hawkins provides the explanation that if the person doing the MT calibrates below 200 (i.e., they are a dishonest person) or the person being MT is below 200 or the thought being Truth Tested is below 200, the Truth Test won't work. That already rules out 80% of the planet but can the other 20% do it?

MT Protocol For Truth Testing

1. Start with a baseline.
2. Ask a question out loud or in your head.
3. Have someone MT you.

A: If strong, don't trust that it means yes.

B: If weak, don't trust that it means no.

In other words, don't trust Truth Testing.

A close reading of Hawkins clarifies that Truth Testing responses are progressively less accurate below cal. 605. According to Hawkins, as of 2006 there were only six people on the planet at or above this level of consciousness (i.e., Enlightenment).

This brings up an interesting question. For those people, or even for the larger number of people who might get one right answer in 50, how it is possible that Truth Testing works at all? How does The Field of consciousness respond to truth?

The Field

Newton's law of the conservation of energy states that energy is not lost and we can infer that information, as a form of energy, is also not lost but merely changes state. This is consistent with the idea that there is a dynamic energy field inherent in **The Substrate of Reality** where information persists after it has transpired in experiential form. Sometimes called the akashic field, the zero point field or simply The Field, this idea provides the scientific basis for Truth Testing and has radical implications in the physics of quantum theory and cosmology.

Further to this capacity of The Field to store transpired information it is also thought to store potential information and universal truth, making it a virtual repository for all knowledge and wisdom. When a scientist makes a major discovery they are thought not to have invented that information but merely tuned into it. At the risk of oversimplification, The Field is where they are tuning into.

If we could access The Field at will, Truth Testing would also work at will. So, the core issue isn't whether Truth Testing is possible but whether we can consciously access The Field. Artists, composers, writers and scientists are thought to access it when they are in a creative state. Whether this is the result of brain waves, genius or intention it is The Field that they are tuning into.

So why can't we all do it? This limitation isn't simply a matter of the separation between Hawkins' linear Reason at cal. 499 and nonlinear Lovingness at cal. 500, it is a function of the delineation between Unconditional Lovingness at 599 and Enlightenment at 600 (or to be precise, 605, since Hawkins specifies in *TVF* p.134 that Truth Testing calibrates at 605). The capacity to consciously access The Field progressively arises as consciousness evolves to the point where the individual self has begun to merge with the universal Self and there is no longer the self-identification with a personal "I"or "me."

So as long as you are still in fact you, you will never be able to access The Field. Only when we merge with the Divinity of existence will the knowingness of The Field arise as a quality of awareness.

At that time (but only at that time), Truth Testing could work.

Who wouldn't want to know the great universal truths? Where do we go after we die? Do we have past lives? What were they? Is there really a Heaven and a Hell, are there angels and demons? What is the form of God? Is there life in the universe? Are there multiple universes?

These are the questions of the ages and we revere our enlightened sages, visionary mystics and great artists for their capacity to provide us with a glimpse of the transcendent field that we cannot otherwise tune into.

An exploration of the nonlinear domain of The Field is not something we can accurately conduct using Truth Testing since we would need to become the thing we are pursuing, but we can rely on Hawkins himself for a lot of this information. His pronouncements are consistent with the bulk of the spiritual literature that we have inherited from the past. His Truth Testing was accurate because like many mystics in history he moved beyond the personal I. What follows is an outline of some of the truths that Hawkins has articulated throughout his own life's work.

God, Angels and the Soul

There is a God. TRUE. Cal. Infinity (*Truth vs Falsehood [TVF]* p.382) LC commentary: *If we define God broadly as all that is, it really wouldn't make sense that "all that is" wasn't there, would it? How we perceive all that is is another matter having to do with the ego.*

We have a soul. TRUE. "It is innate within one's karmic inheritance." (Hawkins, 2003, live lectures: "Realization Of The Soul")

There are angels. TRUE. Cal. 500+ (*TVF* p.383) LC commentary: *It is interesting that some angels can calibrate as low as 500 since according to Hawkins, millions of people calibrate at or above 500. This opens up an entirely new perspective on what type of life form an angel might be, where they come from and how they interact with us in the linear domain. I wouldn't be surprised if the scientific basis for an angel was rooted in their capacity to move outside of the four dimensions we are bound by.*

There are archangels. TRUE. Cal. 50,000 (*TVF* p.383) LC commentary: *Since cal. 1000 is the maximum energy the human form can handle, and only about five people in history have attained that,* *it is intriguing to consider what form a being at cal. 50,000 must have.*

Everybody has guardian angels. TRUE. "That's the good news, folks. Just some of you have pissed them off, that's the problem." (Hawkins, 2008. Live lectures: "Lecture 2")

There are demons. TRUE. "The lower astral realms also include extremely dangerous entities that have the capacity to "take over" the consciousness of weaker humans." (*I: Reality and Subjectivity*, p.260)

Ghosts are real? FALSE. (*TVF*, p.388)

Reincarnation. TRUE.
LC commentary: *I haven't provided a source for this as it is consistently referenced throughout his works. It is notable that the Buddhist, Hindu and Sikh traditions embrace reincarnation as a fact but Christianity does not.*

Reincarnation as lesser species. FALSE. (*TVF*, p.388)
LC commentary: *This contradicts the Buddhist and Hindu conceptions that we can reincarnate as something lesser than human if we have bad karma.*

Animals have a soul. TRUE.
(2008 live lectures) Anyone who has had a dog or cat knows this to be true.

When does the soul enter the fetus? "The human soul or spirit does not enter the embryo until the end of the third month of gestation." (*I: Reality and Subjectivity*, p.268)
LC commentary: *This is a politically charged question and Hawkins' answer to it undermines the current pro-life position that all abortion is murder. Technically only abortion at or after the end of the first trimester is murder.*

When does the soul leave the body? "If death is sudden, it leaves instantly. If death is slow, it starts to leave before actual, physical death. In cases of senility, Alzheimer's or progressive, severe disability the aware aspect of the spirit departs and begins to locate in the spiritual dimensions." (*I: Reality and Subjectivity*, p.269)

When is judgement day? Man extrapolates the ego's qualities to God and then fears God. Judgement day is every day; it is already here and is constant and unending." (*I: Reality and Subjectivity*, p.269)

Science and Cosmology

Microbial life on Mars. TRUE. (*TVF*, p.135)

Organisms on Mars. TRUE. (*TVF*, p.135)

LC commentary: *Hawkins published this in 2003. This answers the question that all astrophysics documentaries start with: Are we alone in the universe? Apparently not. However, the question is even more telling by revealing the fundamental emptiness of a modern science that has divorced itself from religion. The implication here is that it is fine to deny the presence of the radiance of Divinity, leaving us spiritually alone, but then acceptable to determine that we are no longer alone because we have found a tiny microbe on Mars. Really? Come on astrophysicists, you can do better than this.*

Are extraterrestrials real? FALSE. (*TVF*, p.359)

Are UFOs real? FALSE. (*TVF*, p.359)

LC commentary: *This clarifies that aliens didn't build the pyramids. There go alien abductions, the UFO subculture and my planned visit to Area 51.*

Big Bang source of the universe? FALSE. (*TVF*, p.134)

LC commentary: *It should be noted that this doesn't imply the big bang didn't happen, just that it wasn't the source of the universe. So what is the source?*

Divinity as the source of the universe. TRUE. (*TVF*, p.134)

Inflation theory post-big bang. TRUE. Cal.450 (*TVF*, p.135)

LC commentary: *This is where it gets really interesting:*

Are there parallel universes? FALSE. (*TVF*, p.135)

Are there multiple universes? TRUE. (*TVF*, p.135)

LC commentary: *This is still only a theory in modern astrophysics. It will be interesting to see, throughout the remaining 21st century and into the 22nd, whether any physicists are able to design experiments to confirm this fact. A key to the limitations in understanding this issue is that all the thinking is taking place in the calibrated 400s: the Dirac equations–455; chaos theory–455; Schrödinger equations–460; quantum mechanics–460 and relativity–499. It is common sense that measuring another universe would be a nonlinear matter requiring a thought process at least in the 500s.*

Climatology

Earth slowly reversing magnetic poles. TRUE. (*TVF*, p.134)

Global warming due to pollution. FALSE. (*TVF*, p.134)

Greenhouse gas theory of global warming. FALSE. (*TVF*, p.134)

LC commentary: *This is one of the most politically charged issues of the 21st century. The answer above undermines the blame game played by the Davos crowd and climate activists. Hawkins clarifies that while global temperatures are rising, there is no relationship between this rise and carbon emissions from pollution or greenhouse gases. So then what is causing the temperature increase?*

Global warming due to solar magnetic surface cycles. TRUE. (*TVF*, p.134)

LC commentary: *Numerous climatologists have already asserted this fact. Perhaps politicians would give more weight to it if carbon taxes weren't such a convenient revenue source and virtue signaling wasn't so fun. Be free from climate guilt: The Sun is not your fault.*

Conclusions

When we move past the personal desire to be able to perform Truth Testing accurately and make the decision to rely on Hawkins as a source of information about the nonlinear domain, a new vista of awareness opens up. The nonlinear range of 600-1000 is where all the fun happens; the problem is that there is no I or self to enjoy it.

The nonlinear domain is fascinating but also fraught with the perils of misinformation and misunderstanding. Because there is no feedback loop to let you know when you've gone astray, gathering your own information using Truth Testing is not advised. At best you'll end up a little crazy, believing your own self delusions. At worst it can lead to a bad, perilous place that you're not ready to handle without the experience of decades of spiritual work, devotion and the support of a high-calibration (540+) spiritual community.

To better understand nonlinear truth, rather than using Truth Testing it is recommended that you study Hawkins' complete works, watch his video lectures and use him as a trusted spiritual teacher.

Further Reading on the Nonlinear Domain

It has been a focus of mine over a number of years to meditate upon the works of (or about) the great spiritual teachers. These are primarily Jesus, Buddha, Krishna, Zoroaster and Hawkins, but Dōgen, Huang Po and others are also included here.

It is possible to extrapolate from these works a coherent account of the nature of the universe (cosmology) and the nature of reality (religion). I have summarized my understanding of these matters in The Complete Muscle Testing Series: *Book 35 Muscle Testing the Nonlinear Domain.*

Part 1, cosmology, examines the field of advanced theoretical physics and the ways that astrophysics, gravitation, time and chaos theory overlap with consciousness and spirituality.

Part 2, religion, explores the nature of the Ultimate Reality. There is a thread of consistency that runs through all the major religions. The core truths are presented in an account that incorporates the consciousness calibrations developed by Hawkins.

This is more of a summary with some inferences than any theory of my own. It is intended to illuminate the transcendent nature of reality and can be thought of as a foray into the field of unlimited awareness.

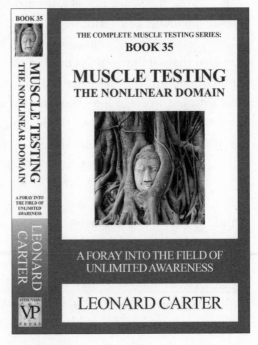

BOOK 35

THE COMPLETE MUSCLE TESTING SERIES:
BOOK 35

MUSCLE TESTING
THE NONLINEAR DOMAIN

MUSCLE TESTING
THE NONLINEAR DOMAIN

A FORAY INTO
THE FIELD OF
UNLIMITED
AWARENESS

A FORAY INTO THE FIELD OF
UNLIMITED AWARENESS

LEONARD CARTER

LEONARD
CARTER

VITRUVIAN
VP
PRESS

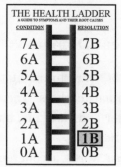

1B. FREQUENCY THERAPY

Eliminates all species of Parasites (1A) from all locations. Clean, quick, comprehensive and free of side effects, it is **the future of human healthcare.**

36

Muscle Testing
Space Age Medicine

To a generation reared on *Stargate, Star Wars* and *Star Trek* the space age is not hard to imagine. But where is the medicine to go with it?

Most of the fictional societies of the future share in common the idea that all illness was cured in the 21st century, that the world entered not only the space age but the space age of medicine, as well. But with our average life expectancy stalled at 80, illness alive and well and medical conditions the leading cause of death, how do we get from here to there? At this stage, we can't even deal with a simple virus. When does this space age medicine begin?

From reading this book, it should be clear that it begins when 3 things happen: 1) We understand The Health Ladder 2) We think in terms of the bioelectric field, and use MT to substantiate this perspective and 3) We learn how to use electricity-based 1B Frequency Therapy to eliminate the parasites that cause illness.

These solutions may not sound glamorous. Certainly, they don't involve lightsabers, starships or wormholes in space. But they do involve worms and that brings us to the truth of the matter.

Foundations

For space age medicine to be integrated into society, it is not simply a matter of inventing a technology. Quite a number of concerns about 1B Frequency Therapy were raised as questions in Pt3-Ch6. Each could have a big impact on how such a technology would be received. We can reduce them to the 3 most foundational concerns:

1. Communication How should the need for 1B Frequency Therapy be communicated to the world? This has been made clear via The Health Ladder. At this stage there is no perfect technology but perfection isn't the issue. The issues are the sketchy history of MT, the laughable state of the antiparasitic FQ generator market, the medical limitations surrounding parasite identification, the entrenched nature of the philosophy of diagnosis as a historical blind spot and the fact that we lack both the nonlinear math needed to mesh an electrical frequency with the human body and the chemical and electrical engineering necessary to develop an effective carrier wave. This really is a can of worms.

2. Evaluation How will the truth of this be evaluated? We may have passed the point where the opinions of scientists and academics are relevant to the average person. Each individual will need to make up their own mind about the validity of this content and MT, the great information democratizer, puts them in a position to do so. Word of mouth will also play a part but will take time to spread.

3. Integration How can 1B Frequency Therapy be incorporated into society? This involves factors like confirming effectiveness, regulatory approval, manufacture and distribution, sales of devices and the management of access to them, what they would cost, what the public should pay for a treatment versus what might be subsidized by governments. Because the focus will be on treating medical conditions, the logistics and management will need to be administered by hospitals and medical clinics. Like an MRI, an effective technology would not be for home use, at least not initially.

None of these factors is insurmountable but they are complex. Such integration may not happen in a decade or even two, but this does have the potential to be the defining technology of the 21st century.

Predictions

The best way to give a new theory legitimacy is to make **a major prediction** or a set of predictions that could only be proved to be true if the core ideas about the theory were accurate.

Einstein made a prediction in his Theory of Relativity about

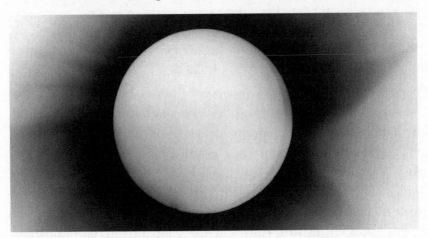

how the gravity of the sun would bend the star light visible at the moment of an eclipse, which the British astronomer Arthur Eddington famously confirmed.

Someone making a major health prediction doesn't need to be called the Einstein of medicine, but the world we live in does deserve and is ready for the major technological discoveries represented by the theory that 1B Frequency Therapy can replace the action of antiparasitic medication and solve The Dosage Toxicity Problem. A prediction is a great way to prove this.

If this theory is correct, based on The Health Ladder implication that parasites ultimately cause the manifestation of medical conditions, then the following major prediction should be an adequate indicator of the coherency of this new science:

It is predicted that a 1B Frequency Therapy treatment, if it is effective and comprehensive, will resolve an admissible medical condition.

Prediction Details

For us to pin down this prediction, it is necessary to define what is meant by the terms effective, comprehensive and admissible.

1. Effective An electrical FQ technology can be said to be effective when it brings about a state where the participant no longer exhibits any evidence (either MT, laboratory or symptomatic) of various parasite indicators. There should be a qualitative shift in perceived wellness and the crisis, if there was one, should have measurably resolved. Some implicit requirements of effectiveness are safety and comfort: there should be no risks, symptoms or side effects.

2. Comprehensive An effective frequency technology might bring about a state where some parasite indicators are eliminated but others are still present. Since a major medical condition is often caused by the parasite that is the hardest to kill, a 1B Frequency Therapy treatment cannot be said to be fully effective until it comprehensively eliminates every last parasite in the host.

3. Admissible Medical Condition It is necessary to differentiate which conditions are the result of permanent damage from parasites versus which ones will resolve or at least noticeably improve (in cases of partial damage) when the organisms are eliminated.

MS and Alzheimer's appear to involve some degree of permanent damage. By contrast, anaphylactic shock to foods like gluten, shellfish and peanuts is temporary and resolves immediately when the parasite causing it is killed, but food allergies are not emphatic enough to bend the light of public opinion.

The medical condition that meets the criteria of being widespread and well-known, emphatic, fatal, easy to measure and is the result of a current, ongoing parasite infection that will resolve or at least noticeably improve once the organism is gone is diabetes. Diabetes is an admissible medical condition.

It is predicted that a 1B Frequency Therapy treatment, if it is effective and comprehensive, will resolve diabetes.

Castles in the Air

It is possible to envision a future where nobody ever has to be afraid of a virus again; where illness is a thing of the past and 110 is the new 70; where the people who reach an age when they can afford to make the world a better place can stay alive long enough to do it; where every person has the health to focus their life energy on living, loving and contributing. How much more happiness is to be found in this world? How much closer does that bring us to finding Peace on Earth? That's a space age I'd like to live in. But is it just a castle in the air?

The phrase "**castles in the air**" is from Thoreau's *Walden*, one of the most interesting books of the 19th century and a must-read. In it, he wrote: "If you have built castles in the air, your work need not be lost; that is where they should be. Now put the foundations under them" (1854).

Are we as a civilization ready to put foundations under the ideas of the bioelectric field and 1B Frequency Therapy?

At an individual level, the way forward is clear. At times like these, when our lack of understanding of health is being leveraged to take away our personal and political freedoms, we must use MT to change the quality of our understanding of health. If you are already using MT, stop using false types of MT as they seriously undermine its credibility and your understanding. Learn to orbit your opinions around what you find in the bioelectric field. Share MT and The Health Ladder with other people. Make these a point in the conversation. Make Truth a point in the conversation.

At an academic level, it is time to acknowledge the reality of the bioelectric field and incorporate MT in the health sciences, particularly in diagnostic medicine, pharmacology and parasitology. It is also time for doctors, scientists and professors to speak out, loudly, against unscientific, totalitarian public health directives.

At a spiritual level, it is sufficient to say may God bless you and bring you joy. Being unconditionally loving will uplift the world.

Gloria in excelsis Deo.

Further Reading on Space Age Medicine

The Complete Muscle Testing Series: *Book 36 Muscle Testing Space Age Medicine* will summarize a set of events that haven't happened yet. They are happening, now, in our time. Chaotic times like these are the perfect setting for symmetry to emerge. This is the natural process of consciousness becoming aware of Reality.

I invite the reader to join with me in creating a society where the principles outlined in this book are a reality—a world where it is possible to be free from illness.

We will manifest book 36 together and in that way, bring the future into the present. This science is yours now too. Try to share it with people you love.

BOOK 36

THE COMPLETE MUSCLE TESTING SERIES:
BOOK 36

MUSCLE TESTING
SPACE AGE MEDICINE

MUSCLE TESTING
SPACE AGE MEDICINE

BRINGING THE
FUTURE INTO THE
PRESENT

LEONARD CARTER

BRINGING THE FUTURE
INTO THE PRESENT

LEONARD CARTER

VITRUVIAN
VP
PRESS

When more information is desired about one of the topics covered here, it may make sense to take further action in the matter, such as:

Books: Reading the book specific to its chapter.

Posters: Ordering a Health Ladder poster for your office, clinic, school or home. It helps the cause, and is a good visual reminder.

MT Kits: Ordering a MT Kit and running your own experiments in MT. This is the pathway to knowledge and understanding.

More information about books, posters and kits can be found at:
www.MuscleTesting.com

Appendix 1:

Appendix 1
Core Concepts cont...

Appendix 2
List of MT Protocols

Appendix 3
List of Charts in this Book

Part 1:

Part 2:

Part 3:

Appendix 4
On the Consciousness Calibrations

Due to Truth Testing not being accurate for non-enlightened persons, none of the consciousness calibrations referenced in this book were derived by the author.

All of them were drawn from the works of David Hawkins. These calibrations can be located in the following books:

Truth vs Falsehood, Hawkins, 2005
-Calibration of the Great Books of the Western World, p.18-19
-Animal Kingdom, p. 32
-Classical Music, p.98-99
-Artists—Creative Works, p.104
-Political spectrum, p.120
-Literary Works of Authors, p.124
-Science—Theory, p.134-135
-Scientists, p.139
-Problematic Philosophies, p.209-210
-Philosophers and Philosophies, p.254-5
-Spiritual Teachers, p.376-377
-Divinity and Avatars, p.382-383
-Other Phenomenon and Belief Systems, p.388-389
-Spiritual Practices, p.397

Reality, Spirituality and Modern Man, Hawkins, 2008
-Great Scientists, p.87
-Relativism vs Reality, p.114-117
-Spiritual Teachings, p.192-193

Appendix 5
Works of David Hawkins

All of David Hawkins' primary works are recommended:

1. Power vs Force (1995)
2. Eye of the I (2001)
3. I: Reality and Subjectivity (2003)
4. Truth vs Falsehood (2005)
5. Transcending the Levels of Consciousness (2006)
6. Discovery of the Presence of God (2006)
7. Reality, Subjectivity and Modern Man (2008)
8. Healing and Recovery (2009)
9. Letting Go (2012)

Index

Index

Index

Index

Index

Disclaimer

The author is not a doctor or medical professional of any sort.

The content of this book is for informational purposes only. It is not intended to be used, nor should it be used, to diagnose, treat, manage, attempt to cure or attempt to prevent any symptom, condition or disease, nor does it substitute for professional medical advice.

Your first recourse should always be to consult with your own physician or some other qualified medical professional, or healthcare provider, if you are seeking medical advice, diagnosis, or treatment.

The publisher and the author are not responsible for any health or medical condition on the part of the reader, or anyone known to the reader, and are not liable for any damages or negative consequences, risks or issues associated with using any treatment, application or course of action based on any information found in this book.

The publisher and the author are providing this book and its contents on an "as is" basis and make no representations or warranties of any kind with respect to this book or its contents. The publisher and the author disclaim all such representations and warranties, including but not limited to warranties of healthcare for a particular purpose. In addition, the publisher and the author assume no responsibility for errors, inaccuracies, omissions, or any other inconsistencies herein.

The publisher and the author cannot provide medical treatment. Please do not contact us requesting medical treatment. Those requests should always and only be directed toward your own doctor or licensed healthcare provider.

You understand that this book is not intended as a substitute for a consultation with a licensed medical practitioner. It does not constitute medical advice.

Your use of this book and any information herein implies your knowledge, understanding and acceptance of this disclaimer.

About the Author

Leonard Carter is a polymath with an advanced understanding of a number of fields, including waveform physics, electrical engineering, chemical engineering, chaos mathematics, bioelectrodynamics, vector biology, parasite biology, cell biology, organ physiology, bacteriology, biochemistry, internal medicine, molecular nutrition, biomechanics, exercise physiology and antiparasitic pharmacology.

He studied English literature, philosophy, logic and Classical Latin at the University of Toronto but dropped out to focus on his health, and because he found group learning to be somewhat limiting.

He was a noncompetitive body builder, spent a few years on Japanese Jiujitsu and kickboxing and has worked as a sales manager in Canada and Upstate New York. In Toronto, he started a national biomechanics seminar company, Vitruvian Training.

He now lives in Vancouver, Canada, with his wife and dog, and runs an international muscle testing consulting practice.

Leonard is the creator of The Health Ladder, a teaching tool used to illustrate the relationship between parasites and medical conditions. He is the director of Muscle Testing Labs, a private research company specializing in bioelectromagnetism and infinite nonlinear dynamics. He is also the founder of Vitruvian Press, a publishing company focused on muscle testing, biomedicine, health philosophy and consciousness-based literature.

His hobbies are book collecting, carpentry (particularly for the purpose of building more bookshelves), modern languages, Latin literature and to unwind, watching documentaries on geology and astrophysics. He regularly travels to India and speaks a bit of Hindi.

Leonard is author of the 36-book Complete Muscle Testing Series, seen below, scheduled to be released between 2021 and 2035.

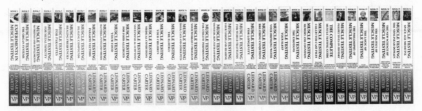